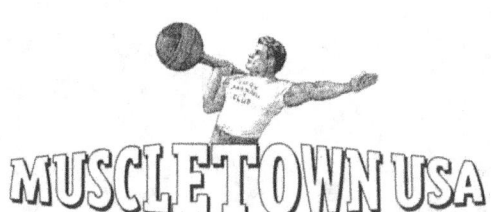

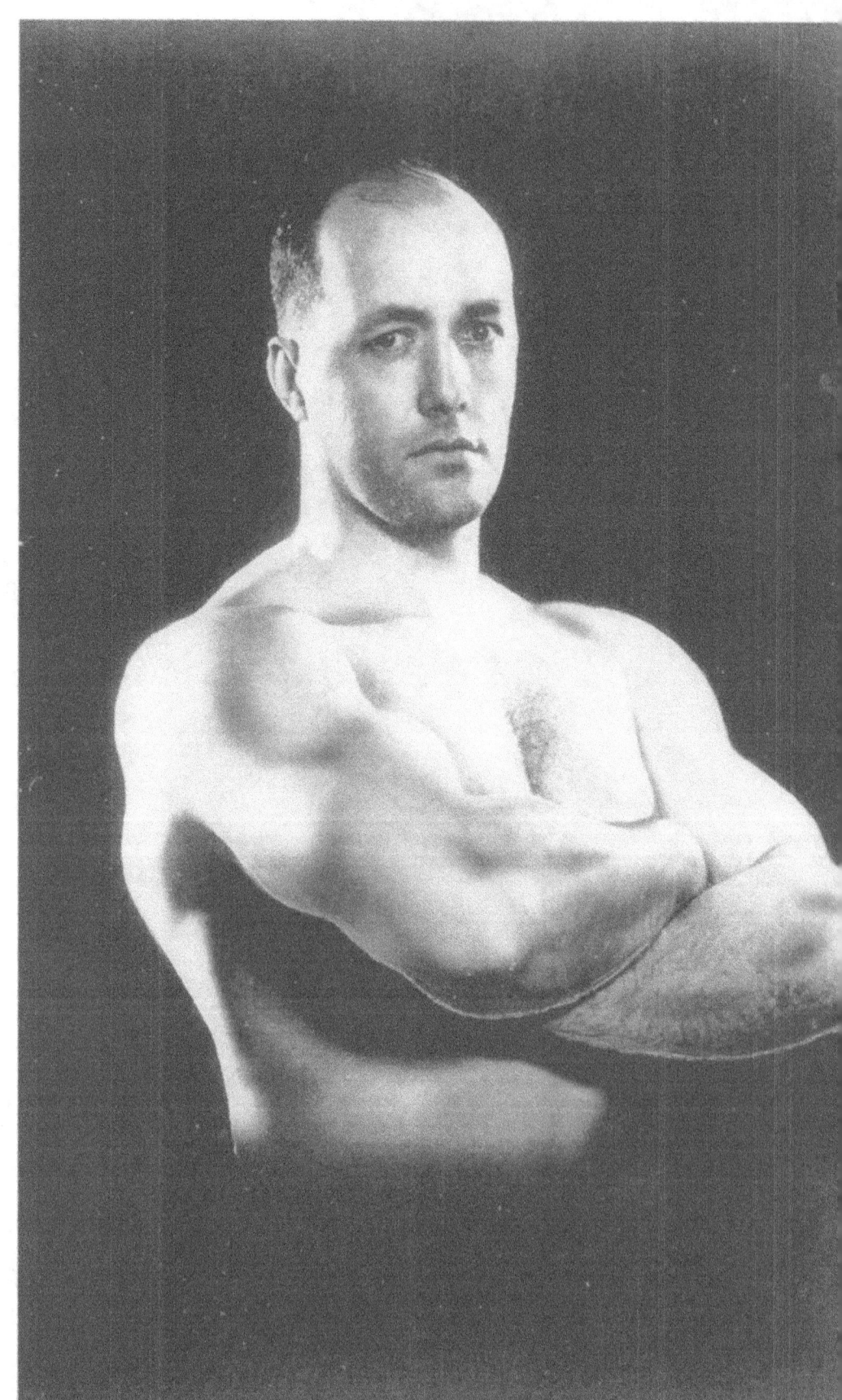

MUSCLETOWN USA

Bob Hoffman and the Manly Culture of York Barbell

John D. Fair

THE PENNSYLVANIA STATE UNIVERSITY PRESS   UNIVERSITY PARK, PENNSYLVANIA

Front Cover: The inimitable John Grimek, whose physique shaped
the manly image of York Barbell in its golden age.

Frontispiece illustration: Bob Hoffman in a 1930s publicity
photograph with enhanced muscularity and hair.

Library of Congress Cataloging-in-Publication Data

Fair, John D.   Muscletown USA : Bob Hoffman and the manly culture of York Barbell
  / John D. Fair.   p.   cm.   Includes bibliographical references and index.
  ISBN 0-271-01854-2 (cloth : alk. paper)   ISBN 0-271-01855-0 (pbk. : alk. paper)
    1. Hoffman, Bob, 1897–1985.   2. Weight lifters—United States—Biography.
                  3. York Barbell Company—History.
                    4. York (Pa.)—Social conditions.
                   5. Physical fitness—United States
                         —History.   I. Title.
                       GV545.52.H64F35   1999
                       338.7'6887641'092—dc21
                                [B]
                           98-39333 CIP

Third printing, 2000

Copyright © 1999
The
Pennsylvania
State University.
All rights reserved.
Printed in the
United States
of America.
Published by
The Pennsylvania
State University Press,
University Park, PA 16802-1003

It is the policy of The Pennsylvania State
University Press to use acid-free paper for the first printing
of all clothbound books. Publications on uncoated stock satisfy the minimum
requirements of American National Standard for Information Sciences—
Permanence of Paper for Printed Library Materials, ANSI Z39.48–1992.

To Sarah, John Oliver, and Philip

CONTENTS

	List of Illustrations	ix
	Preface	xi
	Introduction	1

Ascent to Glory

1	Bob Hoffman's Formative Years	11
2	The Origins of American Weightlifting	23
3	The Old York Gang	39
4	Fitness and Survival in Wartime	71

The "Golden Age" of American Weightlifting

5	Years of Challenge and Achievement	105
6	All Roads Lead to Muscletown USA	155
7	The "New" York Gang	191

Descent from Glory

8	Cultural Countercurrents	243
9	Father of World Weightlifting	293
10	Bob Hoffman's Departure	341

	Epilogue and Conclusion	375
	Notes	389
	Index	409

List of Illustrations

Bob's first business venture.	15
A dapper lad of seventeen.	15
World War I hero.	19
George Fiusdale Jowett.	27
Canoe-racing champion.	31
Hoffman's original barbell course.	41
The York Oil Burner Athletic Club.	45
Sweetheart of the ACWLA.	47
The 1936 American weightlifting team.	55
The House on the Hill.	59
The old York gang.	70
Heavyweight John Davis.	78
Mr. America John Grimek.	80
"Little Gracie."	84
Dorcas Lehman.	85
Alda Ketterman.	85
Bodybuilder Dan Lurie.	91
Abbye "Pudgy" Stockton.	98
John Grimek.	109
Postwar camaraderie.	112
Professor Edmund Desbonnet in Paris.	113
Joe E. Weider.	116
Bantamweight Joe DePietro.	121
Frank Spellman and Pete George.	122
Bob performing a bent press.	124
Chinning contest at Muscle Beach.	126
Mr. America Clarence Ross.	127
Harry Paschall.	132

LIST OF ILLUSTRATIONS

"Bosco."	132
York products at Macy's.	134
Stan Stanczyk at the old gym.	139
Gold medalists at Helsinki.	146
Hoffman and Super Hi-Proteen.	151
Heavyweight Paul Anderson.	161
Visiting the shah of Iran.	163
Light heavyweight Tommy Kono.	163
Dr. Richard You with Hawaiians.	183
York's staunch allies.	185
America's last gold medal winner.	189
Dr. John Ziegler.	199
Mr. America Joe Abbenda.	201
The Hoffman Foundation laboratory.	204
Powerlifter Terry Todd.	214
Harold Poole.	218
Joe Puleo.	221
Louis Riecke's world-record snatch.	226
Craig Whitehead.	231
Bill Starr.	246
Bob Bednarski after his world-record clean and jerk.	255
The 1968 Olympic weightlifting team.	259
Hoffman's 1971 softball team.	284
Bednarski and Dube with President Nixon.	286
Bob with Trudy Engel and Don Bragg.	288
York's rivals.	296
Rick Holbrook at the 1973 Senior Nationals.	300
John Terpak.	304
Bob and Alda doing the polka.	315
Ron Collins.	317
Protesting the FDA.	325
Satire on the Nixon presidency.	327
Bob with Mike Dietz.	332
Lee James at Montreal.	337
Bob Crist.	339
Hoffman in the 1970s.	344
Ben Weider with his physique stars.	351
Mae West with 1977 Mr. America.	351
Jan Todd on the *Tonight Show*.	359
Bob in his dotage.	371
The York foundry.	382
Preserving the York tradition.	384

Preface

"The Strongest Name in Fitness" is the phrase most often used to promote the products and image of York Barbell in the late twentieth century. It is a designation drawn from a long and respected tradition of manufacturing that dates back to the 1920s. The phenomenon that occurred at Muscletown in succeeding decades, however, was more than a successful business venture. It was a sport-and-fitness enterprise that inspired legions of followers worldwide to strive for physical perfection. The movement and its leader, Bob Hoffman, exuded the same spirit of confidence that made America a rich and powerful country in the modern world. For young men who wanted to become stronger and healthier, York was for decades Mecca, where Hoffman served as their prophet and John Grimek as an enduring symbol of muscular manliness. As we pass what would have been the ultimate milestone for Bob, his hundredth birthday, it must be recognized that no one has done more to promote the iron game in this century.

What remains is a bright afterglow. Since Bob's death in 1985 a growing number of devotees—former lifters, scholars, nostalgia buffs, and others—have been trying to resurrect York's rich heritage. This process began with the formation by Vic Boff of the Association of Oldetime Barbell and Strongmen and the staging of his highly successful annual reunions at the Downtown Athletic Club in Manhattan. John Grimek and other aging members of the York gang always held court at these affairs, which often resembled galas once staged at York. Similar gatherings have been held in Santa Monica and London. From 1985 to 1989 Joe Roark produced his valuable "Musclesearch," which focused on accurate research. Terry and Jan Todd's *Iron Game History*, founded in 1990, has provided a much-needed venue for scholarly articles, but it has had a broad readership. The Todds observe that "we get five times

PREFACE

the positive feedback on an article related to Grimek, Hoffman, or one of the other York men, than we receive from articles that do not relate to York." Likewise, features on former York lifters are prominent in Osmo Kiiha's popular *Iron Master*. And Randall Strossen's *Milo* (a name with York connections) publishes the same kinds of articles on strength athletes that made *Strength & Health* so appealing several decades ago. Most important, Susquehanna Capital, the company that assumed ownership of York Barbell in late 1997, has declared that the restoration of York's glorious tradition is an essential element in its business plan. The present account owes much to these laudable efforts. I hope it will stimulate a higher level of interest in iron-game history and perhaps even foster another generation of "*Strength & Health* boys grown up."

This story could not have been written without the assistance of a large number of individuals who have shared in the York experience. I am indebted to many members of the York gang and others who graciously subjected themselves to interviews, some more than once (marked in parentheses): Dick Bachtell, Jules Bacon (2), Claude Barnholth, Clarence Bass, Bob Bednarski (2), Vic Boff, Clair Bollinger, Joe Bowers, Lavern Brenneman, Weldon Bullock, John Coffee, Bob Crist (2), Yolanda Crist, Bill Curry, Winston Day (2), Jan Dellinger (6), Louis DeMarco, Joe Dube, Henry Duey, Jack Elder, Clyde Emrich, David Fortney, Tony Garcy (2), Jim George (2), Gary Glenney, Walter Good, John Grimek (3), Gary Gubner, Gene Heiland, Don Hess, Jack Hoffman, Mike Huszka, Clarence Johnson, Phyllis Jowett, Claudia Keister (2), Alda Ketterman (7), Robert Knodle, Charles Kolchakian, Tommy Kono, John Krout, Murray Levin, Fred Lowe, Bill March (2), Dave Mayor (2), Jim Messer, Gabe Mirkin, Rosetta Morris, Jim Murray, Emmanuel Orlick, Jim Park, Ernie Petersen, Joe Pitman, Richard Pruger, Joe Puleo, Phil Redman (2), Louis Riecke (2), Bill St. John, Norbert Schemansky, Charles Shields, Dick Smith (4), Frank Spellman (2), Vic Standish (2), Bill Starr, Paul Stombaugh, Tommy Suggs, John Terlazzo, John Terpak Jr., John Terpak Sr. (13), Ellen Todd (Hanks), Terry Todd, Harry Utterback, Val Vasilieff, Casey Viator, Donnie Warner, Vern Weaver, and David Webster. I gratefully acknowledge the assistance of these iron-game associates, who not only provided a wealth of information but furnished leads and reconciled contradictions. For assistance in gaining access to sources, I am indebted to Bob Adams, Paul Anderson, Barb Andrelczyk, Ralph Countryman, Bob Crist, Jan Dellinger, Angelo Iuspa, William Moore, Jon Rieger, Charles Spencer, David Webster, Carol Ziegler, and especially to Jan and Terry Todd, whose collection of publications, pictures, and artifacts at the University of Texas constitutes the single most important archive in the world for iron-game historians.

Introduction

> What mudsills are to building, muscular development is to manhood.
>
> —Daniel Eddy

York, a small city situated in the "Dutch" country of southeastern Pennsylvania, is conventionally known for the manufacture of air conditioners, chains, motorcycles, stoneware, caskets, and dentures; and it is frequently touted by city fathers as the first capital of the United States. It has also been headquarters for York Barbell—a Mecca for tens of thousands of physical culturists throughout the world. From the early 1930s to the late 1970s its founder, Bob Hoffman, dominated the sport of weightlifting and the related pursuits of bodybuilding, powerlifting, and weight training. Eschewing the train-by-mail methods popularized by Charles Atlas and other early entrepreneurs, Hoffman promoted barbells and health foods, produced by his company in York, as the surest means to a strong and healthy body. *Strength & Health,* through which he propagated an ideology of success, inspired countless readers to seek not only physical improvement but a greater masculine and American identity.

In the late twentieth century a new cultural dynamic, shaped more by media images, has overtaken muscledom. Today Arnold Schwarze-

INTRODUCTION

negger, the Mr. Olympia contest, Weider Publications, Gold's Gym, and Hulk Hogan are prominent icons in mainstream America, but they could hardly have reached their present level of acceptance without the anaerobic underpinnings established by John Grimek, the Mr. America contest, Bob Hoffman, Paul Anderson, and York, none of which has ever been a household name outside the iron game. Still, these figures will evoke for Pennsylvanians and those whom Hoffman called "Strength & Health boys grown up" a nostalgic feeling for the unique manly culture that once flourished in Muscletown, USA.

Bob Hoffman and York Barbell embraced many of the assumptions of American capitalism as this country developed into a world power nearly a hundred years ago. Hoffman fit the nineteenth-century (Horatio Alger) concept of self-made manhood, epitomized by "industrial work habits, extraordinary moral discipline, and . . . indomitable will."[1] American culture at the turn of the century had a strong social Darwinian aspect, and athletic achievements mirrored the larger game of life. "Ambition and combativeness" were hallmarks of a new passionate manhood that stressed "strength, appearance, and athletic skill."[2] Hoffman subscribed strongly to these congruent images in his youth. As an adult, he projected them to others seeking middle-class acceptance. Central to Hoffman's outlook was his interest in fitness in its broadest sense. During his formative years American sport was relatively immature. Professionalism and specialization were less evident than now, and weightlifting was scarcely distinct from juggling, tumbling, handbalancing, wrestling, and many other fitness endeavors. Hoffman began his athletic career in aquatic sports, especially canoeing, and he was always interested in track and field. Health and fitness, he maintained, were prerequisites to strength and success in athletics. But competition was never pursued for its own sake. It was valued chiefly for the psychic satisfaction it summoned forth, which was always an end in itself. Bob Hoffman was never a great weightlifter, bodybuilder, coach, writer, nutritionist, or businessman, yet he was a great man—chiefly because of his capacity to promote an ideology of success.

The American model of success has often been measured in commercial terms, but no less important to Hoffman and those who subscribed to his ethos was the need to reaffirm sexual identity. The acquisition of health, fitness, strength, and ultimately athletic victory had as its object not only the attraction of the opposite sex but a primal need to acquire domination over the same sex. Maleness, notes a leading sport historian,

Introduction

"seemed most emphatically confirmed in the company not of women, but of other men."[3] Thus seemingly innocent sporting endeavors can be viewed as expressions of sex drive and virility. While sociologist Paul Hoch interprets athletics as reflecting an urge to dominate other males, "the competition behind the competition," psychologists have focused on inadequacy and compensatory behavior.[4] The weightlifter's strenuous feats are merely attempts to overcome feelings of inferiority and "to demonstrate both to himself and to others his male potency," writes Robert Harlow.[5] That Hoffman was gender-conscious is evident not only from his well-deserved reputation as a "womanizer" but from his role as patriarch in the sport of strong men. What more visible way could there be of displaying virility than by asserting authority over the strong?

What enabled Hoffman to advance weightlifting and promote his ideals for a strong and healthy America was the recruitment of a remarkable body of athletes, the York gang, to engage the fitness-minded public. Notwithstanding such early muscle peddlers as Alan Calvert, Bernarr Macfadden, Earle Liederman, and Charles Atlas, performers like Warren Lincoln Travis, or gym operators such as Siegmund Klein, few realized prosperity in the iron game. Hoffman succeeded because he first established an independent financial base in the oil-burner business during the 1920s. Within a decade his passion for sport exceeded his need to produce oil burners. Gradually this business enterprise was converted for use in underwriting and promoting American weightlifting. In the early 1930s the company began to make barbells on the side and to accommodate Hoffman's lifters with jobs. That the training platform was situated in the middle of the oil-burner factory aptly characterized the relationship of lifting to the business. Then, with the founding of York Barbell Company in 1938, Hoffman created a "Muscle Empire" that became the envy of promoters worldwide. But making money, even lots of it, was never more than a means to the greater end of fostering weightlifting and other fitness endeavors, all of which drew attention to himself. His musclemen not only won Olympic medals and physique contests but brought Hoffman fame and fortune by producing his barbells and publications. It was a company of "jocks" trying to be businessmen that emerged from the depths of the Great Depression and helped awaken America to the need for physical fitness.

Most susceptible to Hoffman's appeal was a large body of neurasthenic and hyphenated Americans who were striving for improvement and an entrée to mainstream culture. A common trait of his followers, underscoring their need for virility, was a physical ailment or debility. Often it stemmed from a traumatic experience in childhood and was accompanied by a self-perception of inferiority. To the desire for self-improvement through physical recovery, Hoffman coupled the higher ideal of national regeneration. But he hardly originated this concept. Since the time of Father Friedrich Ludwig Jahn in the Napoleonic era, physical fitness had been an important component of nascent nationalist movements. In America it was epitomized by Theodore Roosevelt, who suffered from asthma and *cholera morbus* as a youth and hardened his body through physical exertion. The indomitable Teddy served as the nation's foremost advocate of the "strenuous life" at the turn of the century. Unique to Hoffman's nationalist embrace was his equation of the aspirations of his company and weightlifting with those of America in its cold-war struggle against the Soviet bloc. A fit America was perceived as necessary to beat the Russians, and Hoffman headed a crusade to defend his country's values against Communism. Success in weightlifting was critical to the triumph of the West.

While Hoffman's ethos, like that of other regeneration movements, appealed largely to individuals with physical deficiencies and low self-esteem, it also had an important sociological dimension. Like boxing and wrestling, weightlifting had a negative image. It was practiced in sweaty gyms, dingy garages, and dirty basements by members of lower socioeconomic and immigrant groups. But "sport has often served minority groups as the first rung on the social ladder," notes Robert Boyle, helping to "further their assimilation into American life."[6] Of the 105 national champions from 1945 to 1960, the period of York's greatest success, at least 73 (70 percent) fell into this category. Of the 28 world champions, 25 (89 percent) were ethnic Americans, and 12 out of the 13 Olympic gold medalists (92 percent) were from recent immigrant families or distinctive minorities. From the East Coast came the Germans, Italians, and Slavs, and from Hawaii and California came various Asian peoples of the Pacific Rim. Hoffman became their father figure, providing largely second-generation Americans with a sense of purpose, inspiration, and identity in an otherwise alien environment. For three decades his teams embraced the ideal of the melting pot. Strong sociopsychological forces were at work inducing the sons of immigrants to strive for success and, through weightlifting, gain assimilation and realize the American dream. At the vanguard of this process was the

Introduction

York gang, the pantheon of iron-game heroes assembled by Hoffman to serve as models for the nation's youth—strong, virile, hardworking, and committed to American ideals.

At least until the 1960s York's formula for socialization and homogeneity worked. But it was chimerical to believe that the comparatively meager resources of Hoffman's company and the minor sport of weightlifting could engage and overcome those of entire nations. At the height of York's powers, British writer George Kirkley noted the predominance of weightlifting's superpowers: "On one side, in America, we have a great weightlifting team gathered, supported and encouraged almost solely by the efforts of one man, Bob Hoffman of York, Pa. On the other there is a huge country of over 100,000 weightlifters, state organized and controlled on a vast scale."[7] When his teams started losing regularly to the Soviet Union and other Communist nations in the 1960s, it was a tremendous blow to Hoffman's colossal ego and the myths he had fabricated about the superiority of the York way.

Likewise, within the American iron game, Hoffman's delusions of grandeur were challenged by a rival organization headed by Joe and Ben Weider of Montreal. The Weiders sprang from recent (Jewish) immigrant stock and staked their success on an alternative commercial strategy. Effectively excluded from competitive weightlifting, monopolized by Hoffman, the Weiders emphasized bodybuilding, and rooted it in the postwar California showbiz culture. The resulting feud between Hoffman and the Weiders, where money, power, and ego were at stake, consumed about two decades, as both parties vied for control of muscledom. Hoffman, with his moralistic and patriotic pitch, triumphed at first. But his failure to keep up with the times and to appreciate the appeal of bodybuilding as America's tastes changed enabled the tenacious Weiders to surpass him by the mid-1970s. It was Joe Weider who arrogated the title "Trainer of Champions" and promoted Arnold Schwarzenegger to international fame. But much of his early inspiration and sales technique was derived from Hoffman. The road that led to the new muscle Mecca of the 1990s in Woodland Hills, California, very likely began in York, Pennsylvania.[8]

Bob Hoffman and York Barbell constitute an important subculture in the twentieth century and a kind of gender construct that has just begun to attract scholarly attention. Recent books on early physical culturist Bernarr Macfadden by William Hunt and Robert Ernst shed light on this examination of Hoffman. Also relevant are Alan Klein's

INTRODUCTION

Little Big Men and David Chapman's *Sandow the Magnificent*, both of which contribute significantly to our understanding of sport and fitness in the twentieth century. In spirit this study resembles the depictions of traditional manhood by John Neuright and Timothy Chandler in *Making Men* and Kim Townsend in *Manhood at Harvard*.[9] But with most current literature in men's studies this book does not readily connect. It is a genre that is highly theoretical, usually informed by a feminist or mythopoetic perspective, and more concerned with the present than the past.[10] Even Michael Kimmel, whose *Manhood in America* deals fully and frankly with self-made men over the past two centuries, seems embarrassed by the concept of traditional masculinity. "Self-Made Manhood is our legacy," argues Kimmel, "but it is not our nature." Much scholarship on males has become apologetic of alleged past transgressions. As Garrison Keillor playfully puts it, "Years ago, manhood was an opportunity for achievement, and now it is a problem to be overcome."[11] Presentmindedness, however laudable for social engineering purposes, corrupts our understanding of the past. This representation of manhood in Muscletown is neither prescriptive nor ideological; rather, it is descriptive and interpretive in the sense of attempting to recapture what Herbert Butterfield calls the "past-ness" of the past.[12] This study therefore seeks neither to condemn nor to glorify Hoffman and his movement but to view them with historical perspective.

Critical to this approach is the use of original sources. Any previous understanding of the York phenomenon has been hampered by a longstanding reliance on oral tradition and an absence of bona fide historical records. To compensate for this void, I have collected information on three levels. First, members of the York gang and others directly linked to Hoffman contributed greatly through their candid observations about the past. Memories, however, can be tricky and not always reliable. Even the most vivid recollections can be distorted to suit current preoccupations or designs. A fuller understanding is possible when oral testimony is anchored to written sources. Such evidence has been notoriously scarce in the iron game, but in the present instance a corpus of such material is readily available in Hoffman's many books and magazines, *Strength & Health* and *Muscular Development*, published for fifty-four and twenty-five years respectively. Furthermore, Hoffman had a keen appreciation of history. Not only did he feature old-timers prominently, but he detailed the accomplishments of himself and his followers with an eye on how they would appear to posterity. He wanted to be the prophet

Introduction

and patriarch by whose hand traditions were set. For this reason, and because of his desire to promote his products and ideology of success, Hoffman extrapolated on the truth. He also wanted to cut a wide swath in history and often stated his intention to reach a hundred and live in three centuries. If this were not possible, he believed he could live forever through his writings. Such cravings for immortality usually mislead more than they inform. However valuable Hoffman's extensive writings might be as a source, they must be used cautiously.

The kind of resource most valuable in gaining an accurate view of the past is manuscript evidence. I asked everyone I interviewed whether he or she had any papers pertinent to York. Almost no one did, but success came unexpectedly from Bob's widow, Alda Ketterman, who led me to a treasure trove of materials at her home in Dover and two other locations. Some of it was filthy and water damaged, but it was unexpurgated, the kind of collection most useful to historians. Also, John Terpak Sr. made available, in successive stages, large quantities of company records—from the Ridge Avenue warehouse, the old Broad Street offices, and the modern plant near Emigsville—that complemented the Hoffman Papers. Eventually he allowed me to obtain whatever I needed from his personal files, enabling me to carry my story through the period of Bob's illness and beyond. The value of the generosity and cooperation of Ketterman and Terpak to the telling of this story cannot be overestimated. With these manuscripts, along with extensive printed sources and interviews, a more revealing picture of Bob Hoffman and the manly culture of Muscletown, USA, is possible.

ASCENT TO GLORY

1
BOB HOFFMAN'S FORMATIVE YEARS

> I have watched Bob Hoffman bloom into herculean manhood. I have ... seen him win many races by the super-human power and endurance of his mighty muscles when other champions were gasping, weary, and exhausted. I have seen him sway multitudes into wildly cheering hysterical masses by the brilliance of his physical mastery. I have seen them spellbound, fascinated as they watched the herculean arc of his oars propel his boat, inch by inch, to sweeping victory. He is the true type of sportsman which the whole world admires. Quiet, cool, compelling—clean and big hearted—utterly fearless.
>
> —"A Famous Writer" (quoted in Bob Hoffman's *Road to Super-Strength*)

Ancestry and Youth

Robert Collins Hoffman was born November 9, 1898, on a 640-acre farm near Tifton, Georgia. His origins can be traced to German and French Huguenot stock. Bob, according to his brother, John L. (Jack) Hoffman, was utterly uninterested in his ancestry. Indeed "one without knowledge might think he was illegitimate."[1] Family lore shows that lineage on his father's side is traceable back to 1613, just before the Thirty Years'

War, when patriarch Abraham Hoffman migrated from Germany to the village of Sissach (near Basel) in Switzerland, where he raised grapes for wine making. A later Hoffman was allegedly an English professor in Bern, the capital. Bob's grandfather, John Hoffman, came to Pittsburgh in 1845 at age seven and enlisted in the Union army during the Civil War. Afterward he worked for the Pennsylvania Railroad and then for Carnegie Steel, where he was superintendent of the Homestead mill. He married Ellen Shanor from nearby Beaver County, and their eldest child, Addison Frederick, was Bob's father. On the distaff side, Bob's great grandfather, James Collins, came to Allegheny City from Glasgow, Scotland, in the 1830s with an infant son named Robert. Bob's maternal great grandfather, named Leone, was a farrier who sold horses during the Civil War to both sides in Kansas. He married a French woman with the surname Linden, and their daughter married Robert Collins, presumably after the war. The Collinses' daughter Bertha (Leone) married Addison Hoffman. Bob Hoffman's heritage was a typical amalgam of the early immigrant strains that embodied American society.

In his youth Addison studied engineering at the University of Pittsburgh, and he was superintendent for a while in the Duquesne mill. Then, in 1892, a depression year, his father bought him a large property in central Georgia from Southern Railway. Addison and Bertha Hoffman cleared the forest, constructed a house and railway siding, built cabins for black laborers, and planted ten thousand peach trees. Their family consisted of a daughter, Florence, and a son, Charles (Chuck), both born in Pennsylvania. Jack, born in 1896 on the Georgia farm, describes his mother as "a trained piano and organ player who loved music," and as "a lady" who adjusted to difficult conditions. Only in the loosest sense of the term could the Hoffmans be classified as "carpetbaggers." Still, they were interlopers. Their ripened peaches were "shipped in refrigerated cars that were supposed to be re-iced at Atlanta but they were not and arrived in Pittsburg in sad condition. There was considerable bitterness amongst Confederates who had lost the Civil War and Yankees did not always fare too well; anyway Bob's father gave up farming." In 1903 the family moved to Wilkinsburg, a Pittsburgh suburb, and Addison became a civil engineer and supervisor of dams along the Allegheny and Ohio Rivers.[2] During this year Bob turned five, and a younger sister, named Eleanor (Booch), was born. Addison spent so much time away from home that family relations became strained. Another woman separated their parents, and Bertha took the children to Chicago. On her return three months later, Bob and Booch moved in with their father, while the other children remained with their mother. Hence Bob had the benefit of a male model. His father married twice again, but at age fifty-six, while working as a chemist, Addison died of radium poisoning.[3]

What Bob acquired from his father was a masculine disposition and some other lifelong personality traits. Bob's foremost childhood characteristic, according to his brother, was his "me first" attitude. "He wanted to be boss. He was the great 'I am.' " Similarly, his father always wanted to be "it" and thrived on the attention and adulation of women. But to ensure compliance Addison sought out lower-class women. "He didn't like educated ones." That Bob's "mother was a lady" was possibly a factor in his parents' marital problems. Bob and his brother Chuck had a proclivity for "uncultured, uneducated women." Jack contends that Bob later married Rosetta "because she was crazy about him and she was trashy. He liked to be on top." Also, like Bob, Addison had an affinity for strength. "He could tense his muscles like blocks of wood," observed Bob. His clenched fist resembled "a sixteen-pound iron shot," and his grip was "marvelous and most unusual." Bob shared the large physical structure of his father, who, unlike his diminutive mother, was 5' 10" and over two hundred pounds. Addison had an affinity for strength and was always asking family and friends to "feel his arm." Bob's common-law widow Alda Ketterman recalls him as "big and strong." She was impressed by Addison's practice of chewing gum to strengthen his jaws. Bob "learned much from him." His father "remembered everything that he read," and his knowledge of medicine, chemistry, and engineering was unsurpassed.[4] Regarding ego and male identity, father and son were strikingly similar.

Apart from the stresses of a broken home, the greatest trauma of Hoffman's childhood was a bout of typhoid fever from drinking contaminated water. In later life he recalled the agony of this ordeal. He was a "real weakling" at age four. "At one time the doctor said I was dead, and when he found that there was a spark of life still in me, he said that I would never amount to anything even if I lived, for my heart and other organs were too badly damaged." His father "syringed him with salt water and saved his life." This experience may have contributed to Bob's lifelong abstinence from tobacco, alcohol, and other harmful substances and his interest in health foods and pure water. Hoffman thus endured the physical debility that lends itself to overcompensation and unrealistic aspirations. His later boast that his "earliest athletic experience" consisted of "running 250 times around a double tennis court" before age five could be a fabrication representative of his having overcome the trauma of nearly dying.[5] He also fostered the notion that he had been "a ninety-seven-pound weakling who would never take his shirt off at the beach." Then Hoffman supposedly "found an old barbell in a dump near Forbes Field in Pittsburgh, and over the years he built up an impressive torso of rippling muscles." The most fantastic yarn about his youthful exploits concerned a modified marathon sponsored by the *Pittsburg Leader*: "My father thought that I was too young [at nine] to enter the race but he didn't tell me that I couldn't watch the race. At the start, two of the boys asked me to hold their street clothes and shoes while they ran the race in athletic costume. I knew they would need their clothes so I ran along with them. At the end of the ten miles I was running beside the winner carrying the clothes and shoes, fresh as I could be and it would have been easy to win had I been properly entered."[6] Such unverifiable stories can be dismissed as the inventions of an egomaniac. But to Hoffman and those later subscribing to his ideas who also lacked self-assurance, they not only compensated for reality but assumed an independent existence that seemed necessary to survival in a man's world. Myth assumed an inspirational quality that truth could never attain.

The real story of Hoffman's childhood and early interest in athletics is far less dramatic. His brother remembers that he rose from bed at 5 a.m. daily to clean streets in the suburb of Oakland. At age eight he hauled trash to the dump in his teddy wagon and delivered spring water to area residents from nearby Schenley Park for five cents a gallon. Hoffman also peddled newspapers, cleaned fish at the corner market, and sold peanuts at Forbes Field, where the Pirates won the 1907 World Series. Later he worked in a brick factory. Even as a youth he required little sleep, one of the hallmarks of ambition, and in later life he could sleep at will, requiring only several minutes each time. He grew to his adult height by thirteen but weighed only 140 pounds and had narrow shoulders. "I was so thin that I just about had to stand twice in one place to cast a shadow. No wonder I was called Chicken Breast and Daddy Long Legs."[7]

Scholastically, Bob was a good student and once skipped a grade. He was a quiet, studious lad who spent much time in solitary activities such as reading. He frequently visited public libraries and claimed to read during summer vacations as many as two books a day. It is not surprising

Bob Hoffman's Formative Years

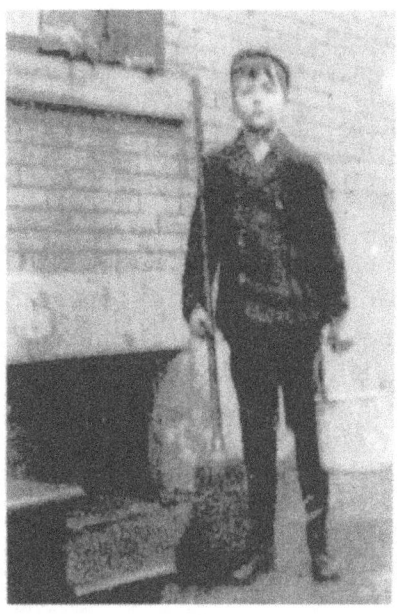

Bob's first business venture—street cleaning in Oakland for a nickel a week.

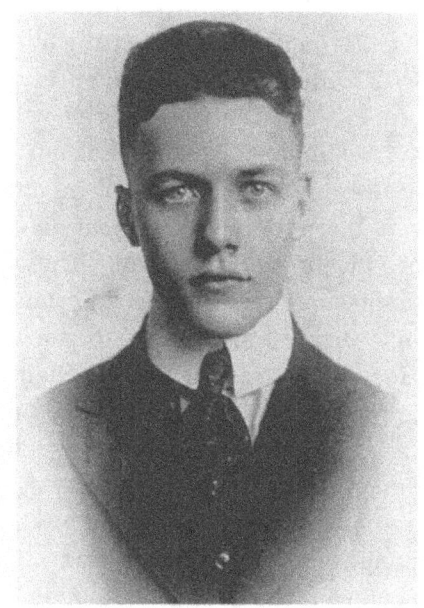

A dapper lad of seventeen—6' 3" and 167 pounds.

that he favored history, particularly stories of heroes. Another choice area was outdoor life and physical achievement. He recalled spending many hours in the Carnegie Library. "I have a retentive memory and I well remember the photos . . . of the strength and athletic stars of the day. The accounts of the early Olympic games are indelibly stamped in my memory as if they occurred but yesterday." Hoffman developed a fund of knowledge that was "well-nigh inexhaustible," preparing him to be, "by a very great margin, the world's leading physical director." His claim that he graduated from Peabody High School in 1914 cannot be verified in school records, and city directories show that his father was not even in Pittsburgh during Bob's high school years.[8] Jack insists that he quit school in tenth grade because he was not learning much and wanted to taste the real world. His first steady job was taking tickets at a movie house in 1914. Just before the war he was employed at Spalding's Sporting Goods, where he allegedly became "their leading salesman."[9]

This occupation reinforced Hoffman's growing interest in aquatics. The Hoffman brothers belonged to the Pittsburg Aquatic Club and competed in various athletic events organized by the *Pittsburg Press*. "Bob Hoffman Stars" reads the heading for an article on the 1916

Press regatta: "The star of the afternoon . . . was 'Bob' Hoffman of the P.A.C. squad, who competed in practically every event on the program . . . and covered himself with glory by taking points in almost every number." In canoe jousting, the final and most spectacular event of the day, Bob eliminated his brother Jack. By the end of the season, through endurance and determination, he earned the sobriquet of Pittsburgh's "Iron Man." These feats enabled Hoffman to pass his first test of manliness—establishing parity with his brothers. Up to this time their maturity and superior strength had made him feel inferior. He was regarded merely as their kid brother, Bob recalls. So during the winter of 1915–16 he trained on the river frequently and did light resistance exercises indoors. At first they ridiculed Bob for seeking "manufactured bumps," but persistence paid off. "Finally I was winning and as the years passed my brothers became Bob Hoffman's brothers in all conversations and introductions . . . at the club."[10] Bob's youthful achievements in aquatics, though based more on stamina than strength, were a powerful stimulus to his interest in sport.

The Great War and Aftermath

These heroics were interrupted when Hoffman enlisted on first call when the United States entered World War I in April 1917. He wanted to enter the "Sub Chasers," but his father insisted it was too dangerous and that he should join the Eighteenth Pennsylvania National Guard regiment. After basic training at Camp Hancock in Georgia and officers' school at Fort Niagara, he earned his sergeant's stripes but was demoted to private for being under age. His account of the voyage to Europe on the *Olympic* is full of references to his physical prowess, acts of daring, and attempts to define his manliness. Boxing was a favorite pastime, and Hoffman says he fought his share of matches. In France he held his own against "Bandsman Rice," alleged to be former heavyweight champion of the British Empire—an entity of four hundred million people! This feat sounds impressive, especially for an untrained pugilist. Bob's self-promotional instincts, however, led him to expand on the truth. Rice was never the British Empire champion, and there is no independent evidence that Hoffman ever fought him. Nor can the assertion that he boxed Gene Tunney "a number of times on the return trip" be substantiated.[11]

Most notable in Hoffman's account of his war experiences is the way he conveys his physical attributes. He describes himself as "champion digger of the American army," a champion marksman who equaled the British army record for accuracy, and a superb human specimen who had "the happy faculty of learning things quickly." He was "far stronger than his comrades . . . always neat and clean," and frequently cited as a model soldier. But his extrapolations on physical prowess were not limited to himself. His romantic notions of robust manhood extended to the American army in general and especially to some Texans in his company who, in Hoffman's estimation, embodied the frontier spirit on which this nation was founded. Their fathers had "grown up on the prairies where a man lived or died, survived or perished," by "courage and his physical ability." The Texans, he thought, were best in hand-to-hand combat. An "unfortunate group of Germans found this out to their sorrow. I wonder what they must have thought to see this wave of huge men, gigantic men, approximately six and a half feet tall, almost as broad as barn doors, for they were built to proportion. Perhaps the Germans were too startled at the size and evident ferocity of their antagonists to fight." Hoffman likened this experience to "a gigantic indian fight" and held the enemy's notion of national superiority in contempt. He had "never liked Germans," and called them "Frankensteins" because of their regimented society. A reason for these qualities, he surmised, was that the Germans were all one race. He preferred America's diverse society, where officers and men "could think for themselves."[12] Much of Hoffman's appreciation for the "melting-pot" phenomenon as a cultural asset was formed during the war.

Many passages in Bob's account describe hard fighting, suffering, and heroic acts, mostly his. During the assault on a German trench in the battle for Hill 204, a grenade exploded in front of him, thereby causing him to lose his hair. "I had hair so thick when I went overseas that I could hardly keep it out of my eyes. . . . I came home with very little hair." Shortly afterward, though wounded and "a mass of blood from head to foot," he claimed to have captured dozens of Germans while gathering batches of souvenirs! He was grazed by bullets in four places—his face, both knees, his left arm—and others hit his helmet, canteen, and shovel. He assures readers that he was one of the luckiest American soldiers in France. He allegedly "led his men where others feared to tread.

He saw his company wiped out to the last man in a hailstorm of lead winged death, but went on alone, capturing single handed thirty-eight prisoners. Time and time again he proved his mettle under fire. . . . He was generally conceded to be one of the most daring and coolest leaders ever to storm an enemy parapet. Such is the value of confidence born of physical mightiness." Decorations commensurate with such heroism were forthcoming, and Hoffman spares nothing in describing them. In addition to three Croix de Guerres (with two palms and a silver star) from France, he was awarded the Belgian Order of Leopold, the Italian War Cross, a Purple Heart, and the Distinguished Service Cross. In the 1930s the latter was disputed by a business rival, who accused Hoffman of using his war record to sell products and reported him to the Federal Trade Commission (FTC). Bob had to concede that it never appeared on his service record, that there had been "a mix-up," and that he was only "recommended for it."[13] To allay skepticism, however, he reproduced a picture of himself in uniform displaying his medals and citation from General Pershing for gallantry.

It would be tempting to dismiss Hoffman's war stories as myth making of a tall order, but there is much truth in them. Official records show that he was in the thick of fighting in July 1918, when his platoon was the first in the Keystone Division to see action near Chateau-Thierry. He was slightly wounded by a shell splinter, and his unit was awarded the Croix de Guerre. His bullet-dented helmet at York Barbell is further evidence of intense combat. Hoffman wrote candidly to his sister about his experiences in the Argonne sector.

> The Major told me that the Third Battallion on our right was having quite a time with it, and needed reinforcements. At the time I thought this was just a new form of suicide. I took the job cheerfully though, and didn't do any kicking for someone had to do it . . . so why not I. I gathered together nearly one hundred men. We were short of non-coms, so had no other sargeant to help me and had to do it all myself. Finally got them together and started over to help the other battallion. The air was literally thick with bullets from the Hun's guns . . . but I got over there with enough men to do quite a lot of helping.

Not only was Bob awarded the Order of Leopold, but he was one of only three sergeants in the 111th Infantry to receive the Croix de

Bob Hoffman's Formative Years

Guerre with palm. There is no mention of a second palm, silver star, or the Italian Cross, but he was cited by Pershing for "gallantry in action" and "brilliant leadership" at Fismette. By the end of two years' service, in August 1919, he had fought his way up four grades to second lieutenant.[14]

The war greatly affected Hoffman's outlook. He ceased to be religious. He had been a believer before the war and taught Sunday school, but he concluded that "a God would never allow such suffering as he had witnessed." Hence his worldview became almost wholly secular, and he remained impervious to all religious solicitations. Belief in self took the place of belief in God. War also affected his sexual maturation. Promiscuity was an integral part of military life, and Hoffman had ample opportunity for sexual experimentation when on leave in Paris. Even in wartime it was a gay city. After visiting the Folies Bergeres he would stroll down the Boulevard des Italiens, where there were thousands of "ladies of the evening." As he awkwardly put it, "I had found a very nice little girl and had enjoyed being with her." Later he collected "French-type" pictures from haversacks of dead Germans, and in captured trenches he observed how the enemy fulfilled their sexual needs. Whether these experiences were new or shocking is doubtful, but the war had an impact on him. Jack, who slept with Bob for two months after his discharge, testifies that "he had terrible nightmares about the war." Despite later claims that "I have never to my knowledge exaggerated or prevaricated," it was at this juncture, with an enviable war record in hand, that he began improving on the truth.[15]

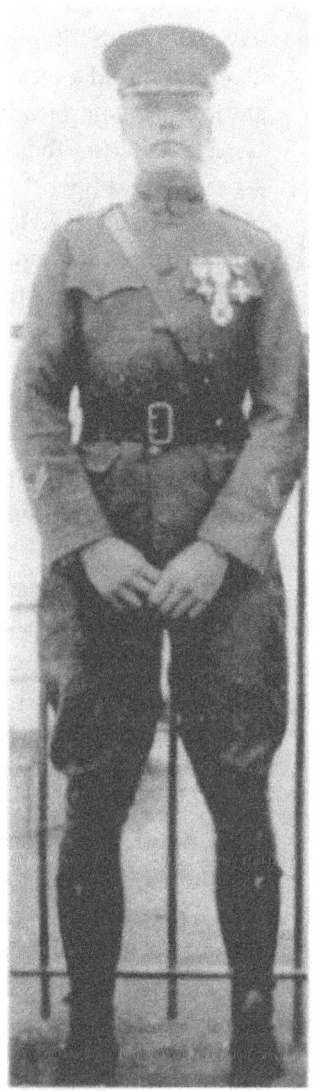

World War I hero—France, 1919.

On returning home Hoffman worked briefly in a steel mill, where he says he drew $150 per month, mainly for boxing on the company team. Then he found a less hazardous way to make a living—sales. Notwithstanding his heroics in athletics and battle, he was confronted with a hard fact of life—that he must sell himself in order to sell his product. As a boy he had been "timid, self-conscious, bashful and retiring," afraid of girls and inclined toward solitude. After being intimidated by various businessmen, he ended up peddling an overpriced medical book, *The Library of Health*, in the small towns of western Pennsylvania. At first he dreaded Monday mornings, but eventually he developed the "mental nerve" necessary for success.

> Some salesmen would carry an expensive silk handkerchief to make themselves feel superior. Others carried a twenty dollar gold piece or a hundred dollar bill. Or a fine diamond ring or dressed expensively and carefully.
>
> But the best system for a man who was an athlete was to make physical comparisons. . . . After going into the inner, private office, having obtained an interview with the prosperous business man who was very likely fat, bald and out of condition generally, I would think of the things I could do better than he.
>
> I would often simplify this procedure by merely telling myself mentally that, I could "lick" him. . . . I was building up a feeling of reliance and confidence in myself. . . . Physical strength and efficiency begets nerve, nerve helps selling and all of life is selling.

He also subscribed to the maxim that in a "country where all men are created equal most men had reached a high place by their own efforts."[16] By such means Hoffman built the self-confidence that became his hallmark. He was a self-made man in an era when people believed that success resulted from effort, willpower, and confidence. Being sold on himself, it became easy for him to sell to others.

Arrival in York

Soon Hoffman graduated from door-to-door salesman to real estate agent, working on commission on the outskirts of Pittsburgh. His transient situation and development of sales techniques undoubtedly affected his approaches to the opposite sex. He developed many temporary relationships, recalls his brother, in which the women were treated as expendable. "It didn't matter if they were married or not.... He didn't have any sexual principles—also no religious principles. Anything went. No second thoughts or remorse." For a man who never smoked, drank, or cussed, it is hardly surprising that he should indulge fully in at least one vice. However selfish and irresponsible such conduct might appear, it was consistent with his growing sense of self; and he never allowed fear or inhibitions to get in the way.

Hoffman came to York in 1920 at the urging of his brother Chuck, who had been stationed at nearby Fort Meade and had married a local girl. At first Bob managed a store that sold tires and automobile fixtures. Then he went into the oil-burner business with his brother. Their venture was unsuccessful, but Bob learned about patterns, castings, and machine work, skills useful later in manufacturing barbells. Eventually he entered a partnership with Ed Kraber, son of a local plumber. Kraber had inherited some money and designed one of the country's first automatic oil burners, but he was "no salesman," recalls an early associate. Bob was a perfect complement. They marketed oil burners from the mid–Atlantic coast to Ohio. According to one of Bob's favorite stories, he was down to ten cents on a sales trip to Baltimore and used it to buy a sandwich. Fortunately he sold an oil burner at the seventh house at which he stopped, and was able to get home. Such a "rags-to-riches" anecdote, true or not, fits the unfolding drama of his success as he perceived it. In any case, the partners soon turned a handsome profit, and their income steadily improved during the 1920s.[17]

A final feature of Hoffman's life in the aftermath of war was his marriage. In York he met Rosetta Snell while installing an oil burner in the grocery store run by her father. Though still in her teens, she already had a child by a previous marriage. When Bob started courting Rosetta, her mother fed him regularly. It must have chagrined him that her fourteen brothers and sisters called him "Daddy Bob" because he seemed so old. They were married on October 20, 1928, in Pittsburgh. Afterward he took her to the Carnegie Tech football game. "I was crazy about athletics, but my wife never forgave me for going to a football game on our wedding day." Still, they appeared happy in their early years of marriage. "To the dearest and sweetest little wife in the world from a man who loves her more than anything in this universe" is the inscription on a picture Bob gave to Rosetta. She recalls fondly the apartment they shared in York. "Before he went out the door he had to hand me a love note." But it was evident that Bob "wanted to do barbell and weightlifting more than anything. Bob wanted it bad."[18] Whether in business, sex, or athletics, satisfying his ego was first and foremost. A strong instinct for survival, stemming from his early bout with typhoid, and a need for masculinity, as defined by his father and American cultural norms at the turn of the century, were critical factors in shaping the founder's outlook in his formative years.

2
THE ORIGINS OF AMERICAN WEIGHTLIFTING

> For men, athletic competition has always been a contest of manhood, a ritual designed to measure strength and speed relative to others. Since the 1920s at least, American men have been transfixed by sports.... More than other cultures, America equated performance anywhere with masculinity everywhere; any failure in the approved masculine world—in the woods, locker room, market-place, or bed—betrayed a disabled man.
>
> —Loren Baritz, *The Good Life*

American Strength Traditions

Sport historians have shown that many games played in the increasingly urbanized environment of nineteenth-century America, though derived from Anglo-Saxon culture, were strongly influenced by immigrants from central and eastern Europe.[1] For strength sports there was also a nationalistic and militaristic tradition. This value system accompanied the peoples who swarmed to the United States in search of economic and political refuge, especially after the failure of the 1848 revolutions. Americans had traditionally relied on medications and electromechanical devices to promote health. The immigrants were preoccupied with "calisthenics, sports, and gymnastics," notes Harvey Green. "Before this, only a few physicians and educational reformers were interested in exercise and physical education, and nearly all of them had studied . . . German or other European systems."[2] Though the German *Turnverein* model was designed to promote fitness through calisthenics and gymnastics, its adherents were also linked to weightlifting.[3] In the strong-man era of fin de siècle America the overwhelming majority of strength athletes were of foreign (mostly German) origin. Hoffman's 1940 book, *Mighty Men of Old,* shows that virtually all strong men from the preceding two generations were either foreigners or first-generation Americans.[4] Significantly, they also often had to overcome a physical deficiency—sickliness, weakness, or underdevelopment.

After World War I a new era dawned in American athletics. "Free from Europe's struggle to recover from the effects of war," writes William Baker, "Americans enjoyed a golden age of sport in the 1920s."[5] Although this observation applies chiefly to such major sports as baseball and football, weightlifting underwent a metamorphosis from strongmanism to more regulated competition. Many old shibboleths and superstitions were discarded. Whereas at the turn of the century Eugen Sandow was advising his readers on how to avoid becoming musclebound, articles in *Strength,* the foremost muscle magazine of the 1920s, discounted this possibility. Also questioned was the "athletic heart," as well as the idea that weight training detracted from athletic performance. "The dilated heart has no place in my mind," wrote George Jowett in 1926, and "is scrapped on the junk pile of unfounded fallacy."[6] Many of Jowett's progressive ideas on heavy training and the harmful effects of tobacco, alcohol, coffee, and tea would later be adopted by Hoffman.

Strength, and to a lesser extent Bernarr Macfadden's *Physical Culture,* served as forums for discussing issues in the iron game as it searched for identity in sports. The former argued that life span was "several years longer than a generation ago" and that this was attributable to "the widespread popularity of sports, games, outdoor life and all kinds of exercise." In 1890 baseball, football, and track were somewhat popular; tennis was "in its infancy and considered effeminate"; golf was "practically unknown"; canoes were "a curiosity"; basketball, tobogganing, and skiing were "unknown"; and hiking was "a mild form of insanity." But by 1922 golf had become the "future 'All-American pastime.' "[7] There were debates about the relative strength of weightlifters as compared to weight throwers and how much climate, race, occupation, and diet contributed to strength. It was once believed, stated a 1922 editorial, that when "the majority of big professional 'Strong Men' were of Teutonic blood," they "derived their power from habitual beer-drinking." Since then virtually every country had "produced physical giants who have equalled or outdone Germany's best." It appeared to be not so much racial as environmental factors that were critical. Climate loomed large, it being noted that California athletes were able to "clean up the prizes in *strength* events in the intercollegiates" even though that state was sparsely populated. Also, the country's foremost lifting team, organized by Al Treloar and David Willoughby and featuring Noah Young, the national amateur heavyweight champion, was based at the Los Angeles Athletic Club.[8] In America generally, but especially in California, the melting-pot effect seemed to inspire what was best from all peoples.

Milo and *Strength*

Strength covered all facets of physical culture and in its heyday carried special features on art, beauty, physique, outdoor life, and women. The magazine's impact on Hoffman is evident from his comment that to have one's photo in it "made any man an outstanding celebrity." It was also an advertising medium for its parent firm, Milo Barbell Company, founded by Alan Calvert in 1902 in Philadelphia. But *Strength* would remain true to its original focus on "weightlifting—the best form of exercise ever devised for the male of the species."[9] That it was able to retain its image as a "man's magazine" stemmed largely from its appeal to readers who suffered physical or emotional inadequacies. Virtually all issues were chock-full of self-help articles, success stories, and solicitations from strong men for readers to purchase books, devices, or programs that would transform them into he-men. Many ads were accompanied by "before" and "after" examples and eye-catching titles: "Are You A Man Or Merely A Coat-Hanger?" (Charles MacMahon), "Re-born Again Through Strongfortism" (Lionel Strongfort), "Are You Changing From A *Man* Into A 'Clothespin'?" (Charles Atlas), "I Make Strong Men" (Earle Liederman), and "Muscles Like Steel For Only 15 Cents A Month" (Bernarr Macfadden). They often included a photograph of the purveyor of the merchandise, attired in breechclouts, with flexed and rippling muscles, testimony to the purveyor's beginnings as a weakling, and a foreign-sounding (usually German) name. The magazine and its products targeted neurasthenic youth seeking virility and self-actualization.[10] Slightly less apparent was their appeal to second-generation Americans seeking acceptance in a society where competitiveness was necessary for survival. From these ideas and promotional techniques Hoffman would devise a unique marketing style in the 1930s.

From 1922 to 1927 much of *Strength*'s virile tone was provided by George Fiusdale Jowett, a native of England who migrated to Canada before the war and later to the United States. Jowett shared the attitude of his compatriots that lifting should be a science and not pursued just for appearance. By concentrating on method and technique, "the Englishman's whole training [was] directed to making records," whereas "the American's [was] aimed more at body-building." Jowett, a disciple of George Hackenschmidt, contended that "development and strength go hand in hand. To become a real orthodox strongman you must have the physique." But "between the two I would choose strength."[11] Jowett's preoccupation, like that of Hoffman, who likely acquired it from him, was with strength, rather than size and shape of muscle. He also developed his body to compensate for a debilitating childhood injury. A beating he took from another youngster during convalescence confirmed Jowett's conviction that heavy exercise was needed. He then devoted all his spare time to "exercises that would make him bigger and stronger," until he finally "licked the hide" of the other boy. Whether such an overt challenge to his manhood ever occurred cannot be verified, but strength pundit Charles A. Smith notes that Jowett was "notorious for drawing the long bow, that what he says is . . . not to be relied on. He always told it to the advantage of George Fiusdale. Nothing he claimed was so." Such an indictment seems harsh, but strong man Sig Klein affirms that "no one ever saw Jowett make the lifts he claimed."[12] It should not detract greatly from the repute of Jowett or Hoffman that what they claimed was not always true. After all, they were promoters. They should be judged by their inspirational effect on youth with a low self-image, who were best served by myths rather than more grim realities.

An indisputable achievement of Jowett is his organization of the first national weightlifting association. Indeed he, more than Hoffman, deserves to be called "Father of American Weightlifting," an appellation

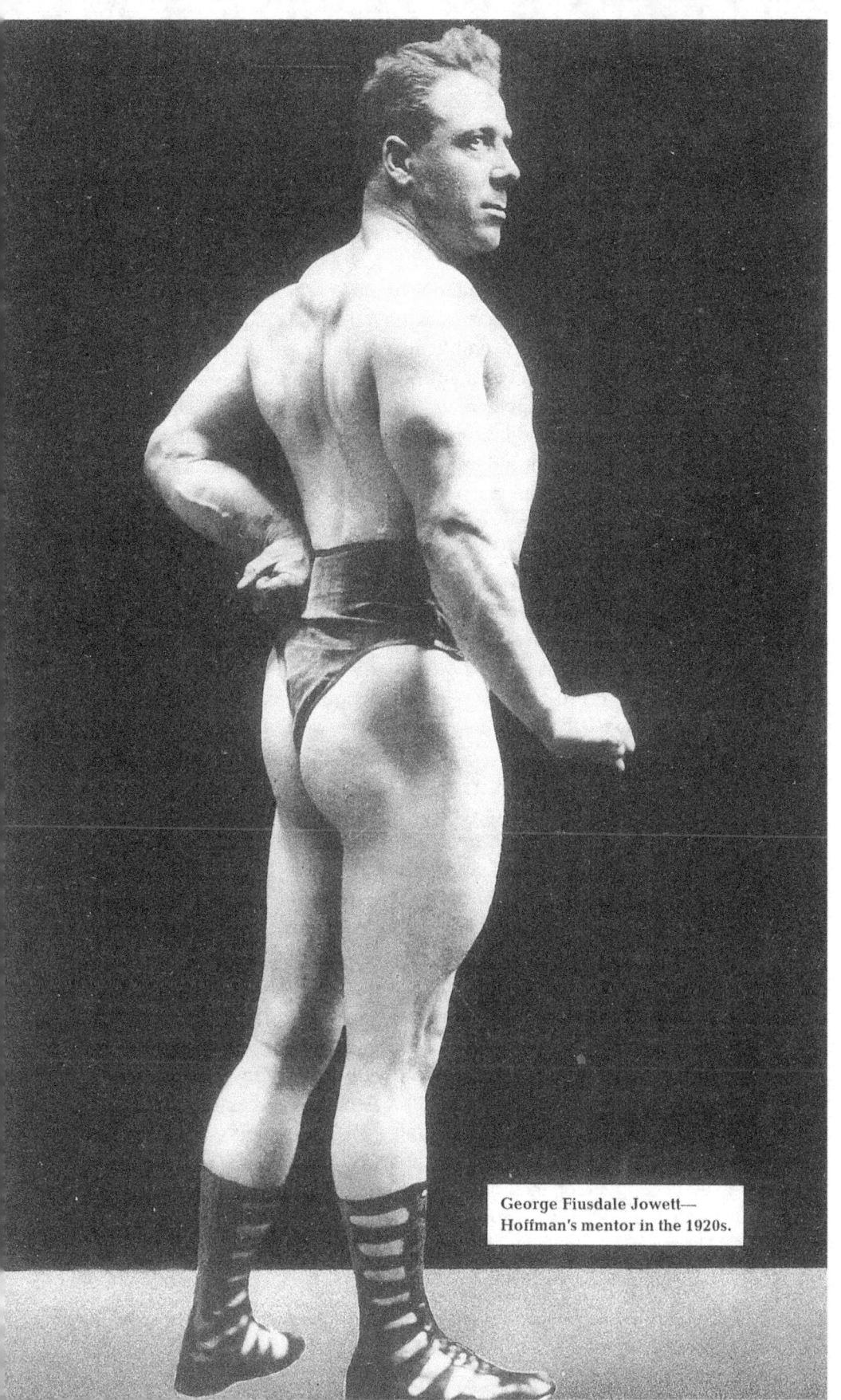

George Fiusdale Jowett—
Hoffman's mentor in the 1920s.

sometimes applied to Jowett in the 1930s. His efforts, however, must be placed in context with organizational trends. Despite attempts to establish rules as early as 1880, there was little regularity in the conduct of weightlifting at the first international championship (London, 1891), the first European championship (Rotterdam, 1896), the first world championship (Vienna, 1898), or the first Olympiad (Athens, 1896). The British Amateur Weight-Lifters Association (BAWLA) was founded in 1901, refounded in 1911, and later complemented by a professional association. The foundation was laid for an international federation at a meeting of German, Italian, and Dutch delegates at Duisburg in 1905. The reorganization of the Federation Internationale Halterophile by Jules Rosset, president of the French federation, at the 1920 Olympics in Antwerp further enhanced the sport's stature.[13] American weightlifting had its genesis with the initiatives of George Barker Windship, William "Father Bill" Curtis, John Babcock, Henry Buermeyer, and Donald Dinnie in Boston and New York. Turnvereins furnished an outlet for gymnastics enthusiasts in New York, but others who were interested in more rugged training in acrobatics, wrestling, and weightlifting formed strength clubs. "It was a common sight during the last part of the 19th century to see these athletes parade through the streets on a Sunday morning with dumbells on a wagon, on the way to their athletic field for training and exhibitions." The New York Athletic Club was a center for strength athletics as early as the 1860s, and in 1884 the German-American Club was formed. At the turn of the century weightlifting was enthusiastically practiced at the Hercules, Carl Abs, Sandow, Anthony Barker, and Cooper athletic clubs in Manhattan.[14] Clearly, German immigrants there had established a solid basis for the sport, and the feats of musclemen could be found occasionally in Richard Kyle Fox's *Police Gazette*.

During World War I Ottley Coulter, a circus and stage performer from Ohio, was in touch with Edmund Desbonnet in France and several German promoters. He knew barbell enthusiasts had had difficulty finding reliable figures for lifts performed during the bygone strongman era. In "Honesty in Weight Lifting and the Necessity of Making Lifters Prove Their Claims," an article in the January 1917 issue of *Strength*, he argued for greater regulation.[15] After the war Coulter renewed his appeal for accurate records and published a list of European and American records in forty-six lifts. With the Amateur Athletic Union (AAU, organized in 1888) preoccupied with track and field, Coulter advocated a separate organization for weightlifting. He was supported by *Strength* editor J. C. Egan, who believed an association would settle the strong-man controversies plaguing the sport. But its driving force was Jowett. Frustrated in trying to form an organization along British lines in Canada, he advised Coulter that it would be better to form one "for the whole American continent." Bernard Bernard, formerly editor of *Health & Strength* and president of BAWLA, quickly seized on Jowett's idea for an American Continental Weight-Lifters Association (ACWLA) and, as editor of a new journal called *Health and Life* in Chicago, actively promoted it. "Oh! for such an organization," exclaimed Jowett, "then an interest would be taken in lifting, we would know how we stood with other lifters and know real lifters from fakes."[16] However questionable his own lifting claims might have been, Jowett appreciated the need for regulation.

During the next several years Jowett and Coulter, with assistance from David Willoughby in California, struggled to establish the ACWLA. It took on new life when Jowett joined the *Strength* staff in 1924. His aim was to secure 250,000 adherents and thereby "unite all lifters." Through existing clubs in Los Angeles, New York, and Pittsburgh, Jowett hoped to stimulate local interest, improve knowledge of proper methods, standardize rules, and promote competition. His "rally call" had a manly nationalistic ring—"Are You A Patriot?" He appealed to aspiring weight trainees "to come in and be with the red blooded men of America. We want you."[17] An accompanying article by Calvert focused on a significant feature in the promotion, governance, and lore of lifting—the superman complex. "There always has to be someone to 'start things,' someone who has sufficient faith in himself, and in the soundness of his own ideas to carry the thing through. . . . I often thought how fine it would be to have all American lifters grouped together in one Association but I knew how much work would be involved, and so never took the trouble to foster such a movement. Such a movement was inaugurated a few years ago by that unquenchable enthusiast, George F. Jowett." Indeed Jowett fancied himself a patriarch of strong men. Writing under a pseudonym, he spoke freely of his own accomplishments and importance—the "corner stone" who supplied the "tangible means" for American lifting success.[18] Hoffman in later years would speak of his own role in founding the sport. But it was Jowett who was the principal instigator of a weightlifting association and served as an avuncular model for Hoffman.

Early York Initiatives

During these years Bob's chief interest was still aquatics, and he returned to Pittsburgh each summer seeking his share of glory. "Hoffman Cleans Up" was the press-report heading for an aquatic carnival in July 1920.

> When "Bob" stood up for the canoe-tilting contest and tripped the gunwhale of the little shell which was to support him, one big gasp went up from those watching.
> With a dexterity which must have come down to him in a direct line from the primitive days of the world, he caught the edge of the canoe between his great toes on one side and the other four on the other side and all his adversaries failed to make him loosen that hold. "The only way you could knock him off would be to sink the boat under him," remarked one spectator, more in earnest, than in fun. In the parlance of everyday slang, "he was good."

To improve his canoeing he trained with light apparatus at home and makeshift weights at the factory. In 1923 he started ordering catalogs from advertisers in *Strength*. Although he could not afford a weight set, he was "convinced that barbell training was the way to gain the strength and muscle I desired." With proceeds from the factory "swear box," Bob purchased a 225-pound Milo set and placed it in the York YMCA, where the new physical director, Doc Bleeker, helped him perform the exercises. Initially an 80-pound press and a 150-pound clean and jerk were all he could manage. By 1925, after two years of weight training, he still weighed only 177 and was not very strong. But soon after 1927, when interest in aquatics began to taper off, Bob passed 200 pounds and by 1933 reached 240. Afflicted with the same "do-or-die" disposition as Jowett's, Hoffman equated size with manliness. According to an early (self-authored) promotional booklet, it was his "cool, calculating practical mind" that "brought him up from a long, lanky, skinny individual . . . to an athletic superman of 243 pounds." As with Jowett, the allure of fulfilling the ideal of the self-made man by expanding on a body of partial truths proved irresistible. "In Bob Hoffman the nation has an honest sincere, splendid example of physical manhood. . . . He breathes leadership, courage and confidence. . . . If any man can make others capable of filling a red blooded he man's niche

The Origins of American Weightlifting

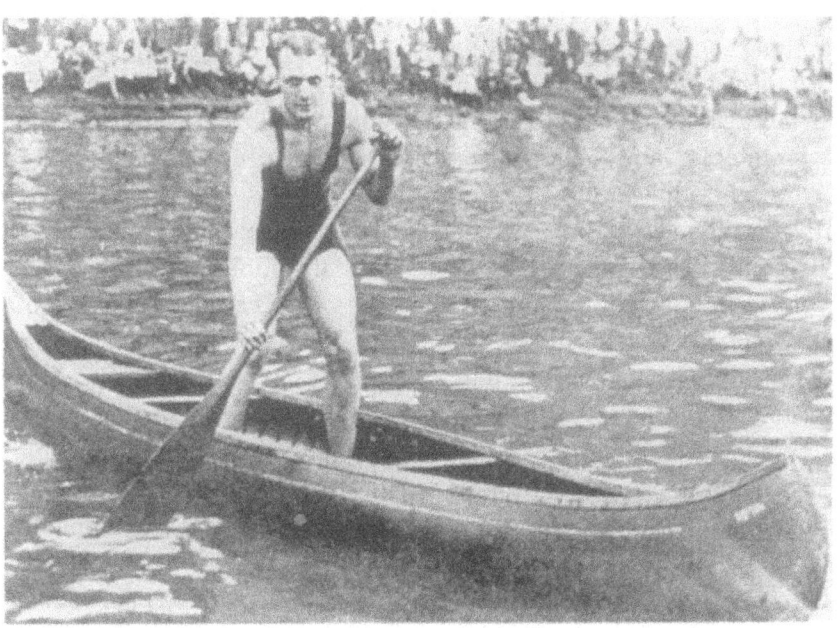

Canoe-racing champion—Bob, after winning a quarter-mile race in 1919. Indentation on inside of knee was supposedly a bullet scar from war.

in this tough old world of ours it is Bob Hoffman—the ace of American manhood."[19] Unquestionably Bob's great size made him noticed and respected, and it gave him a natural advantage in business and sport.

Hoffman, safe to say, was far from being a notable iron-game figure in the 1920s. Yet he later claimed that in 1925 he had organized the nation's first real weightlifting meet. In 1915 there was a meet in San Francisco, and in 1923 the first amateur contest under official conditions was conducted by Willoughby at the Los Angeles Athletic Club. Bob insisted these events were mere exhibitions and that his meet, in number of contestants and kinds of lifts, set a new standard. It was inspired by a local reporter who wondered whether lifters with "manufactured bumps" were stronger than men who developed muscles at work. There were strong men from farms and brickyards, plumbers, machinists and foundry men who had "thrown half of a locomotive wheel in the cupola for melting," firemen, policemen, boxers, and wrestlers—all vying to be "York's strongest man." Not knowing how to run a meet, Hoffman arranged seven platforms and barbells, one for each weight class, at the York YMCA. To lend an official air, he invited Jowett, but belittled his role. "Jowett just sat there aiding us perhaps by his presence, but doing nothing to run the meet, so I had to run from platform to platform . . . trying to help three officials at each platform officiate correctly and trying to see that every man lifted properly." Not surprisingly, despite a creditable showing by Don Pitts of Hanover, Bob won the title of "York's Strongest Man." The glow of victory was lessened by the fact that he edged Pitts by only 2.5 pounds while outweighing him by 60. But Hoffman's chief satisfaction stemmed from the publicity in local papers. "The kids followed me around and a lot of girls wanted dates with a strong man." That he "had more dates . . . the next year than all the rest of my life combined" constitutes a powerful statement about Hoffman's search for masculinity.[20]

Whatever validity may be attached to Hoffman's claims to fame as an early organizer and "York's strongest man," he was never in the same league as such heavyweights as Carl Moerke, Henry Steinborn, or Arthur Giroux; nor was he ever a prospect for international competition. Contrary to later self-serving accounts of his early involvement, Hoffman's activities received scant coverage in *Strength*. His name first appears in February 1926 as master of scales at one of Jowett's monthly exhibitions in Philadelphia, and in later issues he is mentioned in such roles as loader, second, and referee. Otherwise he is mentioned infrequently, and never as a notable lifter, in a position of authority, or as a man of special insight. He was still a novice and not one of the fathers—Oscar Matthes, Jowett, "Teddy" Mack, John Smith, Harry Hall, Mark Berry, and George Blymire—whose group picture appears in the August 1926 issue.

How, then, could he have won the national heavyweight championship in 1927? His success was due to the peculiar way the meet, only the third of its kind, was conducted. Each year, on or before November 5, "national" meets were held at various locations nationwide and the results mailed to *Strength*. In early 1927 Jowett and his ACWLA were displaced by Mark Berry and the Association of Bar Bell Men (ABBM). Still, a national championship was held. One of its staging areas was Philadelphia, and from his performance there Hoffman was recognized as "national champion" by *Strength*. But he was the only contestant in his class, and the description of his lifting assumed an apologetic, almost pitying tone.

> Robert Hoffman, of York, Pa., weighing 205 pounds in light costume, came out next for a trial in the heavy class. The big boy

was not so successful as he hoped to be, and he certainly deserved better poundages for his gameness in appearing on the platform without sufficient time to practice the lifts, having been away from lifting practice for a long time.... Due to his travels he finds it possible only to practice enough to get up on the platform and try his luck. The total he succeeded in making was 843 pounds. The spectators warmly applauded him after he finished.

Hoffman won by default. Remarkably, there were no other contenders in the entire nation for the heavyweight title. Albert Manger won the light-heavy crown, and most other big men were professionals. Weightlifters in the 1920s were diminutive by modern standards. Even the total of Arnie Sundberg of Mayger, Oregon, lightweight champ at 137 pounds, exceeded Hoffman's total by thirty-one pounds. Hoffman later conceded that he won the title "with lifts that the best featherweight can perform today," but he was champion.[21]

For the next several years Manger and others dominated the heavier classes, and the ABBM and AAU struggled for control of lifting. Neither body sent lifters to the 1928 Olympics in Amsterdam, where the press, snatch, and clean and jerk were first incorporated as standard lifts. Hoffman remained on the fringes, professing to acquire lifting knowledge and skill by observing others. Frank Dennis of Birdsboro, Pennsylvania, was an early "idol," despite his liking for beer, and from Sundberg he learned snatching technique. But Hoffman's foremost model was Robert Snyder of Hagerstown, Maryland, recognized by *Strength* in 1917 as "the most finished and skillful amateur lifter in the country to-day." Hoffman could not have chosen a better model. Bob often confessed that it was from Snyder that "I learned more about weightlifting than from any other man. I learned by just looking at his pictures."[22] Another phase of Hoffman's initiation to lifting was his extensive traveling in the late 1920s. Much of it related to selling oil burners, but he tried to arrange trips so that he could attend weightlifting contests and meet the strong men featured in *Strength*. He also engaged, when possible, in other sport and fitness tests. By his own account he continued to win prizes in aquatic events, ran and walked long distances, paddled his canoe along a Mississippi River tributary, and even carried his "tired" 118-pound wife over four miles to the top of Mount Washington! He cultivated the acquaintance of Mark Berry, Sig Klein, Alan Calvert, Harry Paschall, and others who would be important to his future in the strength world. Hoffman describes his role as a sort of goodwill ambassador. He idealized lifters as "a fine bunch of happy, enthusiastic, ambitious, clean-living fellows," men who "always welcomed me and called in all weightlifters in surrounding districts." It was a period of intense activity and observation, during which he trained with "many of the world's most famous coaches." He equates his experience to a "university education," but "desultory" rather than "intense" would more aptly describe his apprenticeship.[23] He had yet to make his mark.

ABBM and AAU

By the end of the 1920s, though there were more meets and interest than ever, weightlifting in the United States was in disarray. The ABBM was run along the same lines as the ACWLA, but it lacked the organizing skills of Jowett and was soon superseded by the AAU. The latter was led by Dietrich Wortmann of the German-American Athletic Club, chairman of the Metropolitan Weight Lifting Committee. In 1927 he presented a set of rules conforming the AAU to international standards and was appointed weightlifting's first chairman. At the 1929 AAU national championships in New York City, virtually all of the contestants either had German names or represented German athletic clubs. Robert Knodle, seven-time national champion from Maryland who won the 112-pound class, recalls that many competitors "could hardly speak English. All they would do was eat and drink. The bartender would be lifting the next day." Knodle "didn't know how they could lift, they ate and drank so much." For many German-Americans, weightlifting was not only a link to their native culture, in which strength was admired, but a means to excel in their adopted land. Americanization, noted Walter Camp, was "more possible through the medium of American sport than almost any other way."[24] Much of the growing stature of the AAU in weightlifting circles may be attributed to the German-American clubs.

Meanwhile the ABBM, never robust, was faltering. Though in 1931 it boasted of having thrice as many members as the earlier ACWLA, it suffered acute financial losses. *Strength* absorbed this burden in the interest of sport but henceforth vowed the ABBM would be administered on "a firm business basis." A year later it announced that response to an appeal for more member support was "disgustingly apathetic." It was, of course, the heart of the Great Depression and many of the estimated half million barbell users in the country were unemployed. Nevertheless *Strength* scolded its readers, insisting that greater cooperation was "absolutely essential." Despite its advertisements and gimmicks, ABBM membership was only two thousand.

> Now contrary to what a lot of you may think, no one is either getting rich or making a penny out of the A.B.B.M. . . . Oh, yes, we are fully aware of the existing belief that the A.B.B.M. is hooked up with the sale of barbells. Well, let us assure you it isn't, and certain parties who should know are convinced that the game of weightlifting is essential neither to *Strength* Magazine or the promotion of barbells. . . . We wonder if you fully realize what would become of the lifting game if those who are behind the A.B.B.M. should decide to drop their support and the *Strength* Magazine editors should become disgusted and decide lifting was too unprofitable. We venture the guess that within several months American lifting would be dead as the proverbial door-nail.[25]

Obviously Milo Barbell viewed *Strength* and the ABBM as financial liabilities, regardless of their advertising value. Money was tight everywhere, it seemed—except in York!

York Oil Burner Athletic Club

Bob estimates he sold 227 oil burners in 1927 and continued that pace for four years. Soon there were branches of York Oil Burner in Philadelphia and Toronto also reporting spectacular gains. By the early 1930s Hoffman was "making money at an unbelievable rate," perhaps as much as $60,000 per year.[26] In 1928 Bob and Rosetta purchased a one-bedroom bungalow on a Susquehanna River inlet. Here he recruited his earliest lifters, devised his barbell courses, and did his first serious weight training. In 1929 Hoffman and his partner acquired a permanent building at 51 North Broad Street to manufacture oil burners *and* barbells. He also purchased some land on Lightner's Hill in north York, where he built a bungalow to house his lifting club and started constructing, in 1931, the multistory "House on the Hill," designed to be Bob and Rosetta's dream home. It is remarkable that Hoffman's glory years began in the depths of the depression, an accomplishment that further fed his ego. With his newfound affluence he could take business interests more lightly and devote more energy to weightlifting. "Finally in 1931," he later observed, "I was so situated that I could go on with the game I had come to love more than any other." The key to his eventual takeover of the iron game was the attachment of his sporting interests to his business enterprise. In 1929 Bob began making barbells from the same facilities used in the manufacture of home heaters, but 1932 marks the real beginning of the operation. "A sale of 22 barbells during the week of fourth of July, 1933, stood as the record . . . for a time," notes Bob.[27] His team, the York Oil Burner Athletic Club (YOBAC), was integrated with the company and trained on the second floor of the factory.

Indicative that Hoffman was instigating a new era of competitiveness was a 1932 article in *Strength* on "The Club Idea." The prominence of the Los Angeles Athletic Club had attracted interest from 1922 to 1926, but German-American clubs in Manhattan, Brooklyn, and Detroit had recently come to the fore. Other clubs were stimulated by Arnold Schiemann in Baltimore, Dick Bachtell in Hagerstown, Arthur Gay in Rochester, Emmett Faris in Cincinnati, and Arnie Sundberg in Portland, Oregon. But most notable was Hoffman, who not only recruited a club but "provided the spark" for competition by transporting it widely. In December 1931, he fielded two teams against a combined Baltimore-Hagerstown contingent. The York teams scored an impressive 7,019-to-6,963 victory over the Marylanders. The winning edge was provided by William Good, recently recruited from Reamstown, Pennsylvania, who pressed 209, snatched 209, and cleaned and jerked 292 pounds at a bodyweight of only 180. In February 1932, however, York lifters were defeated by the German-American Athletic Club in New York City by 4,114 to 4,032 pounds. The former suffered somewhat from their long journey, and the latter benefited from the services of Tony Terlazzo, later one of York's greatest stars, who had the "most remarkable score of the day."[28] A clearer indication of the future of American weightlifting was Hoffman's successful bid to hold both the Middle Atlantic and the National AAU Championships in York the following spring.

By this point it was obvious that Hoffman was appropriating the cream of weightlifting talent in the eastern United States. "At first we didn't mind getting beat," he told team member Walter Good in 1932, "but now we want to have a first team that can beat the best team that can be gotten to-gether."[29] By his financial support, Hoffman was laying a firm basis for American lifting, but his need to dominate it led to some questionable practices. "Some strange matters recently have arisen in official lifting ranks," observed *Strength*. Bob had recently attracted Bachtell from Maryland and Wally Zagurski from Indiana to lift for him despite an AAU rule requiring athletes from another district to compete unattached for a year. It was further noted that the "parties concerned . . . aren't very jovially inclined over the turn of events." Permitting Bachtell and Zagurski to cross district lines might set a precedent for other elite lifters to travel around the country to win titles. This contretemps arose from ambiguities pertaining to multiple membership in the AAU, the ABBM, and affiliated clubs.[30] Given its unprofitability and jurisdictional conflict with the AAU, serious questions emerged over the benefits of the ABBM's continued existence. Underlying this whole process, however, was a subtle shift of power. Berry's ABBM had already been eclipsed by the AAU, and Wortmann effectively applied the AAU's international leverage to his advantage. Now the latter's authority was being undermined by Hoffman's financial wizardry.

Wortmann was using his influence in the AAU to harass Hoffman, but his team's loss to the YOBAC in April 1932 in New York, 5,725 to 5,835 pounds, was a devastating blow. Critical to Hoffman's victory was the appearance of his two "ringers," Bachtell and Zagurski. Hoffman confided to Walter Good that Wortmann and Berry "didn't do any protesting until after we won at New York, but they surely have tried to make it difficult since that time." Not only did they attempt to exclude Bachtell and Zagurski, but Hoffman's opponents protested that use of the York Oil Burner name constituted commercialism, that too many major meets were held in York, and that some YOBAC members had violated amateur guidelines. Hoffman took steps to check his adversaries. "I have been appointed A.A.U. Commissioner in this territory and have been on very intimate terms with the A.A.U. Commissioner in Pittsburgh for the last twenty years. And thanks to Mr. Clarke in Philadelphia, the president of the A.A.U. there, being in favor of the work we are doing here, everything has been satisfactorily arranged."[31] Thus Hoffman wisely decided not to declare war on troublesome AAU regulations but to use its organization and status to advance his own cause.

In the ensuing contests of 1932 Wortmann triumphed in a general sense by assuming titular control over weightlifting under the AAU umbrella. But real authority within the iron game was passing to Hoffman.

In June, Bob's team won its first of many national championships, amassing nearly as many points as all the rest of the nation's lifters. Because of the personal power and prestige at stake, the victory made a deep impression on Hoffman. For the rest of his life his team's winning the AAU nationals became his foremost aim, meaning more than personal comfort or merely making money. As *Strength* observed, "[T]here are just two things he talks about chiefly:—one, the success of his business of manufacturing oil burners, the other, weightlifting."[32] That the latter was becoming paramount was evident in the creation in 1932 of *Strength & Health* to publicize Hoffman's products, glorify his exploits and ideas, and increase his influence in the iron game. Never more than a mediocre lifter himself, he had by the early 1930s enmeshed himself in weightlifting politics to satisfy his craving for success in a man's world. Hoffman advanced almost directly from novice to patriarch.

3

THE OLD YORK GANG

Of the Americans who have come into notice during the past fifty years as poets, as novelists, as critics, as painters, as sculptors and in the minor arts, less than half bear Anglo-Saxon names, and in this minority there are few of pure Anglo-Saxon blood. So in the sciences. So in the higher reaches of engineering and technology. So in philosophy and its branches. So even in industry and agriculture.... The descendants of the later immigrants tend generally to move upward; the descendants of the first settlers, I believe, tend plainly to move downward.

—H. L. Mencken

The New Patriarch

One of the ironies of weightlifting lore is that Bob Hoffman succeeded while everyone else in his field was failing during the Great Depression. In contrast to his obscurity in the previous decade, he could say by the end of the 1930s that he not only was prosperous but had superseded virtually all earlier promoters. "There was Titus, he's gone. There was Strongfort, he's out of business too. There was Sandow and Breitbart, both of whom are dead. There was Zybysco, Matysek, Barker, Arco,

Dryer, McMahon, Leonard, Glick. There was Liederman, the biggest of them all at one time. Bob Hoffman bought his at-one-time Million-dollar-business for just $350. . . . How the mighty have fallen." Hoffman's achievement was remarkable because he sold barbells—a labor-intensive commodity—rather than courses. It no doubt helped that he had already succeeded in the oil-burner business, which required iron, but he virtually revolutionized strength training in the next generation through the widespread use of weights. Though Hoffman was not the first barbell entrepreneur, his buying out the defunct Milo Barbell Company in 1935 and founding his own company in 1938 enabled him to corner the cast-iron-weight market. Along with his firm financial base at York, Hoffman fostered a strength-and-health culture. Outwardly it projected confidence and integrity, and Bob tried to set an example for American youth by molding his own body into that of a superman and assuming attributes of an all-around athlete. Only by portraying himself as a sterling example of manhood could he justify the worth of his products. Just as important was the body of superb athletes who were attracted to employment in the oil-burner plant. They became weightlifting and physique champions and were represented as role models. By 1938 Hoffman could boast that York had "the strongest team in the world."[1] This aggregation constituted the "old York gang." It remained the heart of Hoffman's organization for fifty years, promoting the York way as a corollary to American manliness.

For Hoffman, 1932 started inauspiciously when he and his wife nearly lost their lives in an automobile accident on January 3. They were returning from a weightlifting meet when Bob, a terrible driver, ran their car head-on into another vehicle near Coatesville. Bob's condition was pronounced critical, with a possible skull fracture, and their car was demolished. Nevertheless, he recovered enough to compete with his team against the German-Americans in April.[2] More important, he used this setback to display his physical prowess—to prove that he was the "world's foremost physical trainer" and that he practiced what he preached. He launched a twenty-week experiment to gain bodyweight, raising his total by 102 pounds and acquiring a "much greater shapeliness." By stretching the truth he could claim to be "a great athlete" and "worthy champion." He presumed to show that age matters little, that no special food was required, that weight training with many different exercises was desirable, and that his system was superior to all others. To lend credence to his claims, in 1933 he staged

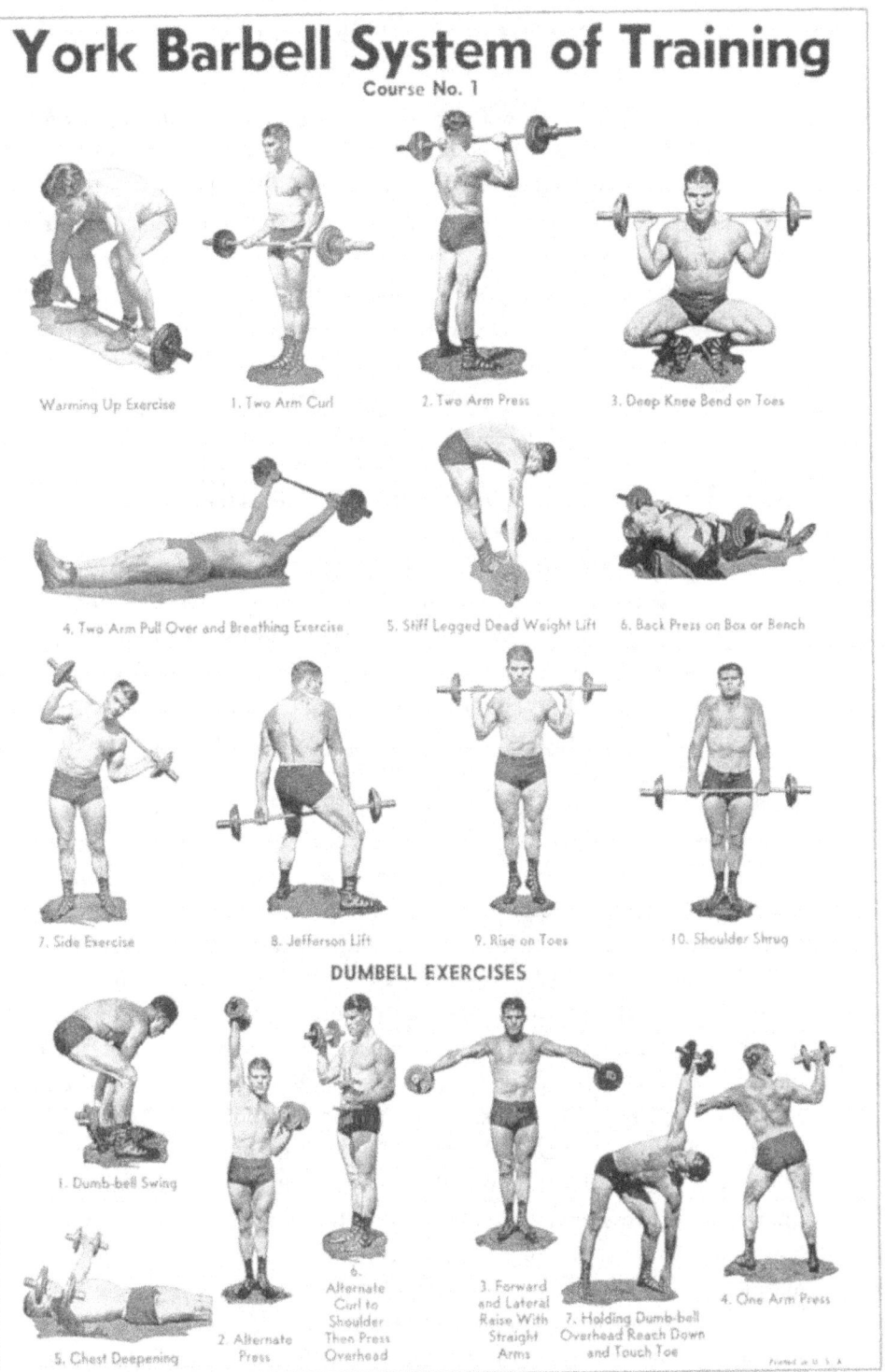

The first of Hoffman's original four courses, included with the purchase of every York barbell—illustrated by Joe Miller.

the first "professional competition to be held under official supervision in America." With three officials and a set of tested scales, Hoffman hoisted a respectable total of 687 pounds, the best of his life. It hardly mattered that Harry Good lifted thirty-five pounds more in a lighter division or that there were no other competitors; Bob declared himself national professional heavyweight champion.[3]

This stratagem worked because Hoffman was by this time advancing in weightlifting politics. Critical to his quest for control was the international perspective he gained at the 1932 Olympic Games in Los Angeles. America's lackluster performance, garnering only two bronze medals, and the strength of the Europeans spurred him to act. The foreign competitors "looked upon the United States team as something of a joke." He resolved to make America the foremost lifting power. An important step designed to enhance Hoffman's standing was his partnership with George Jowett in 1932. "This promotion comes out of the great wrong Berry has done Hoffman," Jowett explained. "He needed me and it was what I wanted so we allied our interests." They created the Strength and Health Publishing Company, with headquarters at the oil-burner factory. Its main pursuit was producing *Strength & Health,* with Jowett as publisher and Hoffman as editor. Though it later served chiefly to propagate Hoffman's ideas and products, it initially reflected many of Jowett's British derivations. The name itself was an obverse of *Health and Strength,* a muscle magazine founded in London by Hopten Hadley in 1902. Jowett also revived the ACWLA, proclaiming that it had left an "indelible stamp" on weightlifting.[4] Another Anglicism was the American Strength and Health League, a curious amalgam of the Boy Scouts and a pen-pal club. Certificates and badges were distributed and medals awarded for physical excellence. A moral and nationalistic tone permeated the league and the magazine. Jowett and Hoffman stressed "physical training for the masses" and the need to make Americans physically superior to other nationalities.[5] Such grand phrases and elaborate organization could easily be dismissed as the gimmicks of two clever promoters out to bilk an unsuspecting public. Desire for money and ego satisfaction was by no means absent in their appeal, but there was also a high-minded aspiration to promote physical fitness and link it to American cultural values.

These initiatives upset the balance of power in the strength world. Hoffman and Jowett protested that they were above the blatant commercialism of earlier promoters, but controversy soon set in. "We anticipated the fight of jealousy and envious competition, and the filthy breath of slander from those who see the finger of doom pointing at them from the sword of our teachings." Every effort was made to revive the ACWLA for its impending duel with the "parasital forces" of Wortmann and Berry, who edited *Strength*. A report of its first meet in March 1933 tried to convey a positive impression, but the ACWLA's failure to mount a national championship in the summer shows that its boasts were premature.[6] Toward Wortmann's management of the AAU, Hoffman blew hot and cold. On the one hand, Bob congratulated him for conducting a "wonderful meet" in "faultless style" at the German-American Club. But on July 4 at Cobb's Creek Park in Philadelphia he was harshly critical. With thirty-five thousand people attending, he believed that those "in charge of amateur athletics should . . . look the part." Wortmann, a former wrestler, had gained weight and was no longer fit. But Hoffman was most critical of his authoritarian manner, referring to "Kaiser Wortmann who ruled with an 'Iron hand' over America's lifters as if they were 'Christian slaves' or conscripts in the German Army. This man Wortmann is riding for a fall." By contrast, Hoffman professed to "treat the other fellow the way you would like to be treated." At the Pittsburgh meeting of the AAU national committee in 1933, the ACWLA decided to compromise rather than fight. "We felt that two bodies could not operate one sport without considerable friction and did not wish to break up American weightlifting," wrote Jowett. Though the ACWLA had a longer association with lifting, he conceded that the AAU should sanction all championships. The ACWLA would "be a fraternal organization like the American Legion" to promote the sport. Hoffman was willing to accept this inferior status only if Wortmann agreed to recommend ACWLA leaders to AAU committees.[7]

Bob's Disciples

Further to dislodge his economic and political rivals, Hoffman recruited the York gang. These individuals largely fit the model of ethnic Americans who had suffered some setback in their youth. Bob initially assembled local lifters of Teutonic roots. From Reamstown, a community of barely a thousand, he found the Good brothers. "They had no opportunity to lift on a team of their own and they enjoyed any sort of lifting activity," he explained. In 1934 Harry Good wrote:

ASCENT TO GLORY

The York Oil Burner A. C. who for the last few years have so completely dominated American weight lifting are about evenly divided among the Sicilians and the Pennsylvania Dutch. My brother Bill, America's strongest man and best weight lifter, my brother Walter and myself, Art Levan, Joe Miller, Dick Bachtell, George Brown, Lou Schell and many other lesser members are the Pennsylvania Dutch. Bob Hoffman is not far removed as his grandfather . . . came from Switzerland 87 years ago. . . . Anthony Terlazzo, Joe Fiorito, Anthony Fiorito, Gus Modica, Angelo Taormine, Harry Thomasillo, and others are the Sicilian members. These Sicilians are small but mighty and have accounted for nine national championships in meteoric careers.[8]

A surefire method of recruiting team members was to offer a $10-per-week job in the oil-burner plant. Bachtell, who had captained the Hagerstown team, told Hoffman "he would walk . . . to York, a distance of 65 miles, on his hands and knees if he could get work" and lift on the team. Likewise Joe Miller, a farm laborer of German descent, was lured by the prospect of steady employment and national recognition. He worked near the Susquehanna River. Each Sunday "Bob Hoffman and his wife would paddle over for me," Miller recalls, and he would spend the day at their bungalow. "We had a fine lifting platform there and used to lift all afternoon." He started to work at York Oil Burner and soon became a national contender.[9]

So closely was the oil-burner business tied to Hoffman's sports interest that "false rumors" arose that Wally Zagurski's job was a sinecure. "He has never taken one minute during normal working hours," protested Hoffman. Rather, he offered other incentives to improve his lifters' performance—good training facilities, traveling expenses to meets, and lots of camaraderie. A gold medal awaited any York team member who broke an American record, and a diamond-studded medal anyone who broke a world record. ACWLA national champions were eligible for so-called Jowett-Hoffman trophies, and membership in the Three Hundred Pound Club assured "undying fame" to any lifter who cleaned and jerked three hundred pounds.[10] According to Walter Good, "you got $15 added to your pay when you won your class, $10 for second, and $5 for third." With such incentives YOBAC lifters won Middle Atlantic and national championships repeatedly in the 1930s. York soon became a hub of lifting, and young men were drawn from all parts of the country.

The Old York Gang

"They hitch hike here, or drive in their own cars to watch the members of the York team," Hoffman noted. "They go home filled with new inspiration and new knowledge. . . . some York pupils write as often as three times a week and always receive a prompt and personal reply."[11] All of this helped make money and drew the kind of attention to York and himself that Bob desired.

Hoffman portrayed his recruits as overcoming their pasts and striving for improvement. Miller, as an infant, "was not expected to live, suffered from waste." At age eight he lacked strength and was no match for his playmates. Bob Mitchell was "the proverbial thin little weakling from which all strong men are reputed to have developed."

The York Oil Burner Athletic Club, 1932: front—Dick Bachtell, Joe Fiorito, Henry Thomasillo, Lou Schell, and Joe Miller; middle—George Brown, Art Levan, Bob Hoffman, Walter Good; back—Wally Zagurski, Bob Pentz, Reed Schwartz, Tony Maniscalco, and Bill Good.

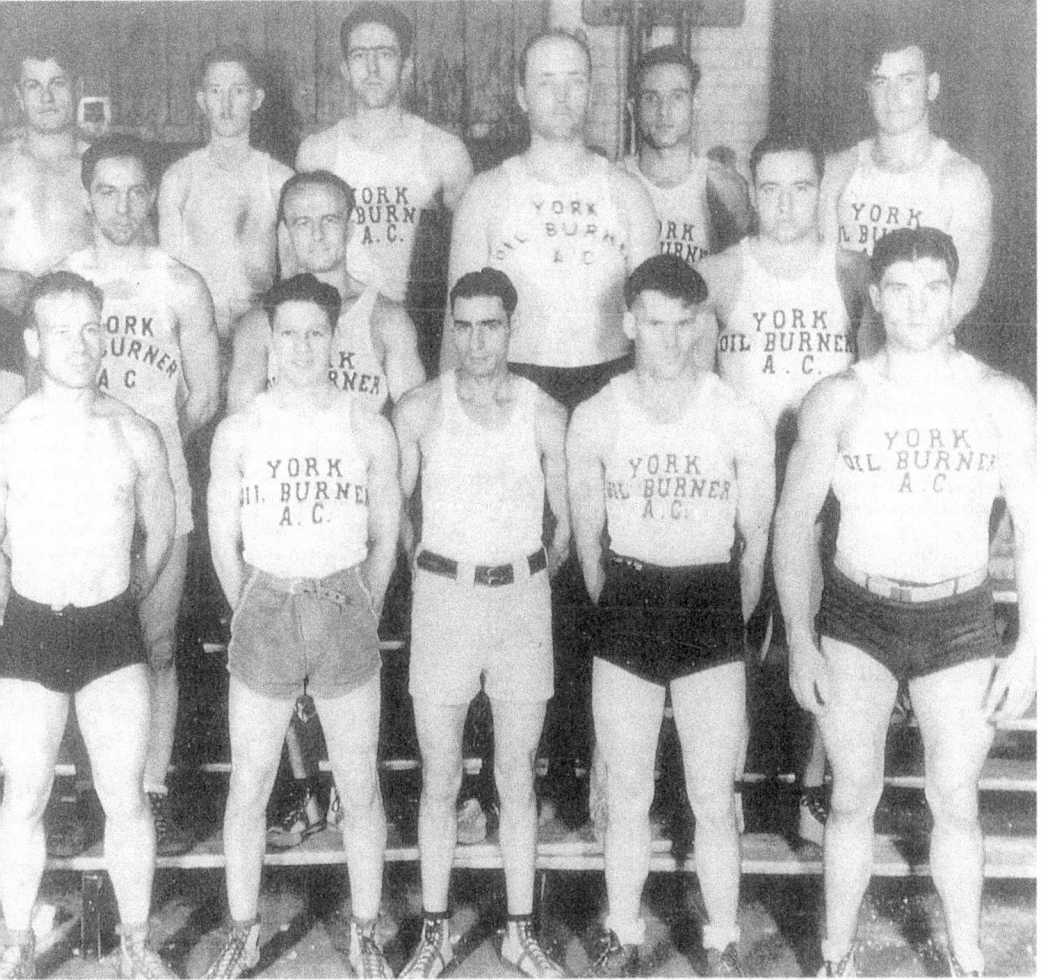

Zagurski was so severely burned at age four that he was hospitalized for six months. "It was thought that he would never recover." Art Levan suffered from a weak heart. In his early youth "running, even hurried walking was taboo." Jowett concluded that "those who have the least chance in the first place to become strong, are the ones that succeed. Their craving is more than a thing of the mind, it is so deep it becomes . . . a passion—which no obstacle is permitted to bar."[12] Harry Good concurred. It was the weakling who "through training obtains a degree of strength which far surpasses those who in the beginning were much stronger." There was "hardly a strong man who did not have to overcome great handicaps." Even Bill Good, then widely regarded as America's strongest man, took up weight training after serious illness. No less notable was the foreign derivation of York lifters. By the mid-1930s eastern Europeans were joining the Pennsylvania Dutch and Italians. These included Zagurski (Lithuanian); John Terpak (Ukrainian) from Mayfield, Pennsylvania; John Grimek (Czech) and Steve Stanko (Hungarian), both from Perth Amboy, New Jersey. Grimek got involved with York at the 1935 national championship in Cincinnati. Hoffman provided a ride back east, paid for his meals, and put him up at the York YMCA for several days. Grimek trained with Bob's lifters and felt a sense of collegiality. What compelled him to settle in York was the opportunity to train with some of the world's best athletes—all of whom seemed close. "That made me want to stick and stay," he recalls. Lots of visitors always came to watch, get information, and lift.[13] Nowhere else was it possible for weightlifters to acquire employment, ideal training conditions, and fellowship in a single organization.

Sweetheart of the ACWLA

This kind of socialization was also promoted in public strengthfests staged by Hoffman. The ACWLA professional championships in November 1933, reported Jowett, included a banquet hosted by Bob's "charming little wife."

> Everybody was welcome, lifter and spectator alike. The festive board groaned with the load of appetizing food. . . . Rosetta Hoffman worked like a Trojan to make the banquet a success, and

she surely succeeded. Numerous toasts were given to this sweetheart of the A.C.W.L.A. . . . . The bonny girl endeared herself to everyone. Throughout the festival, the A.C.W.L.A. Glee Singers sang popular melodies in which all uproariously joined. Good fellowship was everywhere, but then this glorious good time is always the same at the A.C.W.L.A. headquarters in York, Pa.

Another highlight was the strength show in December 1934. The clubhouse on Lightner's Hill was jammed with two hundred spectators who were treated to some fine lifting fellowship. "What a wonderful time, what fun. Good fellowship, records smashed galore, plenty of good eats, visits with old friends, meeting with new ones. A day of days." Completing the activities was a feast of sauerkraut and pork prepared by Rosetta, "the little Strength & Health lady." Everything was free. Hoffman was bursting with pride over his lifters' accomplishments. "It might be the cooking. It might be the enthusiasm. But very likely the training methods have a lot to do with it. For years our group have lifted together, worked together, been friends. Almost lived together and the six records equalled or surpassed at this one contest gives some idea of the heights for which these young fellows are headed." Six of the eight athletes named to the All American Weight Lifting Team by *Strength & Health* readers were from York.[14] Wittingly or unwittingly, Hoffman had hit upon a formula for success. By melding ethnic and neurasthenic youth into purposeful masculine endeavors, he created a distinctive strength culture at York.

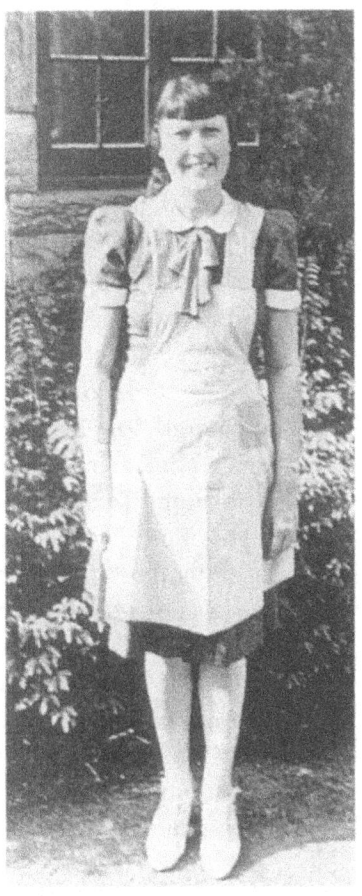

Sweetheart of the ACWLA Rosetta in the smock she to prepare and serve food Bob's strength fests.

Hoffman's portrayal of an ideal family life for himself and his lifters was part of the all-American image he projected. Rosetta was depicted as an exemplar of youthful femininity. In January 1934, *Strength & Health* showed pictures of an athletic looking Rosetta hoisting a set of chrome barbells outside the clubhouse. She was "the true glorified version of beautiful womanhood . . . pulsating with vigorous health and spontaneous youth." Later Rosetta authored a women's section. Ghostwritten by Bob, these articles relegated *Strength & Health* women to traditional roles in the kitchen and bedroom. The first, by the "House of Health Hostess," was entitled "Men Prefer Plain Foods" and featured recipes of "favorite foods that make the STRONG MEN smack their lips for more!" Emphasizing Bob's love of York County cuisine, especially sauerkraut, chicken corn soup, and ham and string beans, these articles were highly sexist and patronizing, with Bob noting that his own exploits were often overshadowed by his wife's cooking. The 1934 Christmas issue featured a wreath cameo of Rosetta on the cover and pictures of her inside peddling exercise equipment. In the series "Beauty Building for Women," she affirmed it was a woman's duty to become fit and healthy to appeal to her male. Accompanying her articles were alluring pictures of Rosetta in wholesome settings—a pensive mood, in Sunday attire, frolicking in the snow, sunning herself on the Susquehanna, and in a tender pose with her husband. She was also featured outdoors, canoe camping on the Juniata and on a Chesapeake Bay fishing trip with Bob's employees. The latter piece not only reported that she caught the most and the biggest fish but, in striking contrast to others in grubby attire, pictured her holding a thirty-one-inch sea trout in her finest Sunday clothes![15]

None of these promotional features, of course, was Rosetta's doing. Remnants of her correspondence reveal that she lacked the knowledge and grammatical skills to contribute materially to her husband's journal. Though Bob was able to capitalize on her youthful good looks, she appeared totally lacking in cultural attributes. "She had a sailor's vocabulary," notes Dave Mayor. In Rosetta's articles there is an incongruity between the feminine subject matter and Bob's masculine egocentric style. Occasionally the narrative lapses into asides on Bob's favorite subjects—feats of legendary strong men and war stories of his exploits in France—hardly attractive subjects to women readers. Bob also employed Rosetta's seven brothers and once even discussed the weight-training prospects of his adolescent stepson.[16] Though Hoffman's use of his wife, her family, and the York gang was transparently exploitative, it was also consistent with his genuine desire to promote health and fitness broadly and to target those groups to which Macfadden's *Physical Culture* appealed.

A Strength-and-Health Culture

Rosetta's features were part of a change in format of *Strength & Health*. In 1934 colored covers replaced traditional lavender ones. The December issue was no longer dubbed "A Man's Magazine for Real Men" but "The Family Health Magazine." This change of emphasis coincided with the departure of Jowett, who told Coulter, "I quit Hoffman because the man is crazy. . . . I did a lot for him. . . . Hoffman has got a big head. He thinks he is the Czar. I told him he was a punk. . . . He copies and cheats and steals other peoples ideas which one of these days will land him in serious trouble." Soon the ACWLA and the Strength and Health League disappeared, and Hoffman concentrated his efforts on bolstering his influence in the AAU. He had learned much from Jowett about promoting, but one organization could not tolerate two such egocentric personalities. In the new *Strength & Health* there was not only a women's section, but adventure articles, human-interest stories, historical features, coverage on general fitness and other sports, and health articles by Dr. Frederick Tilney of Hollywood, Florida, who had formerly worked for Macfadden and Atlas.[17] With these features, the magazine expanded fourfold. A smaller type size permitted more weightlifting coverage without detracting from the overall family-fitness orientation. Most of this material was penned by Hoffman, enabling him to impress his inspiring message on the York system and interpret his movement as the apotheosis of a long strength tradition.

His achievement of a virtual monopoly over the American iron game was facilitated by the bankruptcy of *Strength* and the Milo Barbell Company in 1935. Hoffman acquired their assets and copyrights for $4,000, though Milo had left much more in liabilities, including nine hundred unfilled orders. Jowett seemed perplexed by Hoffman's ability to survive against all financial odds. Not only did he owe York Oil Burner $16,000, but the oil-burner business itself was greatly in debt. "I know he has to pay his P.C. business bills out of Oil Burner funds. He uses their checks. On some he uses S & H Co checks but few. Which all proves he is not making money, but he does things no intelligent man would do. He hates everyone, and is insanely jealous of me. Every kid who pats his back makes his chest swell a mile. He is consumed with ego, and is undoubtedly an eccentric." Even Hoffman admitted in 1936 that his magazine was losing $2,500 a month, but it was indispensable for advertising.[18] Now he was for all intents and purposes the only barbell manufacturer in the country, and with Bob Jones, a skilled handbalancer from Arkansas, at the helm of the client Milo operation in Philadelphia, he could lay claim to a tradition going back to 1902.

Strength & Health expressed idealism and existed, according to Hoffman, to help others gain strength and fine physiques: "I have no desire to be rich"; "everything that appears in S. & H. I believe in." Initially only 2,500 copies were produced, but from June 1934 to October 1936 monthly sales increased from 4,800 to 51,333 copies. What justified its existence was the need to promote a growing variety of York products, including barbells, head straps, a giant crusher grip, spring cables, solid-iron dumbbells, an abdominal board, iron boots, a line of Milo items, and York courses and books, all publicized in Hoffman's inimitable style. Above all, the magazine propagated Hoffman's philosophy and ego. It was pitched to appeal to the middle-class belief that, with sufficient willpower, anything was possible.

His message, accompanied by personal examples, catered to American desires for health, self-improvement, and masculinity. "No writer is qualified to write authoritatively unless he is a positive example of physical perfection," he contended. Hoffman had devised his twenty-week training program and his professional heavyweight championship to validate his credentials as a trainer. He developed proficiency in handball to refute the notion that big men were slow or that weightlifters were muscle-bound. "Like a cat on his feet he has the sock of a trip hammer" was his self description. Though admittedly the "world's worst presser," he created the Three Hundred Pound Club to display his clean-and-jerk ability.[19] He exuded confidence and hope in an otherwise depressed decade.

Naturally Bob's size gave him an advantage over most other lifters. Incapable of winning against his peers, one of his favorite ways of showing prowess was to stage impromptu competitions against lighter champions. So he was able to claim victory over Bachtell by a formula where handicaps of weight (three lift pounds per body pound) and height (ten pounds per inch) were exchanged to Hoffman's advantage. Similar private jousts were set up for Levan, Zagurski, and Canadian recruit Gordon Venables, to prove that Hoffman possessed a champion's ability. These exploits coincided with his appeal for manliness. "Just read the history of this great country of ours and you will see that all the great leaders were great men physically. Sturdy men who could use an axe, plow, sword or rifle. You should strive to be like them. Be alive. Be virile." However quaint these words sound decades later, they appealed to Hoffman's contemporaries. Furthermore, he was striving to create a historical context for himself. It was most evident in published caricatures of him as war hero, handball champion, dispeller of myths about aging and growing muscle-bound, innovator of new exercises, and father figure, a man who "looks after 'his boys' in a paternal manner." Indeed the most impressive aspect of the "boys'" participation in the 1933 national championships in Chicago was "the 'one big happy family' attitude of the York outfit." Each issue of *Strength & Health* carried articles and references to old-time strength stars, all of whom were cast as forebears of Hoffman.[20]

An important aspect of Hoffman's self-idealization, especially after his twenty-week program, was a greater focus on appearance. Back covers of *Strength & Health* featured retouched photographs of Bob accompanied by the headline "What Would *You* Give to Have a Body Like This!" and a pitch for York barbells. So gratified was Hoffman by his improved muscularity that he departed briefly from his emphasis on strength to adopt an alternative line espoused by Sig Klein. "Shapeliness comes first with us," he stated in December 1934; "strength follows and increased bodyweight will result." The two most important things in life were "how you feel and how you look." Even the redoubtable Dr. Tilney was credited with practicing what *Bob* preached, and readers, on facial view alone, were led to imagine he possessed a muscular physique from his "square chin, strong jaw, powerful neck and broad shoulders." Confidence, happiness, and success were traits pertaining to those who followed Hoffman's teachings. Early converts were the Tanny brothers, Vic and Armand, of Rochester. Vic, noting his brother's devotion, wrote to Hoffman that Armand "follows each issue of your . . . magazine and absorbs every word of it." Every argument with his elder brother Armand justified with "Bob Hoffman says that you should do so and so and that's what those guys on the York team do etc." Likewise Dick Zimmerman, a "Dutchman" who lived on a farm near York, read every word of *Strength & Health* "several times over" and "worshipped our great lifters from afar." Bob called Zimmerman his "Newest Perfect Man," a product of his "all around training system."[21]

Johnny Terpak

Hoffman's infatuation with shape was short-lived. He was drawn back to strength, with bodybuilding as a pleasing by-product, by the achievements of his growing stable of lifters. As he began to take his own physique for granted and his strength increased, Hoffman realized that lifting was a more suitable way to display greatness, especially as aspiring young men converged on York to learn the secrets of his champions. In 1935 he observed that "there have been hundreds of lifters in our offices here this summer." What they learned was that "all our men follow the York system, put forth plenty of effort," and "perspire." Hoffman's newest sensation was John Terpak, who displaced Zimmerman as an archetype. This native of the Pennsylvania coalfields became not only a national and world champion but Hoffman's understudy. Bob admired his winning the junior nationals in Philadelphia, making fourteen of fifteen attempts. Afterward Hoffman sent Terpak a letter with a $5 bill inviting him to visit York. Terpak's career at the company began with painting, packaging, and labeling weights and loading them into trucks. He then graduated to a desk job where he answered Bob's correspondence and became immersed in his master's business. "Almost from the beginning, I was Bob Hoffman."[22] A dedicated employee, he most nearly approximated Hoffman's vision for American manhood. "John Terpak is a handsome, manly fellow. He has athletic spirit, a desire to excel, willingness to work hard and train hard to succeed. . . . This lifter has what it takes." He possessed a weightlifter's, not a bodybuilder's, physique, and his potential was not so easy to assess as that of others whose attributes were more visible. Terpak's progress was attributed to a desire to compensate for earlier weaknesses. In his youth he had experienced constant colds, stomach troubles, and rheumatism, and he was undersized. Weight training had improved his health and allowed him to escape the harsh environment of his parents.

Also overcoming physical and cultural disadvantages was Gordon Venables, born of a French mother, who at age eleven had contracted pleurisy, suffered hearing loss, and missed a year of school. Dave Mayor, Jewish, was York's strapping heavyweight at 235 pounds, but at birth he had weighed only four and one-half pounds and had not been expected to live. Survival of the fittest was a doctrine Hoffman applied to his lifters' achievements. "All of life is a fight," he believed, and success in athletics was tantamount to success in life.[23]

The 1936 Olympics

The greatest obstacle Hoffman faced in his struggle for weightlifting superiority in the mid-1930s was Mark Berry. Jim Messer recalls that when *Strength* folded, Hoffman wanted Berry to work at York. But Berry, still important in the AAU, refused and started his own magazine, *Physical Training Notes*. To Berry, Hoffman was an upstart, yet "Bob always thought he should be the big mug because he was putting money into the sport." In 1935 a disagreement between the two men arose from the AAU's substitution of Detroit lifter Stan Kratkowski for one of Hoffman's men, Bob Mitchell, to attend a competition in England. Berry was the obvious culprit, and tensions mounted. Bob also hinted at misrepresentations by Wortmann, but he could not afford to alienate the head of AAU weightlifting with the Olympics on the horizon. Hoffman was eyeing berths for members of his team and himself as coach. To this end he developed grandiose notions of his organization as a world weightlifting power. Having won the senior nationals a fourth time, Bob represented his lifters as the world's strongest club, comparable to the talent of entire nations. Germany had the "strongest team in the world," but the total of its five best lifters exceeded that of York's best five by only eighty-four pounds. Furthermore, Hoffman's men were "comers," their average age being only twenty-four. With his sights on the Olympics, Hoffman was working "hard and long." He would assist aspiring lifters from anywhere to come to York. He paid the expenses of Kratkowski and "carloads" of other lifters to train with his gang. Others he claimed to be training by mail, all to help young strength athletes "make the team and win points for America."[24] He equated the success of his team with that of America.

To ensure a prominent role for himself at Berlin, Hoffman tactfully promoted Wortmann as a "hard worker for amateur athletics." He could afford to be generous, since the old German-American Club was no longer a power. It was trounced at the 1935 nationals by York, thirty-one to seven. At the 1936 junior nationals in Cleveland, however, Berry was named Olympic coach. This was an immense blow to Hoffman, but he made a show of "good sportsmanship," noting in his magazine that "Bob gave no sign of disappointment." Notwithstanding the selection of the wrong person as coach, Hoffman in succeeding months appropriated America's lifters as his own. Even if trained by others, he claimed they had used York equipment and methods. He envisioned the York-trained team as "a happy family . . . who will be training, thinking, breathing weightlifting . . . to win the team title for America in Berlin." Fundamental to its success was fund-raising. Wortmann did his share, but Hoffman's $1,000 was the largest single donation to the Olympic Committee. Bob could also justifiably assert that since 1932 he, rather than Berry, had "coached the lifters of the Olympic team . . . to where they could compete on even terms with the world's best."[25] Disregarding his self-serving accounts, America's lifting prospects had improved greatly, mostly due to Hoffman's efforts.

Unfortunately the York-based team did not perform as well as expected at Hitler's games. Featherweight Terlazzo became the first American to win an Olympic gold medal, but no other American placed higher than fifth, and the United States placed third behind Germany and Egypt. Hoffman was consoled only by his team's scoring higher than perennial power Austria and twenty-four other nations. He was impressed by the Germans' organization and efforts to show they were "a superior race." Bob realized the importance of the Olympics in verifying nationalistic claims, but since his country and team were conglomerates of peoples, he could only subscribe to the obverse of Hitler's doctrines. A mixture of peoples was an asset in Hoffman's estimation. What America lacked was "an understanding of the importance of muscle. But that is the principal work of Strength and Health." Seeing European dictators regimenting their youth and admiring "the power they hold today in world affairs," he implored his readers to "Wake Up America!"[26] It was chimerical to think Hoffman could employ the comparatively meager resources of his company to challenge the strength of entire nations. But failing any greater commitment by his government, he was prepared to do so. At least Bob Hoffman, not Uncle Sam, would receive all the credit.

The Olympics also provided an opportunity for a showdown between Berry and Hoffman. Since 1932 tensions had been mounting, and on the

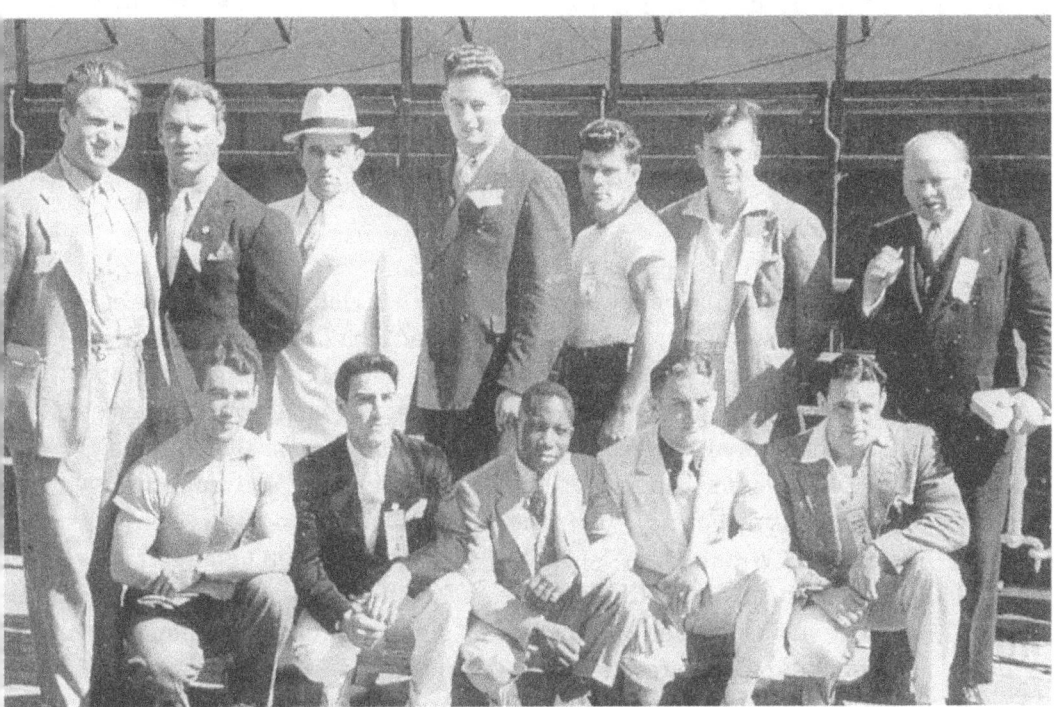

The 1936 American weightlifting team in transit to Berlin: front—Bobby Mitchell, Tony Terlazzo, John Terry, John Terpak, Walter Good; back—Mark Berry (coach), John Grimek, Stan Kratkowski, Dave Mayor, Joe Miller, Bill Good, and Dietrich Wortmann (national chairman).

return journey, at Le Havre, animosities flared. Again Hoffman took advantage of his size. Terpak, who witnessed the incident, recalls that Bob descended on Berry along some store fronts and beat up his diminutive rival. It appeared to be an unprovoked act of cowardice hardly justified by Bob's chagrin at not being named coach. But Hoffman's anger had been aroused by an embarrassing exposure of his business practices in Berry's *Physical Culture Notes* during their absence. Bob explained:

> It would be interesting to know what happened in La Havre, France. The Olympic boat was in port there for a day and most of the team went ashore. When Berry came back aboard he was the worst messed up specimen of humanity we have seen. Blood and mud everywhere. The story went the rounds that he was kicked by a mule, hit by a truck, thrown out somewhere, etc. . . . No doubt retribution caught up with him, for his story appeared in the team's absence. Mails brought it to Berlin. There are men who owe him much and perhaps one of these men caught up with him and paid his debt in part. . . . Berry spent the next seven days in the confines

of his own room, most of it in bed. Perhaps he did a little thinking and may have learned a lesson. If he hasn't, the same mule might catch him again.

This history of the incident was traceable back to Hoffman's purchase of the Milo assets, which, at the time, he assumed included rights to Berry's book *Your Physique and Its Culture*. He thus obtained, advertised, and sold hundreds of copies without giving its author a cent. Berry took legal action and in May 1936 received a favorable judgment on all five points of his suit. Hoffman appealed, but Berry won again, and publicized the fact in his magazine. What must have galled Hoffman was Berry's headline—"I Win the Law-Suit with Bob Hoffman." Bob hated losing, and this must have been the final straw in his attempt to cope with Berry, for many years an irritant. Failing in any other way to relegate him to a subordinate role, Bob resorted to a final physical solution. Berry never recovered his former stature, but Hoffman was forced by the state of Pennsylvania to pay him $544.[27]

Charles Atlas

A no less formidable challenger was the Charles Atlas organization, which registered in 1936 a complaint with the Federal Trade Commission that York was engaged in misleading practices. When his claims for barbell training were questioned, Bob retorted that the FTC building in Washington was "two blocks long and two blocks wide and several stories high. Lots of unemployed men have obtained work there . . . and they have to do something." In succeeding months Hoffman and his lifters attended hearings in Washington and New York. Dr. Tilney, who had devised Atlas's course in 1922, helped Bob deny his adversary's claims that nonapparatus systems were superior and that weightlifters would become muscle-bound. York also mounted a counteroffensive. Bob refuted Atlas's boast that he had built his physique by dynamic tension: "I can prove through a hundred sources that he trained with weights." Hoffman also challenged Atlas's claim to be the "World's Strongest Physical Director" and offered "to pit . . . my muscles against his."[28] Much controversy centered on Hoffman's use of the word "hooey" in describing the Atlas system. It sounded like *chui*, the Russian word for "cock," and Atlas accused him of calling him a "prick." Hoffman tried to prove the superiority of his system by displaying the physiques and skills of his lifters in court. Once he even "stood on his thumbs for the Commission in an ambiguous attempt to prove the superiority of barbells." Interestingly both Hoffman and Atlas held similar views of their respective callings. The latter claimed to be "extremely happy all of the time. . . . My health is perfect and the business no longer has any competition." He regarded himself as the last of the famous strong men who promoted mail-order training. To Hoffman, however, Atlas was "the only Fakir left."[29]

The case ended with neither party victorious. Sanctions, however, were placed on York for misrepresentation in advertising, conflict of interest between York Barbell and York Oil Burner operations, fabrications of Hoffman's military record, and "unfairly disparaging competitors." Bob denounced the report, calling it "trivial." Indeed the FTC case only made him more aggressive. "With all the false claims made for many patent medicines, liquor, tobacco and cigarettes, and so many other harmful products, it would seem that the Federal Trade Commission could spend their time to better advantage." In a tacit admission of stretching the truth, Hoffman observed that Sandow exaggerated to keep up with misrepresentations of his competitors. "But there was no Federal commission in the early days." This inclination of professionals to stretch the truth amused the York gang. On hearing of an outstanding lift, one of them would ask whether it was amateur or professional. "If someone here says, 'I had three hours sleep last night,' or 'I ate twelve crab cakes last night,' the inevitable question is, 'Was that amateur or professional?' The meaning being that something exaggerated is stamped as 'professional.'" "Bob exaggerated just about everything," recalls Dave Mayor. "That was his style." Jowett observed that Bob always assumed more than what actually was, and could distort a meaning of a fact so great one wondered at times whether he was all there in the head.[30] But Hoffman was no better and no worse than others. Like Atlas, he was adept at surviving. Both organizations were thriving in their respective spheres, but Hoffman's emphasis on weight training was the way of the future. His clash with Atlas tested his determination to pursue commercial success through the less lucrative method of selling barbells. It was he, more than any other pioneer in the strength field, who brought about their public acceptance. By this standard alone, he deserves recognition as an iron-game patriarch.

The Patriarch's Paradise Lost

By this time it was obvious that the dingy oil-burner factory hardly fit the grandiose image of his strength community Hoffman projected to outsiders. Therefore he undertook to create a "Strength & Health Center" on his Lightner's Hill property. Hoffman envisioned a "physical Garden of Eden." "A place which could serve as a proving ground to demonstrate certain principles of exercise and right living. Where fresh air, pure water and sunlight were abundant. Where sunbathing, outdoor games and exercise could be indulged in. A place where weightlifting, barbell and dumbell training and all strength sports could be practiced. A place which would serve as a Mecca or center, for all who have come to appreciate the advantage of leading the Strength and Health life." At the entrance to this sylvan retreat was the team clubhouse, completely renovated, with a gym, dressing facility, kitchen, living room, and club room—all to promote socialization. Beside it was Bob and Rosetta's House on the Hill, a "triumph of architectural beauty." The exterior was constructed of Foxcroft stone, brown, gray, and blue, with mica. The roof was constructed of steel and green Vermont slate. The interior featured paneled rooms, stone fireplaces, tile, French windows, and venetian blinds. The basement was to be a museum tracing the evolution of exercise equipment, with a centerpiece enshrining York barbells and dumbbells. Outside on terraced grounds were rock gardens, pools, waterfalls, and a waterway to a pool over which a Japanese bridge was suspended. For athletic endeavors the grounds featured a swimming pool, a field with a 220-yard track, handball and badminton courts, and a lifting platform.[31]

With the completion of Bob's mansion, just when appearances suggested a veritable paradise, his marriage disintegrated. Hoffman's public projection was nowhere more at variance with reality than in his relationship with Rosetta. "Plan to marry and be happy when the right girl comes along," he advised young readers. "And when you pick the little woman as you will some day, make up your mind to be 'true to her.' . . . Married love is a beautiful thing." All who recall the Hoffmans' marital life, however, affirm that both were flagrantly disloyal. Furthermore, Rosetta's penchant for dissipation, in contrast to Bob's emphasis on health and fitness, suggested incompatibility. According to Grimek, "Rosetta liked to drink and raise hell. She liked to go down to the bar on George Street." Yet until 1937 they tolerated each other.

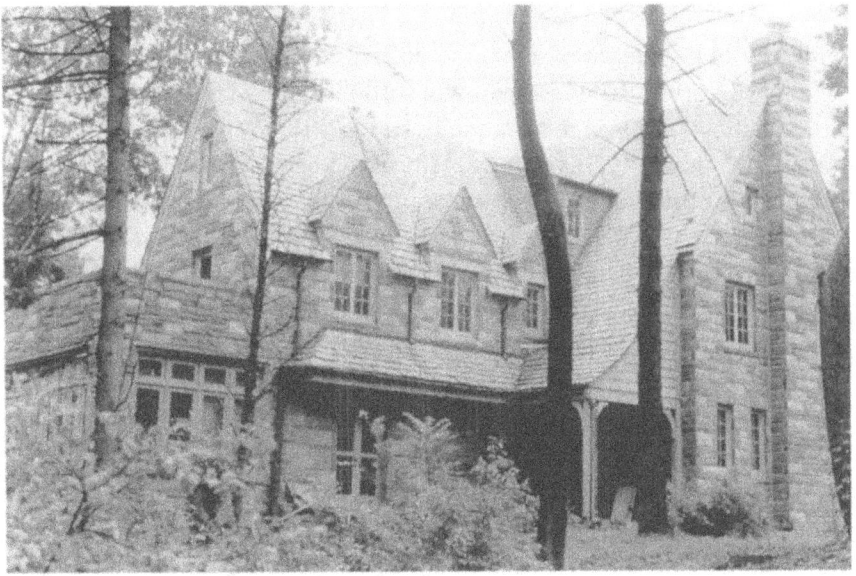

The House on the Hill—intended to be Bob and Rosetta's dream house—later used by Bob to entertain his girlfriends.

Signs of a breakdown appeared in Bob's preoccupation with sex in his articles. He concluded that "development of large and shapely muscles is impossible without the aid of strong and healthy glands and organs" and that "physical strength and sexual strength go hand in hand." Bob believed that "strong men are capable of more sexual intercourse than the average man." Although he espoused married love, he also accepted the amoral view, à la Shakespeare, that "nothing is good or bad but thinking makes it so." Another factor militating against the marriage was Hoffman's total involvement in his work, which fed his ego. He boasted in 1936 that he "worked ten days in a row for twenty hours a day" and drove seven thousand miles in five weeks. "On most of these trips there was an all night drive coming back, five hundred miles or more at times. Three hours sleep while away and little before going. And then a rush of work after I was home." Even allowing for exaggeration, Hoffman, either out of love for sport, which happened also to be his work, or to avoid family responsibilities, was busy. The self-made man thrived on activity. Rosetta less frequently accompanied him on trips and longed for outings on which she could relax. Hints of their separation appear in Bob's statement that a man "may acquire an uncontrollable taste for variety which prevents him from living happily with any one woman." Recalling Kipling's lines, "The more you have seen of the others, the less you will settle to one," Hoffman concludes that the most frequent reason a man strays is that "the woman neglects herself physically."[32] Successive pictures of Rosetta in the 1930s indicate that her youthful good looks were waning, and she was gaining weight.

Rosetta denies being disloyal. "I was a one-man woman." Yet she admits that she was drifting away from Bob. She got "tired of getting up at 3 or 4 A.M. to drive to weightlifting meets. I didn't like going to the army-navy game. I wanted to travel and see something." In 1936 she escaped with a girlfriend to Annapolis for several weeks. Then, in 1937 she was injured in a serious accident. Details are sketchy, but it appears that Rosetta hit another woman while driving drunk, causing Bob much embarrassment and expense. After convalescing "on a lengthy fishing trip by trailer" to Kentucky, Rosetta journeyed to a camp in Santa Monica, where she was treated by a local doctor. She wrote to her husband in despair:

> [S]orry to tell you trouble Dear because you have so much of your own. but I have been layed up this whole week. Just dont seem to get to well there. The Dr said Hes doing all he can to save me from a other serious apperation. he said it would be better if I would but he said Im so young and active it would be ashame to so he is trying all he can to prevent one. . . . watches me every step he wont let me drink dont go to beer places. or do any thing to make it worse. going to try to walk a little tomorrow its a little sore and a great deal of pain in the left side yet. Bob. it pained 2 weeks in succession so you see it isn't much fun for me. . . . I cry every day and pray to God I can go out like Larry and Lois when I see them go out and can have such good fun and think even if you do work hard the good fun you can have in life . . . I love my husband and my Home.[33]

About the same time, Bob received another letter from a woman in Chambersburg named Connie. Addressed to "Mr. Robert William Hoffman" at the York YMCA, it contained several sheets of unprintable sexual doggerel and the following:

> Just saw the cutest picture & am I groggy. One scene was so much like us I had to laff. This girl & boy were on their honey moon &

they stopped at a hotel. Next scene—They were sitting on the bed eating sandwiches & drinking milk. Member—McConnelsburg? I never tasted such good sandwiches. Maybe it was the Burgundy. Gee honey didn't we have swell times together. I miss you & am as grumpy as a bear. *Dam.*

How's York? Did you see in the papers that some one is shooting at buses in Gettysburg. You mite have lost your wife. You'll have a time I'm afraid. Added thot—The guy in the movies wore a pair of silk pajamas like yours—thump thump [picture of heart with arrow] Woe is me. No one to scratch my back. Don't you dare go up any allys. I been thinking about those gals alday. Wot do they do for recreation and do they get a headache? . . . Darn I'm lonely Willyam.

Hoffman thus took advantage of his wife's prolonged absence. His conduct hardly corresponded to the high moral code, "the Golden Rule," he urged on his readers. But many years later he admitted that "I didn't really start having fun until I was thirty eight."[34]

Bob's Managers

Devoid of a stable personal life, Hoffman lavished attention on members of his gang, whom he portrayed with all-American masculine virtues. "Personality" was their foremost attribute, but being ambitious and hardworking were other desirable traits, and of course being a good weightlifter. Hoffman urged employers to hire weightlifters, whom he idealized. "They have good habits and are nice fellows to have around. No headaches or time lost through sickness or bad habits. They fill a man's place in this world. All of the York Bar Bell lifters are getting ahead in life. They attend night classes at the Y.M.C.A. or business college." Although most lifters performed menial jobs with the company, one rising star took charge of the finances. Mike Dietz, like many others, was Pennsylvania Dutch. He was hired to fill in at the office while Bob attended the Olympics. Dietz started training and impressed Hoffman at his annual birthday contest in 1936 with a creditable 185-195-230 as a lightweight. His steady improvement led Hoffman to observe that none of those he had hired from the business school had "heard of a barbell," yet they all became lifters. "It's contagious." Dietz did not win a berth on the world-championship team at the 1937 senior nationals, but he earned a feature article in *Strength & Health*.[35] The feature gave Hoffman an opportunity to tell another Horatio Alger story—a young man who by his own effort and ambition was destined to succeed. Dietz had proved his manhood and earned an important niche in the organization. His adroit handling of the books allowed Hoffman time for other pursuits. But his role in company affairs did not lessen Hoffman's regard for Terpak. After Terpak's victory at the 1937 nationals Bob referred to him as "the mystery man of weightlifting. Where he gets the power to make such lifts few people can realize."[36] Hoffman seemed in awe of it. Furthermore, Terpak's approach to business and sport coincided with Hoffman's conception of "the York Way." He complemented, without threatening, his boss's formidable ego and, as general manager after 1939, served as a counterweight to Bob's more Olympian notions. Bob was always the moving force, but Dietz and Terpak were his managers. This pattern was set by the end of the 1930s.

While Terpak and Dietz became permanent fixtures, the fortunes of others waned. Sporting competition symbolized life. Tony Terlazzo and Terpak, as Hoffman noted, were "the closest of rivals and best of friends," and as they pounded typewriters outside his office, they challenged each other to private contests. Hoffman was amazed by their intensity. Little else was talked about, and it seemed as if "both lifters were more nervous, more thrilled than before the competition at the Berlin Olympics." The resulting showdown, with Terpak yielding a thirty-pound handicap, was a tie, and Terpak and Terlazzo shared the November 1937 cover of *Strength & Health*. But Tony eventually bowed out and went to California to open a gym and sell exercise equipment. Bill Good also severed ties with York. When his brother Harry left the business to sell his own products, Bill quit the team, and Hoffman began criticizing his lifting. In contrast to Terpak, Good was entering the downside of his career. Thus at the 1937 senior nationals he "squeaked through" to win his class, but Hoffman noted that at "each contest he gets just a bit weaker. . . . He's through as a champion after this year."[37] With lots of recruits coming to York, "old-timers" such as Miller, Mitchell, and Zagurski were expendable, and, unlike Dietz and Terpak, they did not develop a stake in the business. It was survival of the fittest.

John Grimek

Size was a foremost characteristic among Hoffman's newer stars. Dave Mayor of Philadelphia, unlike Good, was a full heavyweight at 250 pounds. When he beat Good at the 1937 Middle Atlantics, Hoffman exclaimed, "I could have kissed Dave. What a man!" Another physical superman was the inimitable John Grimek. "John stripped for action makes any group of enthusiasts or disbelievers speechless. There is only one John Grimek and the more I see of him, the more convinced I am that he is the most extraordinary physical specimen in the world, past or present. John is powerfully muscled; probably all of you know that he holds the highest military press record in America, that he was heavyweight lifting champion, that he made the highest U.S. total in the Olympics, yet he is as flexible as a contortionist." At Bob's 1936 birthday show Grimek's performance climaxed the festivities. "He is a master of muscle control and has more to control than any other man. Heavily muscled, he has smooth, much desired muscles when in repose, he can bring them out like whip cords . . . and make them as hard as a block of wood. He has a huge rounded chest and a very slender waist. He pulls this waist in until he looks more like Ringling circus' 'man without a stomach' than the man without a stomach does himself. His huge, powerful, finely proportioned limbs cannot be described by words."[38] It was Grimek's classic physique that brought visibility and financial success to York, but it is also true that much of his appeal was due to Hoffman's promotion. York was the vehicle by which Grimek became an inspiration to virtually all subsequent bodybuilders. In his heyday, he became almost a cult figure. Grimek's was the image that sold magazines and fired the blood of the young men of America. But his place in the organization became somewhat anomalous as Hoffman's orientation gravitated toward weightlifting. By the end of the 1930s the lifting feats of Steve Stanko and John Davis exceeded Grimek's; still, his physique was in a class of its own for at least a decade.

The Melting Pot

What brought about phenomenal performances by the York gang was a combination of factors—Hoffman's encouragement, superior equipment and training environment, and natural ability. But Hoffman also tapped the subliminal sociopsychological forces of low self-image, both personal and cultural, endemic to many of his strength stars, and a compulsion to enter mainstream America. Hoffman's awareness of this dimension was enhanced by Hitler's declarations about German racial superiority. Germany and Austria had traditionally been lifting powers, but he believed strength was not peculiar to one race. Bob was especially intrigued by the abilities of black athletes and subscribed to Abraham Lincoln's maxim that "all men are created equal." Citing strength stars John Terry and Carleton Harris as examples, Hoffman contended that "in Africa when only the strong, the brave, the capable, the enduring became the fathers of their race, physical superiority was being born." Likewise "the little brown men of Burma, Java, the Malay Peninsula, the men of China and Japan, men of all races, creeds and colors, unite in one common desire to excel physically."[39] He was far in advance of views of his day by judging nonwhite athletes on the basis of performance and not skin color.

Hoffman believed that people of all nationalities could be forged into world-class athletes by adhering to his training methods and his vision of the self-made man. He attributed spectacular accomplishments to weight-trained men and equated ability in lifting to expertise in other sports. He even pitted his champions against other athletes in transit to the Olympics. Hoffman also sought to show his own versatility. In 1937, after little training, he exceeded several personal lifting records and won three handball games against the local York champion. "The best proof that barbell work . . . keeps one's coordination at the top, the muscles which can put up 225 pounds with one hand can also pitch ringers in quoits and put the little handball where the other fellow can't return it." Likewise the object of the so-called Four Hundred Pound Club was to show that a lifter could excel at both the snatch, a quick lift, and the slowly executed bent press. He admired "real power" and the all-around development that comes from a balanced routine. "To build a superman, slow movements and quick lifts are required." No longer was shapeliness enough—"a chorus man is shapely, but he is not strong and he loses any cause for admiration." Hoffman desired strength and was fond of splendid proportions, "but if this strength and shapeliness cannot be converted into athletic ability, I am not satisfied." All current champions, he contended, possessed utility.[40]

The Manly Art

The best way to prove the superiority of Bob's barbell-trained athletes was by demonstration. To this end he chose boxing, a sport he had always viewed as the most manly of endeavors. Bob, believing "any man can be big, strong and fast at the same time," set up a boxing gym on North George Street to develop pugilists as outstanding as his lifters. For Hoffman, training for boxing meant practicing the Olympic lifts, the assumption being that boxing form would naturally follow. "The regular press builds power in the punch, the two hands snatch and two hands clean build many desirable physical qualities.... Weightlifters easily master the correct boxing positions." The York boxing team included Joe Fiorito (118), Lou Schell (126), Art Levan (132), Hooley Schell (148), Walter Good (165), Joe Miller (181), and Bill Good (HWY). There is no evidence that Terlazzo, Terpak, Venables, Mayor, and Bullock ever did more than spar, but Hoffman rated their prospects as good. Terpak was deemed "an ideal type." Boxing never materialized, however, probably owing to its costs in time and money. At a match with a Harrisburg team in March 1938, the outlay for expenses, including $97 for boxers' fees, was $183, while gate receipts totaled only $55.[41] Such losses were hardly justifiable, even to service Hoffman's masculine ideals, and the boxing fees paid to the lifters jeopardized their amateur standing.

Furthermore, boxing was not necessary to sustain the socialization inherent to his organization. On Saturdays the York gang gathered round the platform at the Broad Street gym to engage in limit lifts and minicompetitions. Other regular gatherings included Bob's birthday show and an annual strengthfest in August, later known as the Strength and Health picnic. In 1937 it was held on Lightner's Hill, where cars were parked three-quarters of a mile in every direction. Dubbed the "greatest event of its kind ever staged," the picnic began drawing visitors in midweek, and the weights at the gym were in constant use. "There wasn't a time Saturday night, before the contest and Sunday morning that someone was not lifting weights." Among the performers were Olympic gymnast Connie Carrucio, handbalancer Bob Jones, acrobat Carleton Harris, strong man Sig Klein, bent presser Bob Harley, contortionist Frank Ebersole, and of course the York gang. Hard put to conjure up feats others had not performed, Hoffman bent-pressed the 217-pound Cyr bell and broke chains with his chest. In what Bob called a "real step forward in American lifting," lifting, he declared, had ceased to be just a cool-weather indoor sport.[42] He always exaggerated his innovations, but it is still remarkable how vigorously he promoted such ideas as weight training's benefits in other sports, the baselessness of the muscle-bound myth, and fitness possibilities for women, children, and the elderly.

Gracie Bard

What was lacking from these convivial gatherings was a woman who could be placed on a pedestal. Women were important to Hoffman, and the absence of the "Sweetheart of the ACWLA" left a void. Her articles still appeared in *Strength & Health,* but beginning in March 1938 they were illustrated by a local model/dancer named Gracie Gerzetski, whose stage name was Gracie Bard. Bob became infatuated with Gracie, but his story of how she had converted to the Strength and Health way of life appears fanciful. Formerly she had been "staying out much of the night . . . drinking and smoking too much with friends and patrons of the clubs where she danced," getting little sleep and eating only sandwiches. Her reform was pronounced total—"at least two good meals a day, cream and eggs, good solid food, more than enough sleep, and a great deal of exercise made a difference. And she was happier when she found a new interest." Few readers probably realized that Gracie's "new interest" was as much Hoffman as his philosophy of health. "It is possible," Jan Todd observes, "to follow Hoffman's marital and extra-marital arrangements via the pages of *Strength & Health* in its first two decades."[43] Increasing pictures and endearing references to Gracie indicate that Bob had found a new "sweetheart" to bolster his virile image.

As cheerleader/mascot, Gracie began accompanying the team to meets. In reporting the 1938 nationals in Woonsocket, Rhode Island, Hoffman dwells as much on her personal attributes as on the lifting. She "won the hearts of all those present. . . . The world little knows what an important part this little lady has played in helping and encouraging a host of American weightlifters." In the upcoming dual meet with the German national team, the United States would go into action

> fortified with some of the world's finest cooking prepared by this little strength athlete and dancer. A promise of a dish which sounds

ordinary at first thought, baked beans, helped Stanko win. For Gracie's beans have become a legend with all who have tasted them. The writer defeated Weldon Bullock, Dave Mayor and John Grimek in an eating contest, consuming seven heaping dishes of these beans while the best my able rivals could do was six. All the other dainties were passed up to eat beans and the ten pounds of bacon and pork they contained.... Gastronomic history will probably be made when the United States team and the German team put their feet under a table literally groaning with beans, at Gracie's beautiful country home.

Thus Gracie's beans replaced Rosetta's sauerkraut as the inspiration for American weightlifting. At the subsequent match with Germany, Gracie was much in evidence, not only serving beans but dressed in an "attractive little uniform," selling souvenir programs. On Thanksgiving 1938 Hoffman, Grimek, Stanko, and a young Philadelphian, Jack Graves, were marooned by a snowstorm at Gracie's country home. They disposed of the turkey and some of Gracie's chickens before Venables and Terpak rescued them. When the York gang went to Cuba in 1939, Gracie was pictured prominently in their frolics.[44] She seemed indispensable.

Reaching for the Heights

Socialization undoubtedly contributed to the success of Hoffman's lifters in national and international competitions. The York team was so strong by 1937 that while its best lifters were competing in the world championships in Paris, a second team was winning the Canadian nationals. The world was not yet Bob's oyster, but the following year's national championships provided a harbinger of hope—heavyweight Steve Stanko, who would give America a chance to beat the Germans.

> Quite the finest weight lifting contest ever held in America went out with a thrill filled finish that rivalled the stories of Dick [sic] Merriwell or those written by Horatio Alger. The heavyweight class was contested last and the championship was not decided until the very last lift. The next to last lift equalled the American record, the last lift broke that record by six and one quarter pounds.

And the man who made this lift was an almost unknown, a man who flashed to the top of the American weightlifting firmament, with dazzling speed only equalled by the heroics of story books. . . . This clean and jerk of 347¼ pounds was the highest lift ever made on the American continent.

Hoffman regarded Stanko as "a fighter, a real man," but there was also Gracie, "sitting at the officials table coaching him," and she "reminded him of the beans." Hoffman also attributed Stanko's success to his training with the York gang. "He's the most remarkable lifter in the history of the world." In the first dual meet with the Germans in Baltimore, featherweight John Terry hoisted a world-record snatch of 214 pounds and Terlazzo, Terpak, and Kratkowski handily outscored opponents in their classes. But the Germans won, solely as a result of heavyweight Josef Manger, who, with a gigantic 302 press, outlifted Stanko, 946 to 847 pounds. Hoffman, though frustrated, was satisfied that his team had shown the world its great potential. He also believed visitors would take home a warm feeling "for America, the lifters and enthusiasts here, for Gracie and for her beans and other gastronomic dainties." He even speculated that Gracie's beans had helped the Germans win! In New York the German victory margin was even greater, but only because Terry missed all of his clean and jerks. Had he made the 275 he did in Baltimore, the United States would have won. Bob also dwelled on how the Germans had government jobs and thrived on the nationalization of Hitler's autarkic regime. But most of America's lifters either had jobs in Hoffman's company or benefited in some way from his paternalism.[45]

The kinds of loyalties fostered by Hoffman within American weightlifting were not unlike the patriotic sentiments promoted by nation-states. While most of the lifters Hoffman sent to the 1938 world championships in Vienna were not members of his team, all of them lived and trained in York. His object was to make America the leader, and *his* team was America's team. "Our men are going over there with the determination to win the championship for me and for America." What confounded him was that the Anschluß in March 1938 had brought about a combined German-Austrian team, and the United States was relegated to second. Hoffman was especially proud of John Davis, the African-American lifter who won the light-heavy class. It was gratifying too that his team won another first (Terlazzo), a second (Stanko), and a third (Terpak), a gain over the previous year and enough to have beaten

Austria or Germany separately. To ensure that his team would win in 1939, Hoffman arranged for the world championships to be in New York City.[46] Unfortunately the war intervened, and Hoffman had to wait eight years to display America's weightlifting superiority.

The basis of Hoffman's bid for international supremacy was his business. By 1938, however, the oil-burner company, though it had nurtured his teams to success, was no longer thriving. Bob was devoting so much effort to his fitness enterprises that oil-burner sales were dwindling. For a decade he had been milking oil-burner assets to support his sideline interest in barbells. Now, with profits down and an imminent separation of financial interests mandated by the decision in the Atlas case, it was time to bail out. In June, York Oil Burner was sold to Thomas Shipley, Inc., for an estimated $380,000, with Bob receiving $125,000 and his partner double. Hoffman thus reaped considerable financial gain as well as the freedom to indulge fully in his chosen sport.[47] Company records indicate that the barbell business, if not lucrative, was at least doing well. Monthly cash and mail orders increased from $6,526 in December 1935 to $18,422 in December 1939. With this, along with income from his farms, grocery stores, and rental properties, Hoffman felt confident enough to sever his oil-burner ties. Expenditure data are scarce, but materials, foundry costs, and shipping accounted for most expenses. Weekly payroll averaged $455, and Hoffman gave Rosetta $95 every two weeks, presumably part of their separation agreement.[48] Altogether Hoffman and his company were making about $78,000 yearly before taxes, a sum sufficient to finance his grandiose intentions of making America a weightlifting power.

By this time the old York gang was virtually complete. The inner circle included such talented performers as Bachtell, Terlazzo, Terpak, Dietz, Mayor, Grimek, Venables, and Stanko. Hoffman and his women—successively Rosetta and Gracie—occupied a special position. All were engaged not only to make money but to validate Hoffman's need for manliness. "Nature intended that all of us of the masculine gender become real men, ready, able and unwilling to be a bunch of weak, spineless, fat incased Mollycoddles." This urge to conform to American ideals summoned forth responses from his growing body of followers, who were also compensating for personal or social inadequacies. After witnessing the first Mr. America contest in 1939 in Amsterdam, New York, Hoffman concluded that nearly all the contestants "had taken up weight training because they were inferior physically, usually in poor health, skinny, fat, flat chested, narrow shouldered." Likewise he was aware of the need of ethnic Americans for self-esteem and acceptance. When war broke out in 1939, Hoffman realized that if the members of his team of many nationalities were still in the Old World, Venables, Levan, Grimek, and Mayor would be fighting against Terpak, Terlazzo, Stanko, and Fiorito. But they had come together in the melting pot of "Lucky America,"[49] and Hoffman had socialized them into Americans.

The nucleus of the old York gang—Tony Terlazzo, John Grimek, Gord Venables, Steve Stanko, and John Terpak.

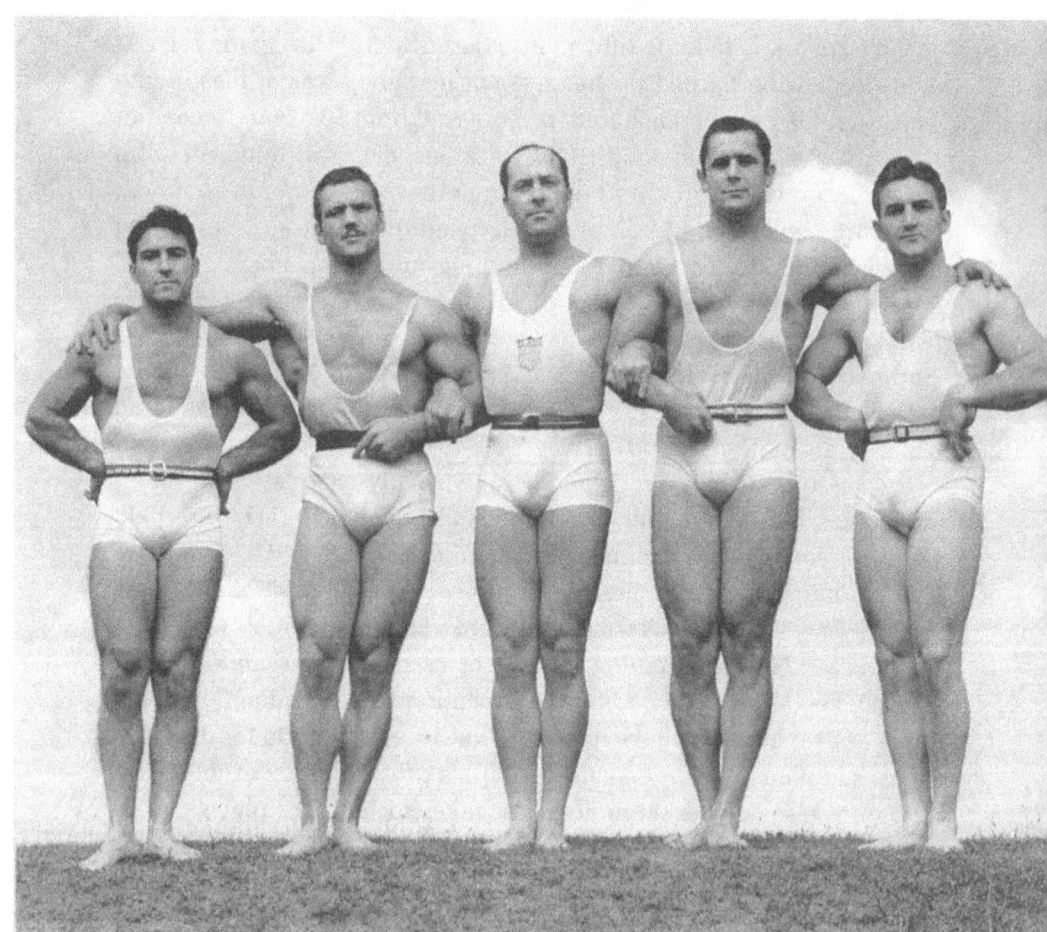

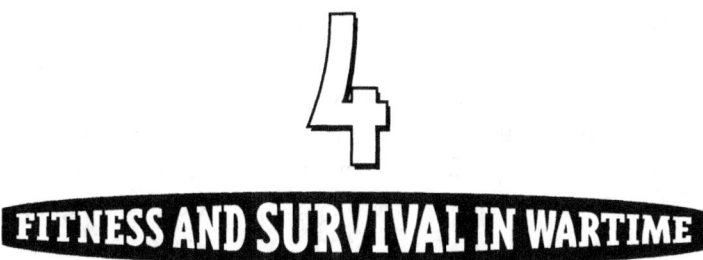

FITNESS AND SURVIVAL IN WARTIME

Only strong muscles can make men great and nations free.

—Father Jahn

With the outbreak of war in Europe, Hoffman had to seek other, less lofty ways to promote his ideology of success. He had excelled by collecting the finest strength athletes in America, exhibiting physical prowess, achieving business success, and conquering the opposite sex. Now he was beset by some disturbing circumstances. National service endangered the York gang, and the need to perform war-related work threatened his business. Equally ominous was the possibility of personal failure. As he entered his forties, he needed to reaffirm his manliness, either by athletic feats or a vigorous lifestyle. The dissolution of his marriage, far from daunting him, led to multiple relationships. Typically he overcame challenges through acts of will, aggression, and overcompensation. Hoffman survived by personalizing the national crisis and making America's cause his own. By resourcefulness, strength of character, and stretching truth to its limits, he successfully promoted the idea that the Strength and Health way of life was crucial to victory.

Bob's First Books

In 1939 the York Barbell Company comprised three interrelated operations, the most important being the manufacture and sale of barbells. Close kin to it was York Athletic Supply, which marketed various ancillary items. Combined sales for these two product lines increased from monthly averages of $13,496 in 1939 to $18,931 in 1942. Magazines and advertising brought in another $4,200 per month.[1] Also contributing to Hoffman's financial success were ten books he published between 1938 and 1941. Drawn from themes familiar to *Strength & Health* readers, each volume averaged about 250 pages. They are an amalgam of Bob's personal experiences, his commonsense approach to health and fitness, and scientific information—the kind found in medical encyclopedias. It seems incomprehensible that he could have written all of them himself. Dave Mayor calls Bob "a prolific repetitious writer" who filched much from Mark Berry and others, but garbled a lot of it. Hoffman, on the other hand, boasted of having "read every book procurable on health, exercise and physical training" by age forty. He was most inspired by the works of Sanford Bennett, a health enthusiast who became young at seventy by exercise, Horace Fletcher, who became healthy at fifty by correct diet, and Luigi Cornaro, a sixteenth-century nobleman from whom Hoffman borrowed the concept of using himself as a guinea pig. By revealing time-honored concepts, he claimed to be "the world's leading physical director."[2]

Hoffman's foremost statement on health, fitness, and well-being is conveyed in *How to Be Strong, Healthy, and Happy*, which he claimed to have written in ten days. In four hundred pages he advocated the importance of eating plain natural food, getting sound sleep, maintaining a tranquil mind, developing "mental strength," and avoiding medicines and habit-forming substances. He also advocated continence before marriage. Not accidentally, explications of his philosophy of life always coincided with promotion of himself and his business: "Every strong man worthy of the name has trained with adjustable weights" and shunned train-by-mail physical directors. Hoffman advocated irregular training—subjecting the muscles to heavier loads from different angles—and dismissed any notion that weightlifting would strain the heart, lead to rupture, induce atrophy in old age, or cause early death. How was it, he asked, that he had surpassed all others in his field? "Much of the reason is sincerity, a desire to help others, a good system, a host of star pupils who have startled the world by their deeds." Most important, "we practice what we preach."³ He also convinced others of his integrity by constant reiteration. Virtually all of Bob's subsequent books elaborated on topics addressed in his first one, known as "Bob's Big Book."

Weight Lifting was his fondest book, full of pictures of York champions and other strength athletes from past and present. His opening statement was classic—"I am a weight lifter. I like weight lifting and weight lifters." He lovingly traced the development of American lifting from its affiliation with the AAU in 1929 through the decade in which he raised it to international supremacy. In support of his claim of responsibility for this supremacy, he pointed out that all twenty national (and sixteen world) records were held by York lifters. Less credible was his statement that weightlifting was gaining popularity and that more than a million Americans regularly used barbells. *Guide to Weight Lifting Competition* was a primer for neophytes wishing to compete. In a self-serving and inspirational tone, Hoffman insisted that he witnessed virtually all of his gang "start from a very ordinary beginning, and right in our York Barbell gym attain the heights of the lifting world."⁴ The message for the average weight trainee was that by using York methods and products anyone could succeed.

In *Secrets of Strength and Development* Bob portrayed himself as a human dynamo and "leading contender for the title of 'world's healthiest man.'" Hoffman perceived himself as the quintessential "self-made man," who, by dint of his "energy, ability, and initiative," achieved the pinnacle of success. Undoubtedly Bob's size gave him an edge over other ambitious people. As he would say, "[A] good big man is always better than a good little man."⁵ But most of what he had achieved came from hard work.

Another theme in Hoffman's writings is all-around development, which forms the basis for *Big Arms*. Contrary to popular belief, he maintained that large muscular arms were not the result of concentration on that body part. He believed that "men who never specialize in arm development have the best arms," while those who do so "never have a much better than average arm." The secret to big arms, he argued, was sound health and a program of all-around training. *The Big Chest Book* contains a lot of physiological detail, but again the emphasis is on overall health and strength. The text is enlivened by hundreds of photographs and drawings. The foremost image is that of Hoffman's own development and how he increased his chest size from thirty-six inches in 1919 to fifty-two inches by 1940. One photo depicts him proudly displaying his chest to strong man Henry Steinborn, an attempt to show how the sport's legendary figures respected him.[6]

Hoffman's books on sex also had a doctrinal base, namely his four rules for healthful living—correct eating, sufficient rest, a tranquil mind, and "the greatest essential of all,—PROPER PHYSICAL TRAINING." Many letters he received revealed inhibitions and ignorance on sexual matters. By discussing such subjects as nocturnal emissions, masturbation, and venereal disease in matter-of-fact terms, Hoffman sought to dispel misconceptions about sex and assure adolescents and young adults that they were not abnormal. But much of what he wrote was inaccurate or naive. Masturbation, for instance, was said to cause circles under the eyes, make one thin, irritable, and weak, and inhibit virility. He also argued that most men, unless they maintained good health and trained regularly, became impotent after forty. Hoffman believed one could sublimate sexual desires and that the best rule was to avoid the first step. To avoid licentious thoughts, he advised redirecting one's energies elsewhere.

> If you have the power to concentrate, reading of an interesting book may serve. The solving of a difficult problem is another escape. But something vigorous in the physical line will be most helpful. Stand on your head, or your hands. Turn a cartwheel or a somersault if you are acrobatically inclined. Take a bout with the weights. . . . You can, if you live in the country or a small town, make a hobby of raising chickens, either for their beautiful feathers, for their meat qualities or for eggs. Keeping pigeons, rabbits or any one of a multitude of pets will give you an interest. You could save coins, collect stamps or relics. . . . You can build an airplane, a boat, kites, windmill. . . . Read biographies of famous men. . . . There are Boy Scout activities, the Y.M.C.A. and church interests. Music offers great possibilities. A young man is always popular who can entertain the group of his friends with music of some sort. The accordian is an especially fine instrument.

The problem with such well-intentioned advice was that these wholesome pursuits were better suited for sissies than he-men and ran counter to Bob's own pursuit of virility through sex. "The approval of young ladies" was "the real power behind the desire of so many young fellows to excel physically."[7] Weightlifting, to Hoffman, was a form of sexual expression.

Sex Technique featured an explicit treatment of taboo subjects, but because of revealing advertisements for this volume, *Strength & Health* was banned in Canada, and the title was changed to *Successful-Happy Marriage*. Nevertheless, much sound information was conveyed on such topics as the advisability of premarital physical examination; the necessity of foreplay and of variety, frequency, longevity, and completion in coitus; and problems of frigidity, impotence, and inadequacy. There was also a graphic explanation of the sex organs. But the essential ingredient to sexual power and happy marriage was the same as that for developing big arms and a shapely chest—Hoffman's four rules for healthful living. Heavy exercise with right living was nature's way of replenishing the body's sexuality. "Men and women who are strong sexually retain their youth until an advanced age." Why this bounty could only be achieved after marriage remained largely unexplained. Still, Hoffman was more enlightened on sex and its relation to health and fitness than many writers of his generation. *Better Nutrition*, unlike Hoffman's other works, is highly technical and reads like a textbook. There is little in it about himself, his training philosophy, or his lifters, and its bland style shows nothing of Bob's ebullience. Indeed, large portions were lifted, without acknowledgment, from the Department of Agriculture's 1939 yearbook.[8]

Sales of Hoffman's books show that he was filling a real need, particularly in sex education. His two books on that subject accounted for 51.4 percent of his total book sales from 1939 to 1942. Clearly, sexual confidence and virility were foremost among the needs of individuals who took up weight training. *How to Be Strong* accounted for 18.4 percent of sales, his books on weightlifting 11.7 percent, his bodybuilding trilogy 15.5 percent, *Better Nutrition* 2.6 percent, and *I Remember the Last War*, a history book, only .3 percent. These percentages, indicating that only a quarter of his readers opted for titles directly related to weightlifting and bodybuilding, suggest that Hoffman's emphasis on health and fitness was a wise business decision. Hoffman's other major publication was *Strength & Health*. At the outset of its eighth year he boasted that about 110,000 copies were sold monthly. By 1940 the magazine had expanded to sixty oversize pages garnished with many pictures and illustrations. The addition of special features, such as "Incredible but True" by Venables, Bosco cartoons and fables by Harry Paschall, a column by Sig Klein, success stories, self-improvement contests, and personality sketches, generated much reader interest. Hoffman staked his standing as a promoter on *Strength & Health*'s success. The future of "the entire York gang," he asserted, depended on his readership. "When the amateur lifting days of these men are over . . . they intend to spend their lives right here working with this magazine."[9] *Strength & Health* had become an inspiration for many thousands of weight trainees seeking male identity.

Paragons of Manhood

These successes led to further promotional efforts. In November 1939, Bob staged a show to commemorate his forty-first birthday. He claimed that two thousand visitors from twenty-five states jammed the York YMCA. Some were "hanging to the rafters" to witness Terlazzo press 250 pounds, Stanko break the world clean-and-jerk record with 370 pounds, and other spectacular feats from "the world's best men." The highlight for many was the physique show. In contrast to recent Mr. America contests, Hoffman's object was to see that the man with the best physique won, "not a 'tall, dark and handsome man.' " The contest showcased the physique of John Grimek and reinforced Hoffman's view that muscles should be useful and not just for display. This outlook underlay Bob's respect for William Curry, a young lifter from Georgia who won the light-heavy title at the 1940 junior nationals. When the York gang toured the South later that year, Bob got Curry selected as " 'The South's Best-Built Man' by convincing judges that he was a good lifter." Though he was never a bodybuilder and had a lifter's build, he was a "finished athlete" to Hoffman, and his physique, flanked by two Southern beauties, graced the cover of the hundredth anniversary issue of *Strength & Health*.[10]

It was this stereotype of strength with pleasing form that Bob idealized in Terpak, and had Curry been a member of the York gang, he would have been raised to mythical status. Bob projected an image of his protégés as possessing more than just muscles. "Who Said: 'All Brawn but No Brains'?" was the title of a 1939 article portraying York lifters as having both "he-man muscles" and "brain power": Hoffman showed versatility as a publisher, author, and agriculturalist; Terlazzo was a singer of opera, Bachtell a skilled archer and craftsman, Venables an artist, and Grimek a philosopher, ballet dancer, writer, and photographer. Stanko, Hoffman admitted, was somewhat coarse when he arrived at York but endeared himself to others as a champion lifter and reliable employee. "Modest, but confident, handsome in a manly way, neat, well dressed, and now that he has acquired a Buick car, he'll get around even more." John Terry was unique because of his color, but Bob seemed no less eager for him to fit the Horatio Alger mold. He brought Terry from New York City and set him up in business with the Yea Man Cafe. Hoffman outfitted an adjoining training room and donated a 310-pound barbell to the black community. Terry was portrayed as a real success story—a strength athlete, an entrepreneur, and a young man with wholesome pursuits whose hobby was collecting "shootin irons." "He is an idol of the colored boys. Member of the Olympic team, national champion, world's record holder, a real big shot—they hang on his every word and do as he does and as he says." The irony in this portrayal was that Hoffman was supporting an enterprise that catered to consumption of alcohol and tobacco.[11] But however much Hoffman's philanthropy smacked of paternalism and even hypocrisy, it coincided with his vision of American success.

John Davis

No less striking was John Davis, who won his first world championship in Vienna at eighteen. He never knew his father, and was raised by his mother in Brooklyn tenements. He became for weightlifting what Grimek was for bodybuilding—unbeatable. Hoffman recognized his ability, brought him to York, and helped finance his schooling. The fact that Davis was black seemed not to deter Hoffman, but the strength of his convictions was tested by a reader's challenge to use Davis or Terry on the cover of *Strength & Health*. Hoffman responded by featuring, in January 1941, a view of the muscular back and buttocks of Davis. The following month J.W.B. of the Harlem YMCA praised his appearance. But from C.V.C. of Mobile, Alabama, came the following: "Can you imagine my extreme repugnance and indignation when I went to purchase my favorite magazine and found J. Davis' Gluteus Maximus staring me in the face. I nearly went stark raving mad with insult and

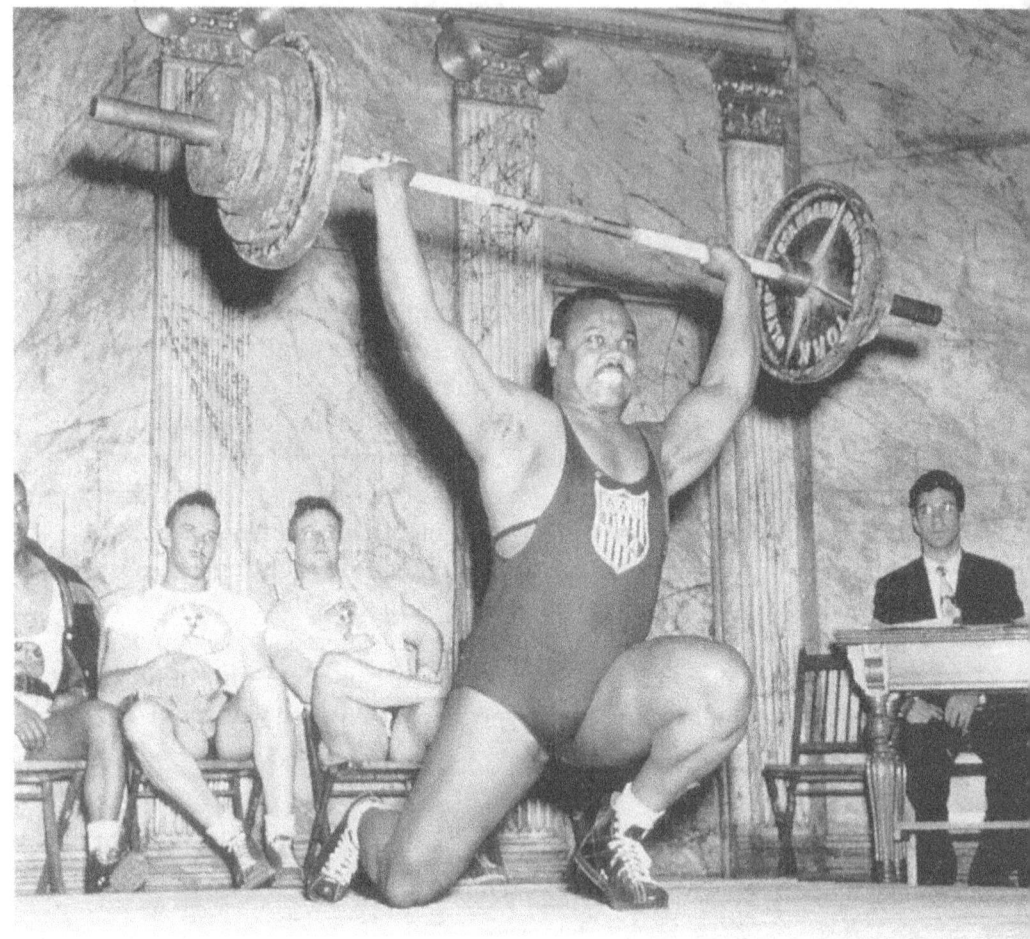

John Davis—York's unbeatable heavyweight from the late 1930s to the early 1950s—shown here performing a heavy snatch at the 1948 Middle Atlantic Championships in Philadelphia.

horror. A most absurd blunder no doubt. I said to myself: 'In the name of the God of Goona Goona, why in the H——ll do you have to put a $%&O* on the cover?' " "Because John Davis is the world's best weightlifter and this is still a Democracy," Bob retorted. The effect was enhanced by an accompanying caricature of Davis extolling his many achievements. The next issue included a letter from M. Wade of Gainesville, Texas, written in reaction to Bob's stalwart defense: "If sticking a nigger's a—— on the cover of a popular magazine is democracy, then it's time we tried something else. . . . so far as I'm concerned, turn your magazine over to the jigs. I'll never have it in my home again." "Tsk! tsk! Mr. Wade" was Hoffman's smug response. Alda Ketterman recalls that the Ku Klux Klan was active in York before the war. Local citizens, outraged by Hoffman's sexual escapades, were even less delighted that he befriended blacks. At the 1942 Mr. America contest in Cincinnati, Bob observed that "John Davis is more than extraordinary. He much prefers to have a good physique to being world's weightlifting champion." Hoffman believed Davis's physique was as good as that of the winners, that "were it not for the handicap of color, he might have been 'Mr. America.' "[12] Nearly three decades before it became a reality, Bob was ready for a black Mr. America.

York on the Move

Though Hoffman was disappointed that the European war prevented him from displaying his champions on a larger scale, their achievements before America's involvement were considerable. At the 1940 national championships in Madison Square Garden, York men won every division, and Grimek was the unanimous and popular choice as Mr. America. He appeared to Sig Klein as "the reincarnation of Hercules, with the grace of Apollo." At the 1941 nationals in Philadelphia, though York lifters won only four of the six classes, they scored 40 percent of the points registered by twelve teams. Davis's snatch of 317 pounds exceeded the heavyweight world record by 21 pounds and the Olympic record by 38. And Grimek captured the Mr. America title a second year. "His posing was magnificent, his muscularity unmatched, his proportions symmetrical, his appearance majestic." He stood so far ahead of the others that a rule was adopted prohibiting previous winners from entering the contest. Hoffman was quick to point out that these unprecedented achievements were the result of his patriarchal influence.[13]

Hoffman's fatherly role included sponsorship of lifting activities in York, whose public display was facilitated in 1940 by the acquisition of Brookside Park on thirty-two acres of woodland near Dover, seven miles northwest of York. In these sylvan surroundings he hosted a strength show in June 1940, at which his eighty-one-year-old mother and sister

ASCENT TO GLORY

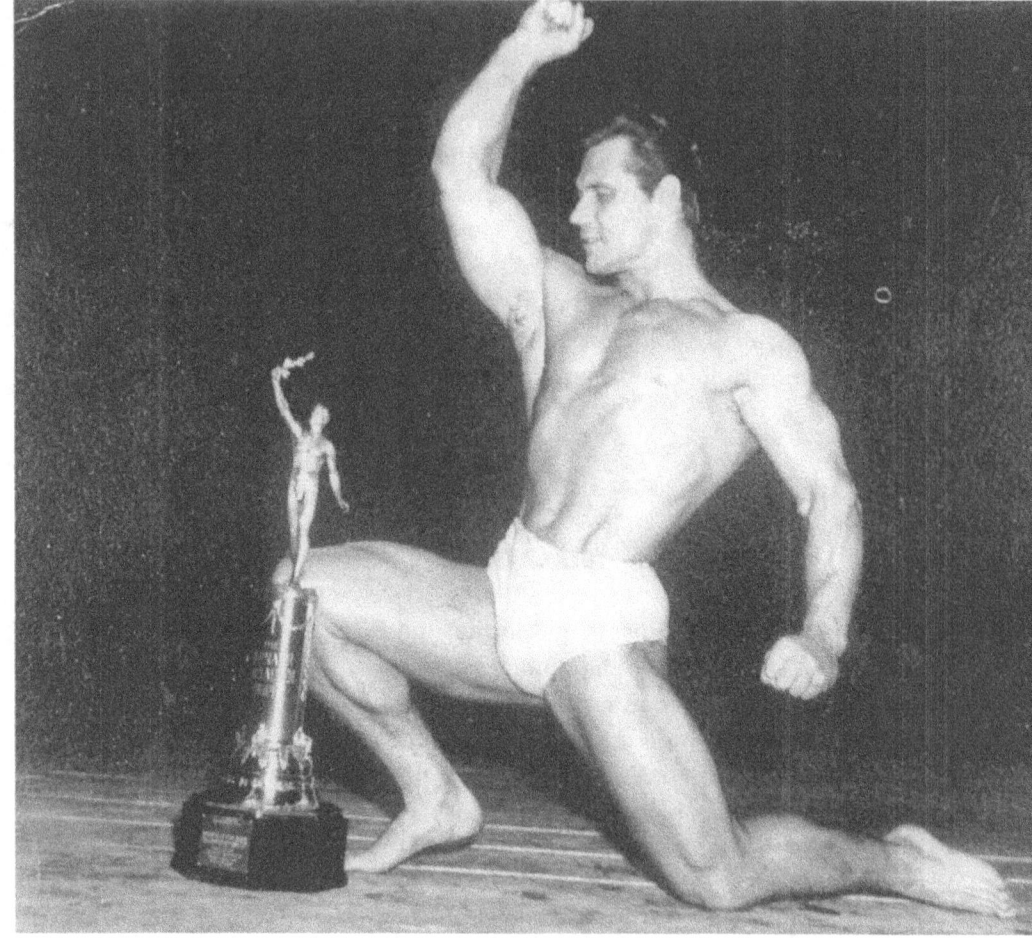

John Grimek winning the 1940 Mr. America contest at Madison Square Garden.

Booch were among the alleged two thousand visitors. It served to exhibit Bob's new property, his organization, and, above all, himself.

> Bob Hoffman put in the busiest day of any man present, he was of course the largest and the oldest competitor. With visitors coming in late he was up most of the night, out of bed early and busy with details all day long. Bent pressing, chain breaking, entered nearly every event on the outside program, performing well in every event, was in charge of the meet, the announcer and covered plenty of ground taking care of details, entered the dancing

competition in the evening and at midnight when some were so tired they almost needed to be carried away he was still fresh as a lily, went for the day's mail and read it until 3 A.M. 365 letters in all.

In addition to strength exhibitions there were competitions in rope climbing and chinning, a handstand race, a wheelbarrow race, and a jitterbug contest, won by Gracie Bard and Elmer Farnham. To display his own speed, strength, and dexterity Bob devised an event in which he carried over his head, on one outstretched arm, a lifter weighing 150 pounds over fifty yards in 12.1 seconds. Grimek did not perform, but his presence caused a sensation. He was surrounded by "gangs of beauties" all day. "Little Gracie" entertained visitors at her home and later allowed the entire Mallo Athletic Club of Akron to sleep there: "in the sun parlors, in the attic, on the floor, studio couches, every bed was doing double or triple duty." Even allowing for Hoffman's embellishments, it was obviously an enjoyable gathering in the tradition of earlier strengthfests. One visitor, on returning home, thanked Bob and conveyed his impressions of the York gang: Stanko, "A Powerhouse"; Hoffman, "friendly, a swell guy"; Terpak, "the weight lifters delight"; Bachtell, "modest"; Venables, "humorous, versatile"; Bard, "vivacious and versatile"; Farnham, "Full of Pep"; Terry, "Power Galore"; and Terlazzo, "cool as a cucumber."[14]

There were many more convivial gatherings, but the most energetic York promotion was a series of trips to the South and West. In October 1940 Hoffman, Grimek, Terpak, and Stanko headed to Chattanooga for an exhibition, then to Atlanta for another big show. Through arrangements made by Karo Whitfield, Bob addressed students from Georgia Tech, high schools, and the National Youth Association. Then they traveled to Birmingham for a meet, followed that with shows in New Orleans and Shreveport, and stopped finally in Kilgore, Texas, for a contest held by Jack Elder. Elder describes Hoffman, whose exhibition barbell was made of a nonferrous material painted black and carefully guarded from the public, as "a real snake-oil salesman." Still, Bob displayed extraordinary stamina, which he likened to that of Wendell Willkie during his energetic speaking tour in his recent run for the presidency: "He made a half dozen speeches a day. I made as many, but Willkie didn't have to lift weights too, to lift 250 or 260 overhead night after night in the one arm bent press."[15] Surely he noted Willkie's death four years later at age fifty-two, but nothing could restrain Hoffman's drive or desire to prove his manliness.

In December Bob, Grimek, Gracie, and Terlazzo embarked on a fourteen-thousand-mile western trip. York's oldest revolving bar, made in 1929, was strapped to the front bumper, and the car, with Bob's typewriter in tow, was packed full. The gang presented exhibitions and clinics in Columbus, Denver, Boise, Spokane, Seattle, Portland, and various locations in California. The most dramatic event of their sojourn occurred while Grimek was preparing to press 270 pounds in San Francisco. Members of the audience began shouting that a forty-eight-year-old Norwegian fisherman in their midst, Karl Norberg, could press more than Grimek. The challenge was accepted, and the reluctant Norberg mounted the platform to have it out with Mr. America.

> Grimek agreed to go first and press 240, which he did with absurd ease. Norberg took the 240 but *with his hands in the palms out position, like in a regular curl!* With very slight effort he *fast curled* the 240 to his chest! . . . He continental pressed this poundage. There was a deafening applause and some of the crowd shouted for Grimek to try a press in that fashion. Without hesitating Grimek made a fast regular curl with the 240 and military pressed it! More deafening applause. . . . The exhibition that Grimek was to give was turning into a contest. Norberg curled and continental pressed 250. Then 260! Grimek took his next attempt with 270 pounds which he likewise curled and military pressed. Norberg told John that 255 was the most he had ever lifted but he wanted to try that 270. Grimek says that it was incredible the ease with which he fast curled 270 to his shoulders but in pressing it he had great difficulty, there was considerable back-bending, leg bending and jerking but he made it.
>
> John then took 280 which he curled and pressed to terrific applause. The audience shouted for the fisherman to take a turn, his friends wanted him to retire in view of his age, but Norberg was enjoying the contest . . . He made a wonderful try but failed.

Hoffman's tour was followed by several miniswings westward by Terpak, Terlazzo, Bacon, and Louis Abele (of Philadelphia) to reinforce the York line. Unfortunately these expeditions, especially when copies of *Strength & Health* were distributed, aroused AAU suspicions of commercialism. Hoffman protested that his motive was to spread the weightlifting gospel. Beyond that, "we are patriotic and wish to . . . build up the strength of the people of our nation."[16] Whatever degree of truth was conveyed in this statement, it was not the whole truth. In succeeding months the number of York sales representatives nationwide grew dramatically.

Gracie Moves On

Gracie Bard, York's "Sweetheart," figured prominently in these promotional endeavors. She accompanied the York gang on trips, helped host shows, and modeled for Hoffman's exercises and products in the magazine. Her picture in a dancing pose with Grimek, on the April 1940 cover, was the most popular to date. As formerly with Rosetta, the woman's role, according to the magazine, was to satisfy her man with food and sex. Soon Gracie was placed in charge of the women's section, her first article being "The Smart Woman Plans Her Meals." That Bob wrote all of Gracie's articles is evident from his rambling style and references to such figures as George Hackenschmidt and Stanislaus Zybszko, of whom she could have known little. Hoffman rewarded Gracie with money, a farmhouse, and cars.[17]

By the spring of 1941, however, she was becoming restless. She began performing with a dance band in Philadelphia, then consorting with Orville Grabeel, a lifter she had met in California. Grabeel, a muscular light heavyweight, soon showed up at York, where he got a job with Bob and became part of the gang. His relationship with Gracie blossomed as they developed an acrobatic act called the "Hawaiian love dance." Hoffman tried to tolerate their partnership and even featured them in the magazine, but when Grabeel tried to lure Gracie away, Bob realized that vital issues impinging on his manhood were at stake. As with Berry, he resorted to violence. He explained to a friend that "a pretty husky weightlifter decided to kill me the other day because Gracie Bard decided to keep her job here instead of going away with him." Aside from bruised hands, Hoffman claimed he "didn't get hurt at all and as they often say, you should have seen the other fellow." But Gracie could not be held against her will, and several months later she eloped. From Los Angeles "Little Gracie," as Mrs. Grabeel, sent

Bob some photos and wrote, "I notice you are still using my name & articles in the magazine. If you wish to continue I would be glad to have you do so providing you pay for it." All of this must have bit deeply into Hoffman's ego. Gracie's articles suddenly ceased, but Bob needed to believe he was still attractive to women. He claimed to overhear, at his forty-second birthday show, the remarks of two girls during his bent-press performance: "One said, 'Why, he doesn't look like he's forty.' The other said, 'I should say not, he looks like a young man.' "[18] Hoffman may have desired to be father of American lifting but hardly relished being old.

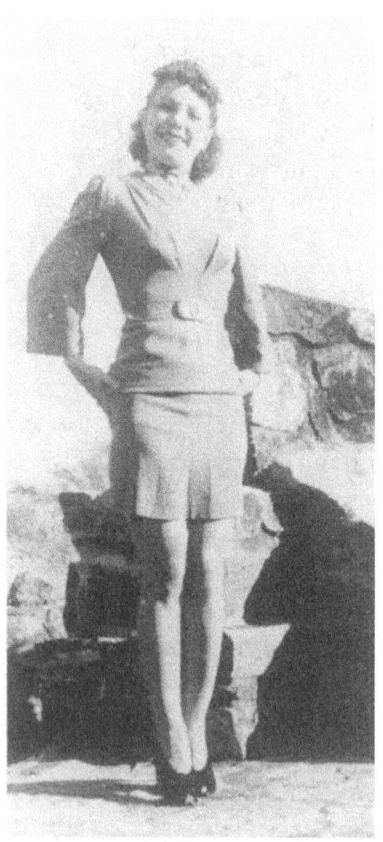

"Little Gracie," as Mrs. Orville Grabeel, Los Angeles, October 1941.

Dorcas and Alda

Bob quickly rebounded from Gracie's rejection by developing relationships with several women. One was Dorcas Lehman, whom Bob introduced as "a leading contender for the title of 'American Venus,' or 'America's strongest woman.' " As daughter of a local grocer and raised on Pennsylvania Dutch cuisine, Dorcas's weight once rose to 201. With Hoffman's inspiration and courses, she lost over fifty pounds. Like Gracie, Dorcas reformed her life of rich food, drinking, and smoking, and now "never cease[d] to marvel at how wonderful she [felt]." A feature article showed her on Silver, once dubbed Gracie's pony. And as Gracie had been the "strongest woman for her size in the world," Dorcas, having pressed 125 pounds, was "the strongest girl we have ever seen." She supposedly leg-pressed 566 pounds twice. A picture from the gym shows her supporting a

Fitness and Survival in Wartime

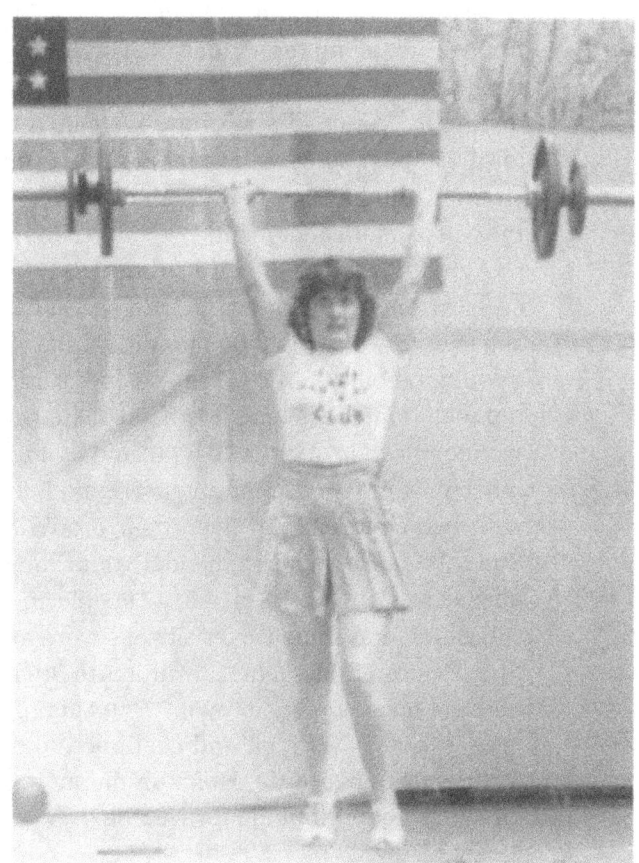

Alda Ketterman, in high heels, performing an overhead lift with 130 pounds.

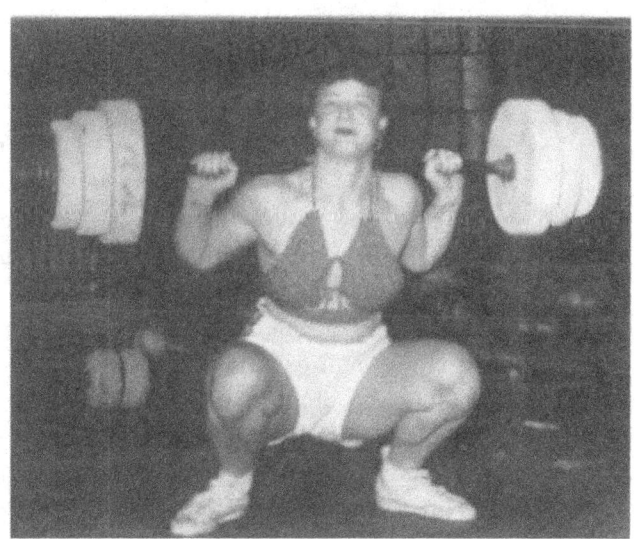

Dorcas Lehman performing a full squat with a York ersatz barbell in 1942.

245-pound barbell and 180-pound Jules Bacon on her shoulders. Soon Bob was extolling the virtues of oversized women. He ascertained that Dorcas's dimensions were roughly those of the Venus de Milo. "Undoubtedly Venus was a strong woman" and "must have weighed at least 150 pounds." He thought many readers preferred "a girl who has strength and muscle" to the slender "undeveloped" type epitomized in the Miss America Pageant.[19]

Alda Ketterman was also strong, and Venables featured her in "Incredible but True" for having pressed eighty-five pounds the first time she ever saw a barbell. Bob predicted she would attain "world fame for her lifting ability." In 1943 she set a "record" for "swinging a 50 pound dumbell from the floor to overhead 30 times with her left arm. Everyone wondered where a girl who is tall and slender, 135 and 5-7 could have so much power." Alda recalls first meeting Bob in 1940. She was divorced, with two children, and lived near Brookside. It was a miserable day. She was depressed and suicidal when she met Bob on a country road and went for a ride with him. "People in York disapproved of him," she states, and some Dover citizens were even going to tar and feather him. "He can bring in his prostitutes to Brookside Park," they said, "but he can't have one of our own." But Alda regarded Bob as "the nearest man to God I ever met, and continued to date him."[20] By enlisting his girlfriends to his cause, Hoffman did more than any other promoter to advance weight training for women.

Before the Deluge

As America gravitated toward war, Hoffman felt beleaguered by charges that he was merely a business tycoon. Therefore his rhetoric assumed a more nationalistic tone—blending business, sport, and patriotism. After visiting Berlin in 1936, he feared the United States was falling behind. In editorials he drew on his survival-of-the-fittest doctrine, warning that to "avoid having our own country invaded we must be strong." American life was "too easy, the vast majority of the people are soft." The obvious remedy was to buy Hoffman's products and follow his methods. The York way became synonymous with national preparedness. To anyone who questioned his motives, he pointed out that Hitler's regime was anathema to the "league of nations" of lifters he had recruited, which included blacks and Jews. Two *Strength & Health* issues in 1940 were devoted to physical readiness and featured a full-blown plan. When President Roosevelt appointed Philadelphia civic leader Jack Kelly to devise a Physical Preparedness Campaign, Hoffman attended an organizational dinner and set to work establishing clubs nationwide. "Before long there will be groups in every city and suburb, every town and village. . . . Be ready when the movement spreads. But we can't force the authorities or the people to train with barbells. We can show them the favorable results. The Strength and Health show at Brookside Park last Sunday was advertised as a part of the Preparedness Program. The long trips which will take Terpak, Grimek, Stanko and myself around the country will be advertised in each city as a part of the Physical Preparedness Program." Hoffman provided elaborate instructions on how readers could organize a "Strength and Health Preparedness Club." Weightlifting, of course, was the principal activity prescribed, and Hoffman pointed out what apparatus would be required and its cost! His involvement in the campaign was a clever mix of business with patriotism. "Awaken physically, America," he beckoned.[21]

In succeeding months Hoffman's appeals became more intense, with articles on German/Japanese threats and regular features on barbells in the armed forces. "If you know congressmen or senators, write them that you are in favor of weight training," he advised. In the spring of 1941 he began listing names of servicemen who had access to weights. He also made trips to Washington, where he discussed with congressmen, War Office officials, and military leaders the merits of barbells, and he arranged demonstrations at West Point, Springfield College, and Mitchell Field on Long Island. Further to project the preparedness image deemed so necessary to his company and America's survival, Hoffman arranged a series of fitness outings for his men—at the beach with Mr. America, canoeing on the Susquehanna, and hiking in the historic Pennsylvania countryside. In the latter the York gang conducted military-style calisthenics, not with fire arms or dummy guns, but with barbells and sandbags. He encouraged readers to write to Kelly and recommend that *Strength & Health* be the official organ of the new fitness movement, known by 1942 as the Hale America program.[22] Attempts to combine his company's commercial endeavors with national security culminated in the "Victory Issue" of March 1942, dedicated entirely to physical readiness.

Wartime Austerity

In the fall of 1941 York Barbell began gearing its operations for war. Hoffman boasted that 200,000 York sets had been manufactured and shipped worldwide. But it was evident that foundries in Lebanon and Hamburg were no longer able to supply the hundred tons of iron needed monthly, owing to defense contracts. Therefore Hoffman purchased a foundry in Marietta, enabling his firm not only to produce more barbells, "but do a great deal of defense work besides. We are pleased to do this, for we are helping our own cause." It was true that he was helping to build a stronger nation, but the real point behind his purchase was to ensure that business, up 46 percent over 1939, would not be jeopardized so much by war work. At first there were problems. Neither supervisors nor workers had experience with heavy castings, and none could pour more than six hundred pounds daily. Hoffman set out to correct matters: "We proved that more weight could be turned out. One day Bob Hoffman put up 152 molds containing 25 pound plates, over 4000 pounds of iron. . . . In time we had a group of molders turning out 150 molds a day, one man produced 173 25 pound plates. The production rate went up, past 25,000 pounds weekly, past 50,000; at this point we had a big party, plenty of food and drink (a barrel of lemonade for those who liked it, a barrel of beer for those who preferred a stronger beverage), music and dancing on the concrete floor of our foundry." Once all back orders were filled, immense quantities of iron were stored in "every available barn and shed in Marietta." Hoffman began stockpiling 1.25- and 2.5-pound plates in case the company had to resort to concrete for larger plates. He stored 100,000 small plates and a supply of steel bars that would "fill many railroad cars."[23] Hoffman delighted in outsmarting the laws of supply and demand.

It was, in any case, a struggle to maintain business as usual. To sustain manufacture of cast-iron plates, Hoffman secured from officials in Washington occasional shipments of pig iron with the justification that barbells would be sent to armed-forces units. The remainder had to be made up in scrap, and Hoffman combed the countryside for it. He salvaged an old pipe line from under the river and procured over two thousand old automobiles. He reported: "These cars have been purchased at backwoods garages where the steel mills, other foundries and junk men had overlooked them. 70 miles from York, up in the mountains our men worked 14 weeks to tear 436 cars apart and transport the material to the foundry. We bought an old abandoned quarry way down in the 'sticks' of Maryland. 125 tons of iron, but necessary to build a road and hire a steam derrick to get the heavy castings out." There were labor problems too, owing to the higher wages paid at a government plant nearby. After a "walkout," Hoffman had to help in the foundry, observing that "it takes a man to do that work." Unlike Milo Barbell, which suspended its operations in the previous war, Hoffman was determined to stay in business, notwithstanding shortages of rubber, paper, and high-quality iron.[24]

Adversity for Bob inspired creativity. He was leading a "high speed life from morning until night" and admitted once that he had not trained for an entire month. Therefore he devised a new routine of "three to seven exercises while shaving and performing his ablutions in the morning. Program consisting of ten or twelve pull ups and press behind neck with 100 pounds, place the shaving cream upon his face, 10 repetitions with continuous pull up and press in front of neck, 100 pounds, shave half his face, then ten repetitions with 100 pounds in the high pull up. At times repeat these three exercises, sometimes as many as seven times 10 with the pull up and press." Needing to train for short periods, Hoffman conceived his "Simplified System of Barbell Training": "Lack of time is no longer an excuse, for this barbell can be used in any space large enough to stretch the arms side to side, front or overhead." This booklet was followed by similar ones on dumbbell and swing-bar training, all of which generated money and ego gratification at a time when the war effort was making extraordinary demands on his resources.[25] Consistent with his patriotic thrust, this new "10 minutes a day" system was free with the purchase of each 100-, 150-, or 200-pound set, now termed the York Victory Barbell. When supplies of iron were depleted, the Victory set was made from concrete. "It's Patriotic to Purchase and Use the Victory Type Barbell" was Hoffman's line.

The Human Element

Human resources were also short. By mid-1942 some of the York gang—Elmer Farnham, Eddie Harrison, John Terry, Jack Ernst, and Harry Utterback—had enlisted. But a strong nucleus remained. Hoffman and Bachtell were too old to serve, while Terlazzo, Terpak, and Venables were married, with children, before the war and therefore exempt. Stanko and Grimek became less eligible when they married in 1942, and both suffered from physical disabilities relegating them to 4-F status. Stanko was afflicted with a weakness in the legs, later diagnosed as phlebitis, and Grimek, according to Terpak, had high blood pressure. The fact that Mr. America had flunked the physical was not publicized, but when bodybuilder Dan Lurie, winner of the "most muscular man" trophy at the 1942 Mr. America contest, was rejected for having a heart murmur,[26] newspapers leaped on this opportunity to show the futility of bodybuilding. An article in the *New York Journal American,* with a large photo of Grimek, was entitled "Athletic Supermen Unfit for War Service." "Hardly a week passes when some mountain of muscle whose name is a byword on the sports pages isn't rejected as unfit for military service while flabby muscled, hollow-chested, ex-clerks who have never competed in anything more exhausting than a game of checkers, march off to defend their country." Although Hoffman denounced the article as "filled with glaring lies," he admitted that Jules "Little Mr. America" Bacon was rejected because of old injuries. Even at the 1942 AAU convention in Chicago, a respected physician scoffed at the idea of national rejuvenation through barbells, noting that weightlifters have small and fast-beating hearts and that big muscles were not a sign of good health.[27] Hoffman's views on the efficacy of weight training were still much in the minority.

It is hardly surprising that performances of American lifters, owing to the war, deteriorated at the 1942 senior nationals. Nor could the York gang sustain its prewar level of performance. Lack of competition, war work, and schooling hindered progress. Terlazzo, after taking a machinist's course, worked at the *Strength & Health* office from eight to four and then on war contracts from four to midnight. "When he trained, except on Saturday, I do not know," remarked Hoffman. His lifts of 240, 235, and 285 in 1942 were down from 250, 240, and 310 the previous year. Likewise Terpak attended night school in ordnance inspection twenty hours a week in addition to his ordinary work. Later he held the equivalent of two full-time jobs, with war work in the day and company work at night and weekends. His lifts also declined. The only inspiring performance of the 1942 championships at Cincinnati occurred purely by happenstance. Light heavyweight Frank Kay was drinking in a local dive with Venables and Paschall when he heard that John Davis was ready to start his presses.

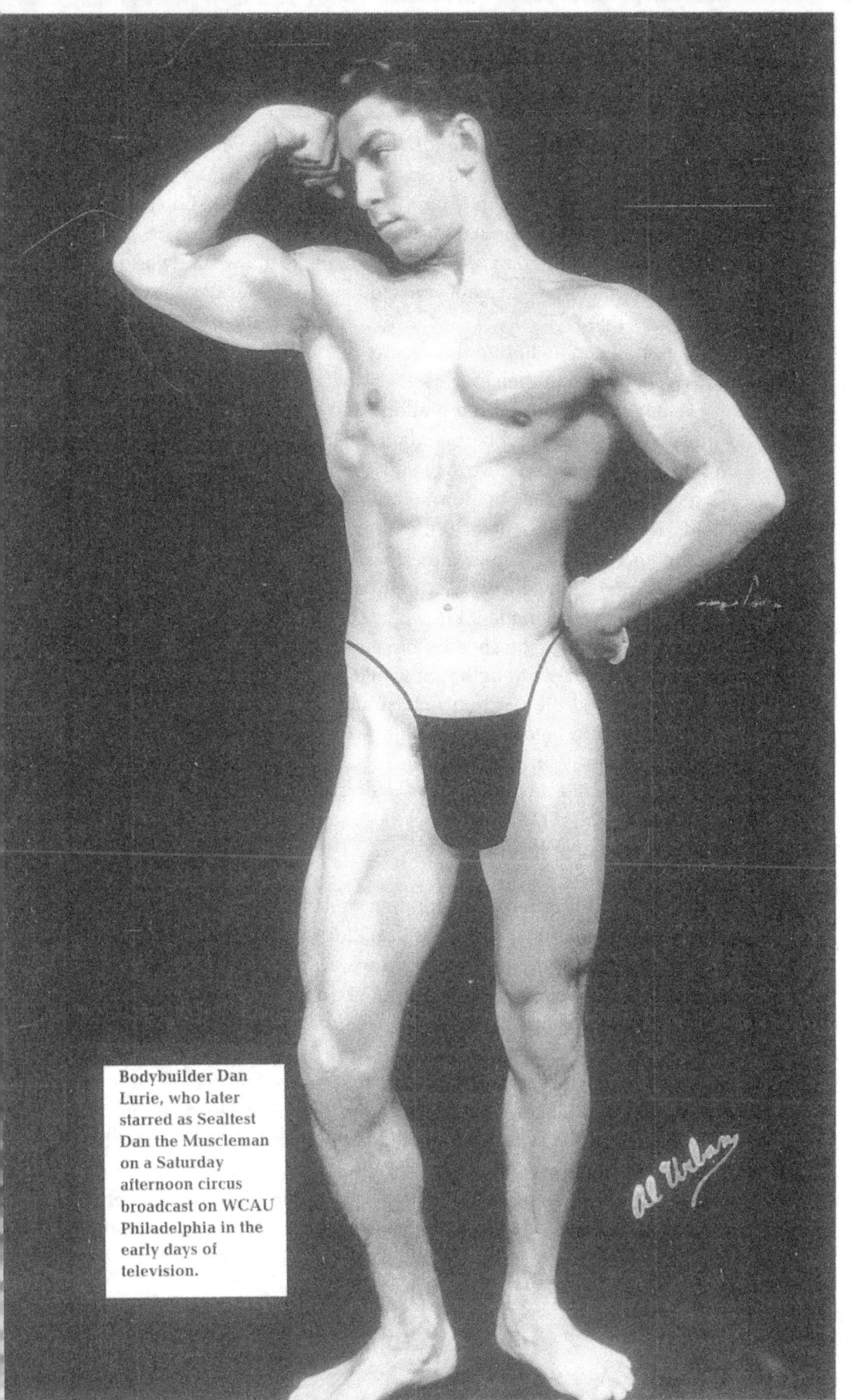

Bodybuilder Dan Lurie, who later starred as Sealtest Dan the Muscleman on a Saturday afternoon circus broadcast on WCAU Philadelphia in the early days of television.

Suddenly, Frank pushed through the crowd to the Officials' desk. He asked to try 275 while Davis was resting! Perhaps the officials were amazed at his audacity for they just looked blank. Bob Hoffman was M.C. He managed to stutter:

"Frank are you crazy? Why, 275 pounds is above the world's lightheavy record, you've got your clothes on and besides . . . well, it's impossible."

"I think I can do it, Bob."

"Well, go ahead then."

Frank walked out on the platform fully dressed (no coat) and grasped the 275 pound barbell. Immediately up sprang [meet director] Emmett Faris who tried to get Frank off the platform claiming such a thing was out of order and not permissible. This made Faris decidedly unpopular with the audience which started to stomp and whistle. They wanted Frank to try. Maybe a 275 press on first try by a light-heavy was impossible, but they wanted Frank out there and they made it known in no uncertain terms.

Bob told Frank to go ahead. Conventions be damned if we were to witness a feat of strength that would go down in lifting history.

Frank pulled the bar to his chest and with a slight back bend pressed the 275 pounds! The weight exceeded the world's record and he made it on his first try! To say that the applause was deafening would be a prodigious understatement.

Think it over; Frank had a few beers and was smoking a cigar less than ten minutes before.

The feat hardly accorded with Hoffman's rules for healthful living, but it was remarkable in an otherwise lackluster lifting era. As Terpak reported to Vic Tanny, the nationals were "quite dry. . . . Not many entries . . . a lousy place . . . and a punk of a sponsor."[28]

Similarly, the quality of *Strength & Health* began to suffer. A reader stationed in California pointed out that previously it was his favorite magazine. Since the coming of the war, however, it had "changed completely." The 1942 Victory Issue contained "not an article of interest for the barbell man. Every article directed at the non exerciser, or in other words for people who don't read S & H." But serious lifters made up only a small portion of readers, and it is obvious from his correspondence that Hoffman was addressing the needs of his more health-minded followers. Advice was most frequently sought from those who were

Fitness and Survival in Wartime

either underweight or flabby. Others suffered from such afflictions as scrawny neck, knobby knees, prominent buttocks, stomach rumbles, tumors, varicose veins, hernia, bad nerves, poor eyesight, pimples, swollen testicles, bulimia, baldness, stiff wrists, poor bowel movement, smoking addiction, nocturnal emissions, spastic colon, and insomnia. Another area of concern was sex, especially masturbation and homosexuality. Some cases were extreme.

> I believe from self diagnosis that I am afflicted with homosexual sadism. The thoughts of torturing men keep running through my mind until I sometimes fear that this is going to force me to perpetrate some terrible crime. Often I find myself planning methods of luring men into secluded spots and there inflicting some inhuman cruelties on them. The great physical culture magazines that once gave me such inspiration now only seem to incite this sexual desire to torture. Instead of seeing the body beautiful I imagine mutilated victims of my mad desire.
>
> In seeking to relieve this desire I at one time found myself resorting to masturbation. This soon became as great an evil and I have since stopped. I have even gone to the extreme of self torture. My body still carries the scars of cigaret burns, red-hot wires and gouges made by a razor.
>
> You may wonder why I am unloading my soul to you. It is because I must find a solution to my problem now before I do something I will be sorry for. I am desperate. I am alone. I need your help.[29]

The distress of such individuals was beyond the capacity of Hoffman or his staff to relieve, but a surprising number of letters received sincere responses. Even during the war years Hoffman remained true to his philosophy of "personalized instruction." Notwithstanding underlying commercial motives, many young Americans were helped in their struggles with life's adversities.

Winning the War

Hoffman tried repeatedly to convince Washington officials that he was not in business for personal gain. He explained that York was aiding the war effort by filling defense contracts and promoting fitness, the latter through supply of weights to the army, navy, and colleges for preflight training. Most galling was an Internal Revenue Service regulation that classified barbells as gym apparatus, rather than health equipment, and therefore subject to luxury tax. Lifting weights was no leisurely pursuit, Bob argued. It was "no fun to train with barbells. A man pants, puffs, and perspires to improve his body, particularly his health." Despite numerous appeals, Hoffman was unable to alter bureaucratic views. Eventually he paid the government, "under protest," $5,298 in back taxes, a sum made more hateful by the fact that it had never been charged to his customers. It was one thing to exhort citizens to be patriotic by dissemination of Victory issues, Victory barbell sets, and "Hale America" programs, but sacrifice with no concomitant returns was unpalatable. Hoffman waged other struggles with the government over draft deferments for valued employees. He described Venables, for instance, as "a key man in our plant" who could operate any piece of machinery and lay out work for others. He was "irreplaceable." The Marietta foundry and machine shop were alleged to be doing 100 percent war work.[30] This included cargo winches for the Maritime Commission, cranes and submarine parts for the navy, castings for diesel engines, parts for antiaircraft guns and landing craft, hand grenades, and even vegetable slicers. Unsuccessful in securing government permission to hire more workers, the number of York employees dwindled from 233 in early 1943 to 114 by the end of the war. Hoffman claimed that Terpak, Terlazzo, Stanko, and Venables were devoting over forty hours a week to war work. "Visitors to York have been surprised to learn that these men . . . arise at 6 o'clock or earlier, ride over to our big plant, work their eight hours, drive back, train for an hour or two, and then spend the evening catching up with the strength and health work." Bob even enlisted his girlfriends. Dorcas was on the payroll, and Alda was driving a truck with loads of twenty thousand pounds to Trenton. Jules Bacon, Mr. America for 1943, was pictured in *Strength & Health,* muscles bulging, doing heavy work in the foundry. Thus Hoffman was able to sustain production *and* a physical plant that eventually would "be turning out barbells in unprecedented quantities."[31] Clearly his sights were set not just on winning the war, or even survival, but on expansion.

Despite restrictions and inconveniences, the company did well, and after problems were overcome at midpoint in the war, profits increased. By 1945 sales recovered, allowing York to surpass prewar totals:

Fitness and Survival in Wartime

1939—$232,356	1942—$227,174	1945—$282,900
1940—$248,030	1943—$215,364	
1941—$288,197	1944—$222,064	

The large profit potential for weights was evident. Only material shortages hampered sales during the last six months of the war. "We are filling these orders very slowly because parts for the barbells come to us in a trickle," Bob explained. "Stuff is scarce." As much as a third of sales from 1942 to 1945 were devoted to supplying training bases, especially the navy, and service hospitals, where the wounded were using weights to recuperate. These contracts made little profit, but Hoffman used these kinds of sales to justify his company's existence. The War Department, he concluded, finally realized that weight training was "the best way to build strength and muscle."[32] There was also the prospect of future profits from servicemen who received *Strength & Health* and whose pictures and letters graced its pages during the war. Despite paper restrictions, Hoffman claimed in 1944 that there were "far more sales of S & H than before the war." Even wartime barbell sets were selling at the rate of twenty a day, or over seven thousand per year. "A lot of barbells." Many regarded the magazine as an important link with home and to their manly aspirations. Toward the end of the conflict came a typical letter from a soldier "somewhere in Burma." He was

> one of the many thousands of your proteges whom you've never met or even dreamed that we conscientiously, yes, religiously take all your instruction and advice. . . . I can also say that I've never had one issue which wasn't read & reread by so many others that I wished it was made of leather. . . . When we all return home after the war you'll have to open up a few factories & printing shops to handle the orders for apparatus & subscriptions for Strength & Health. This is no mere hearsay. I've seen endless numbers of soldiers working out daily with home-made bells of all types & descriptions (my best method is to tie bricks on the end of bamboo sticks). Nearly all of these men expect to order your courses and sets of apparatus as soon as they're home & settled.

Even Tony Terlazzo, who moved to California in 1944, could feel his York ties tugging. "Now that I'm out here I take time to read the old 'rag' where before I hardly looked through it," he told Terpak. There is truth in Hoffman's claim that because of barbell men stationed in such distant places as Java, the Penang Straits, and the Canal Zone, he was becoming "York's best known citizen" and "the world leader in weightlifting."[33]

The Social Scene

Throughout the war the nuclei of the York gang, despite the draft, defense contracts, and economic uncertainty, remained intact. Socialization, an inherent part of Hoffman's organization before the war, continued but at a lower key. In lieu of strengthfests, Hoffman staged weekend outings where health, fitness, and patriotism were emphasized. Bicycling was stressed over car use, and parsimony over extravagance, in articles entitled "The Ride to Gettysburg," "Strength and Health Goes to the Circus," and " 'Mr. America' Goes on a Picnic." Regional and national championships, where York had excelled before the war, lacked their usual luster, but Hoffman was confident that there would be a revival of American weightlifting. Responding to a reader stationed in Egypt, Hoffman regretted that the Egyptians "don't believe the records we have made over here. But some day after the war they will be convinced when our boys 'clean up' in the lifting world." By early 1945, noted Terlazzo, Bob was "collecting lifters again." The organization was poised for growth, and Bob, announcing the York Barbell Club picnic in June 1945, first used the appellation "Muscle Town."[34]

Women remained central to Hoffman's image during the war. Pictures and articles of Dorcas and Alda frequently appeared in *Strength & Health*. Alda, who managed Brookside Park, was featured in an article on swing-bells, ersatz dumbbells Hoffman was promoting owing to material shortages. At an exhibition at New Castle Army Base in 1944, Bob offered her a dollar for each swing with a seventy-five-pound dumbbell over five. She made fifteen and went on to clean and jerk 140 pounds in high heels. In July 1944 "Pudgy" Stockton, a West Coast female strength athlete, initiated a "Barbelles" column in the magazine. Dorcas was featured in August. At 160 pounds she was "super powerful, well muscled and so well developed that she has been called a female John Grimek." Anxious, however, that she should not be perceived as hefty, Bob boasted that she could "pull in her waist until it is 24 inches. . . . When she pulls in her waist, one expects to see the backbone come through."[35] Bob was divorced from Rosetta in 1944, but she still occupied one of his farmhouses and held a lien on the "Strength and Health Center of the World" on Lightner's Hill. Rosetta remained a personal and financial strain on Hoffman, and the irregularity of his personal affairs continued to alienate York citizens. Once, when asked by a *New York Times* reporter about records he held, Bob bragged that, having made love sixteen times in one night, he was world champion for sexual intercourse. "He has a greater interest in sex than most of us," observed Ottley Coulter, who ascribed this "quirk" to Bob's need "to prove to himself his masculinity."[36]

York Survives

His failed marriage and unorthodox sex life were not Hoffman's only liabilities. A much greater concern was a challenge, from distant Montreal, to his authority in the iron game. In 1940 Joe Weider began publishing *Your Physique*, which presented a new slant on weight training by emphasizing bodybuilding. Any advantages it might have had over *Strength & Health* were not immediately obvious, but a reader in 1944 thought York's publication was becoming monotonous. "I have heard of a Canadian publication ('Your Body'?) spoken of with favor and am sure it is only because of the fact it has different authors which gives it a fresh approach." Only in retrospect can it be seen that the enterprising Weider had slipped into two areas of the iron game where Hoffman enjoyed less than complete control—Canada and bodybuilding. From this power base Weider would build his rival empire. By the end of the war Weider's promotional activities were reinforced by Dan Lurie, who, perhaps resentful of being perennial runner-up in Mr. America contests, was eager to strike out on his own. According to Charles Smith, Weider used Lurie to market his wares in the United States, while Lurie used Weider publications to satisfy his ambitions for stardom. The 1945 Mr. America contest was won by PFC Clarence Ross, a virtual unknown from Oakland, California. Lurie did not compete in it, but instead reached for instant fame by issuing a public challenge to Grimek, boasting that he could beat Grimek in a most-muscular-man contest. Ross became incensed over this bravado and told Terpak "that Dan Lurie sure must

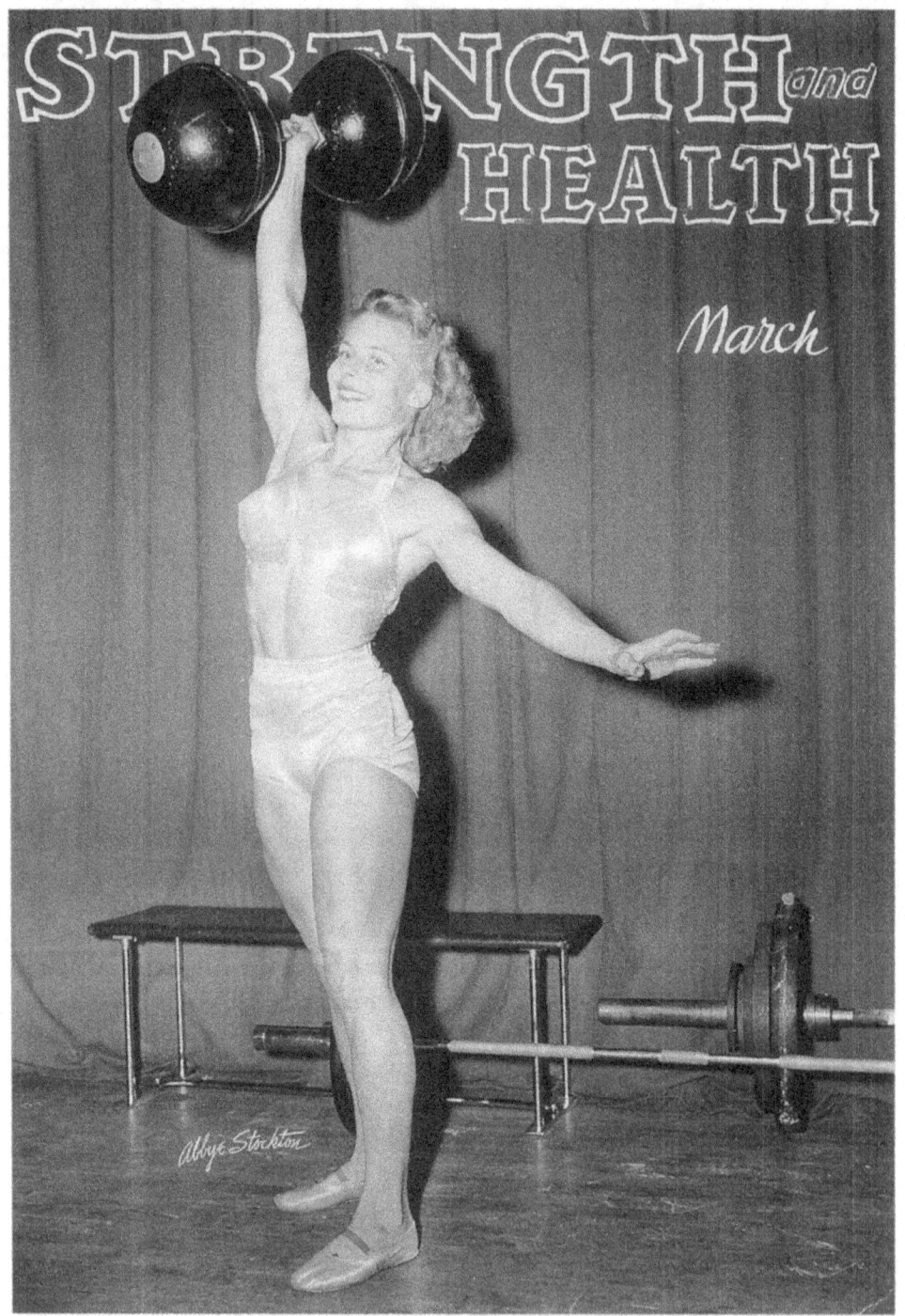

Abbye "Pudgy" Stockton, a Californian who collaborated closely with York for several decades. America's first female bodybuilder.

think a lot of himself to be going around challenging Grimek to a contest. I don't think Grimek can be beaten."[37] Ross's high opinion of Grimek, as well as Lurie's challenge, indicates how far the York star outdistanced all rivals. With three Mr. Americas—Grimek, Bacon, and Stanko—and the allegiance of Ross, Cliff Byers, Joe Lauriano, Kimon Voyages, and others, York was the center for bodybuilding as well as weightlifting.

Most physique stars, even those who later became "pupils" or proponents of the Weider system, were firmly in the York orbit. According to Terpak, Ross had started "with 'the best way,' barbell training the York way." Like so many York followers, Ross adopted weight training because of an inferior self-image. Just before the war Franklin Henry, a California professor, had found that those who engaged in rigorous sports had an inadequacy. Weightlifters were "significantly more introverted, hypochondriac and neurotic, and suffer[ed] more from inferiority complexes, hypersensitivity, and self-consciousness." They were trying "to compensate for their lack of self-confidence." These results coincided with the message Hoffman conveyed about champions' being made rather than born. More than ever, he employed the "ninety-seven-pound-weakling" syndrome as a basis for his success ideology. He also understood how the strength culture appealed to immigrants' sons. For Hoffman, America was a land not only for those of white Anglo-Saxon Protestant heritage. In response to a reader's letter pointing out the predominance of Slavic names among weightlifters and a possible association with atheistic beliefs or "some weird form of religion," Hoffman rose to their defense, dispelling the notion of atheism and flaunting the "league of nations" character of his team. From 1928 to 1938 Italians, French, Germans, and Egyptians won world team titles, and now Americans, representing many nationalities, were supreme. Success, not race or creed, was the means by which he measured his lifters' worth, and he chided those promoters or regions of the country infected with xenophobia or discrimination. When Emerick Ishikawa, a York lifter/employee of Japanese-American origin, was denied the right to compete in the 1945 senior nationals, Hoffman was incensed. He was later allowed to lift, but not in the stadium.[38] Admittedly Bob might not have felt so strongly had Ishikawa not been in his club, but he also protested vehemently about the treatment of black lifters at the 1944 nationals in Chattanooga. On racial matters he was far ahead of his time, and his views were an enormous asset in developing American weightlifting.

Wartime Heroes

During the war years Hoffman's appreciation of cultural factors in sport was subsumed under the rubric of manly support for one's country. Much of what Hoffman had written in the 1930s had played on nationalistic themes, but the war provided a focus for these sentiments. In lieu of combat heroics by his gang, he appropriated leading war figures to exemplify the benefits of physical training.

> Gen. MacArthur was a great athlete, an extraordinary physical specimen at 64, active, he exercises at every opportunity. General Eisenhower was a fine gymnast, can still chin with one hand. . . . General Stillwell and General Chennault of the Flying Tigers still play softball with their young officers. . . . General Mark Clark, only 48 years of age, is strong, young and as vigorous as a man who trained with weights. General Rider, my commander at the first officers training school at Fort Niagara in 1917, is an all around athlete as well as a war hero. . . . Admiral Halsey was a star football player at Annapolis, Admiral King a crewman. Henry Ford still exercises and runs from building to building.

Hoffman claimed that Eisenhower used weights in his youth and that Stilwell carried a pair of dumbbells with him through the jungles of Burma and China. He did not mention that both were also heavy smokers. Field Marshals Alexander and Montgomery of Britain were portrayed too as "regular users of dumbells." He did not attribute barbell use to the founding fathers, but if weights had existed then, they *would* have used them.[39] The right way to emulate these masculine role models, Hoffman exhorted American youth, was the York way.

The war presented an obstacle to Hoffman's ambitions. Although in 1939 he was on the verge of raising America to the top echelon of weightlifting, he was just able to keep the York gang intact through the ensuing struggle. Similarly his company, which monopolized the sale of weights before the war, was nearly put out of business by material shortages, labor problems, and government restrictions during the war. And the manly culture he had created nearly disintegrated. As Hoffman protested in 1944, it should not be the intention of Uncle Sam to "put people out of business who do not interfere with the war effort. The country must go on." By dint of his imagination and perseverance

Fitness and Survival in Wartime

York Barbell survived. Typically he turned his greatest adversary—the United States government—to his advantage by melding his philosophy, company, and organization to the war effort. He argued that physical-fitness training, using York methods and products, was the greatest guarantor of victory. His magazine became an organ of national service, his products were targeted to military bases and hospitals, and his company engaged in work that directly aided in the fighting. Hoffman not only survived but laid a firm foundation for success after the war. By 1945 the business included a foundry, sales were recovering, and York lifters were ready to become world champions. An indication of things to come was Bob's adroit handling of the senior nationals held in Los Angeles in June 1945. To preserve his team's unbroken streak of victories, he gutted his workforce. While Ishikawa, Bachtell, Terlazzo, and Terpak made the long trek west, Bob picked up the slack.

> We are desperately busy, desperately short of help, so short that I just can't get out of pouring three or four thousand pounds of iron every afternoon.... Yesterday I had the hardest day I ever had in the foundry. I poured iron continuously, over 5000 pounds of molten iron in nearly two hours. It was the hottest June day in history, 106 unofficial reading.... like the gallant 600 who had guns all around them as they rode into the valley of death I had hot iron all around me in front of me where I was pouring iron, in back of me where the ladles were already poured, beside me in the pouring ladle, under my foot at all times, many men gave up, but someone had to keep going and I poured the last pound of iron.[40]

Bob thus fulfilled a hero's role. As he approached his forty-eighth year, he had to keep proving that he could sustain his physical and mental capacity to practice what he preached. However great the demand for barbells may have been, Hoffman's intense activity and portrayal of himself as an activator was intended not so much to fill any business requirement as to satisfy the infinitely greater demands of his ego.

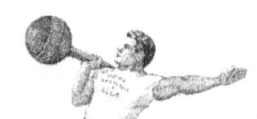

THE "GOLDEN AGE" OF AMERICAN WEIGHTLIFTING

5
YEARS OF CHALLENGE AND ACHIEVEMENT

> There was a time in United States history, back in the pre–World War II era, when sports knew its place in American culture. It was a pastime, diversion, leisure, recreation, play-fun.... But after World War II, sports assumed an extraordinary significance in people's lives; games became not only a reflection of changes occurring in the United States but a lens through which tens of millions of Americans interpreted the significance of their country, their communities, their families, and themselves.
>
> —Randy Roberts and James Olson,
> *Winning Is the Only Thing*

At the end of World War II, all strands of Hoffman's strength-and-health endeavors seemed to converge. The next decade would be his reckoning with destiny, the midlife hinge on which all previous and subsequent activities would turn. The very magnitude of his achievement, however, called forth new challenges. Bob had assumed near absolute authority in the iron game, superseding Atlas and other early muscle culturists and arrogating authority from Berry and Wortmann. Now he encountered an even more formidable adversary in Joe Weider. Put in simplest terms, it was the "Trainer of Champions" vying with the "Father of Weightlifting" for control over America's musclemen. Hoffman, however, broadened this struggle for power. The German weightlifting program, dominant in the thirties, was devastated by the war, but the Soviet Union began to employ the same forms of socialization Hoffman had developed, only on a larger scale. Hoffman viewed Weider and the Soviets as a single enemy, to himself and America.

Building a Muscular America

People in the United States had been experiencing an acculturation to American values at least since the end of the nineteenth century. It reached a climax during the war and included a patriotic awakening, as well as more emphasis on physical fitness, a greater acceptance of weight training, and an unprecedented boom in barbell use. Manly self-esteem was seen as a patriotic virtue, and Hoffman encouraged such thinking by preaching that physical fitness was the key to national superiority and that victory had been achieved largely by barbells. "Our country was saved through the physical ability, the courage, the strength, the endurance that was built on the football fields, baseball fields, and in the gymnasiums, back-yards, and homes of those who trained with weights. Many of our heroes were barbell men."[1] Thus his company's prosperity reflected the spirit of a muscular and confident America as it emerged from World War II.

Most evident by mid-1945 was a tremendous pent-up demand for weightlifting information and equipment. From the far corners of the globe, letters flooded into York, and many personal stories were related in the "Barbell Men in the Service" section of the magazine. Servicemen proudly described how, inspired by York, they improvised weights out of train wheels, airplane armor plating, water pipes, cement blocks, and gun-carriage wheels. Some were York followers before the war. Former champion Bill Curry promoted barbells at postings throughout the South. On opening a training facility for the Second Army in Kentucky in 1945, Curry vowed, "If I ever get an opportunity to exercise with weights regularly again I'll never stop." Sergeant Dick Falcon, from Columbus, Ohio, had set up four York-equipped gyms, where he "trained hundreds and hundreds of young men," most of whom vowed "they were going to buy York weights." In his 1945 report to the Middle Atlantic AAU,

Years of Challenge and Achievement

Hoffman noted that weightlifting, "after years of hard and intensive promotion, finally came into its own with the armed forces." Indicative of this popularity was the availability of *Strength & Health* on Iwo Jima and Okinawa during "the heat of the fighting" and the adoption of Bob's simplified training system by soldiers during battle lulls. Also, many tons of York equipment were shipped to veterans hospitals for rehabilitation. In a visit to one in Martinsburg, West Virginia, Bob observed that each cot was equipped with a chinning bar, York dumbbells, and rubber cables. "It was proven that an average of one month was saved with each hospital case by including our form of exercise, one hundred thousand patients a month, one hundred thousand months saved." The York gang promoted barbells among disabled veterans, and Hoffman engaged an advertising agency to reach the public.[2]

Company records confirm that a great swell of business consumed York in the immediate postwar period. Gross sales leaped from $282,900 in 1945 to $558,419 in 1946. The highest for a single month was $59,557 for August 1946. More business could have been done, but it proved impossible under lingering restrictions. Especially sensitive to the production shortages was Tony Terlazzo, who was building a gym in Los Angeles and wanted to sell York weights. In January 1946 Terlazzo reported that rival manufacturer Walter Marcyan sold weights at his machine shop. During a ninety-minute visit he witnessed five two-hundred-pound sets being sold. "People are buying weights left and right. All they have to do is walk into places like Marcyan's, Paramount's, Kline's, Sid's, and others and take their sets home with them. . . . Three of the local barbell manufacturers have offered me very attractive commission to sell their sets for them. But I have turned them all down though it hurt. With everything going out and nothing coming it takes a helluva lot of will-power to keep saying 'No.' But I'll keep turning them down no matter how much it may hurt!" Vic Tanny had less reason to stay with York. Yet he also was resisting the temptation to sell other brands, despite being offered as much as 28 percent (as opposed to York's 10 percent) commission. Only residual sentiment for the York gang and the prospect of *Strength & Health* advertising kept him steadfast. When the war ended, York, after having its own way for years, was suddenly confronted with other barbell companies. The "flood of business," Hoffman observed, "placed us many months behind . . . and gave a number of competitors a chance to make headway in selling weights." Yet the very existence of other concerns may be attributed to an acceptance of weight training creditable to Hoffman.[3]

Through the lean war years Bob sustained public interest in physical culture through his publications. Book sales peaked in 1945. This was also the year Hoffman was sued by the postal service for obscenity in his sex and marriage books. He contended, however, that they were intended to benefit the "sexually ignorant" and to build "better families." Ultimately the judge agreed that the books were "authoritative discussions of sex and healthy living" and "not obscene, lewd, lascivious, or filthy." But as so often happens, sales increased with this hint of scandal. In 1946 Bob published *Broad Shoulders* to complement his *Big Arms* and *Big Chest*. In typical Hoffman style, readers were enticed by the prospect of greater masculinity. "And there is nothing which stamps a man as being stronger, more manly . . . than broad, well developed shoulders." The contents were again a combination of autobiographical lore, physiological description, and exercise advice, accompanied by photographs of strength stars. But his formula for broad shoulders was the same as he prescribed for big arms, a deep chest, or anything else— "an all around body building program."[4]

Strength & Health sales at the end of the war coincided with book-sale trends. Subscriptions quadrupled, and newsstand sales reached 86 percent of production by 1945. Further advances were sparked by the September cover, featuring a sitting pose of Grimek, "the greatest muscle picture ever shown," according to Hoffman. With the growth of rival publications from Weider, the readers market was being saturated. But York was by far the leading purveyor of goods, as indicated by increased orders and catalog requests and over five hundred letters a day that required answers. Hoffman must have been comforted by Terlazzo's observation in 1945 that Weider's *Your Physique* was virtually unavailable in Los Angeles.[5]

Postwar Camaraderie

The postwar mood in the iron game was one of optimism and collegiality. Strength enthusiast Frank Giardine, who attended Ray Van Cleef's New York City show in September 1945, told Hoffman that his emceeing made him feel "like it was ole times and all the fellows that graced

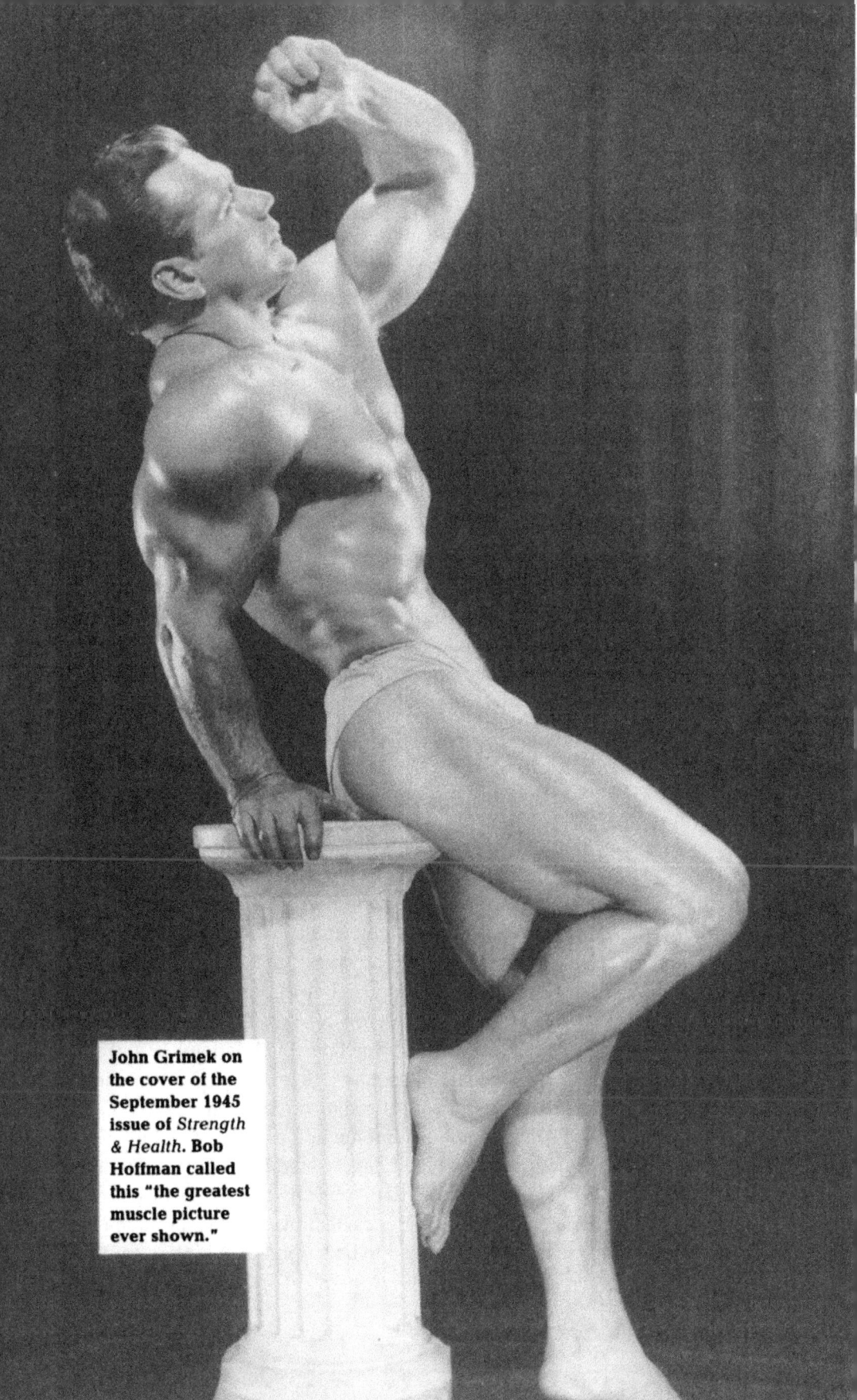

John Grimek on the cover of the September 1945 issue of *Strength & Health*. **Bob Hoffman called this "the greatest muscle picture ever shown."**

the pages of S & H . . . before the war, were all together again and one big happy family." One of the first things future champ Frank Spellman did on returning from service overseas was to "buy one of the mags. It really was a good feeling to see my name." Hoffman's birthday show at the York YMCA in November was a great success. "We were proud to have with us many of the nation's heroes," Bob reported. "There were many oak leaves in the audience," made up "largely of men still in uniform." Included among the performers were remnants of the old York gang and such new recruits as George Shandor and Pete George. Shandor, a promising heavyweight from the Pennsylvania coal region, was recently discharged from the tank corps. Hoffman thought he would be another Stanko. George was truly a "boy wonder." Only sixteen, he cleaned and jerked three hundred pounds as a lightweight. At Bob's home, after the birthday show, contestants and spectators were treated to a feast prepared by Alda and her friends. John Fritsche staged a similar spectacle in Philadelphia in March 1946, leading Bob Jones to observe that "it affords real thrills and satisfaction to the 'early birds' of the iron game to see the popularity which is finally coming to this grand old exercise-sport."[6] Hoffman, from the same generational perspective, was also pleased that York seemed destined to revive the socialization so evident in American lifting before the war.

Symbolic of Bob's hegemony over weightlifting was the restoration of his team's competitive standing. At first he fretted over the availability of lifters. Terpak was the only sure winner from the previous York team that would have beaten the world at Helsinki in 1940. Featherweight John Terry, though back in York, was overweight and not training. Terlazzo had turned professional, Stanko's leg condition prevented him from ever lifting again, and Bachtell, at thirty-eight, would retire soon. On the horizon, however, were some interesting prospects, including Richard Tom of Honolulu, Fred Curry of Santa Monica, Bob Higgins of Indianapolis, Frank Schofro of St. Louis, Pete George of Akron, Stan Stanczyk of Detroit, Frank Kay of Chicago, Frank Spellman of Philadelphia, and Joe DePietro of New York. Hoffman also hoped that some unknown might come forth from the thousands of returning servicemen. "Fellows, it's up to you to make America again supreme in the world of weights."[7]

At the 1946 seniors in Detroit Hoffman wanted to secure his fifteenth team victory, but his "most important objective [was] to produce a strong U.S. national team." To these ends he provided transportation for twenty-one lifters. The lifting proved to be surprisingly high in caliber.

Years of Challenge and Achievement

DePietro and George showed great promise, while Davis, whose 917-pound total was below his best, was still far above anyone else. The real surprise came in the middleweight class, where three top performers vied for honors. Spellman astounded the lifting world with a 257 press, a 252 snatch, and a 322 clean and jerk for a 831-pound total, superseding identical 816 totals by Terpak and Stanczyk. All were tops in the world. Though overall standards were below prewar levels, the cumulative total for America's five best lifters in 1946 was 3,976 pounds. Still, a team from the Soviet Union had recently done 4,079 at a meet in Prague and was widely regarded as "the world's strongest weightlifting team." It was therefore with utmost surprise and delight that an American team of six defeated a highly touted Russian squad of eleven and a strong Egyptian contingent led by Khadr El Touni at the 1946 world championships in Paris. Technically, America's triumph stemmed from Stanczyk's ability to lose bodyweight and win the lightweight class and from the unexpected second-place finish of Kay as a light-heavy. But it was also a personal achievement for Hoffman, whose team registered a cumulative total that was two hundred pounds more than the same lifters had hoisted in the nationals. According to French journalist Leon See, America arrived with a

> united and perfectly trained team. The Russians, like the Egyptians and all the other lifters, came "separately." . . . Spectators and officials alike marvelled at the manner in which the American team worked, how they were handled, how every man had his work to do, to help the man lifting in every possible way when he himself was not in action. . . . Perfect synchronization, efficiency such as had never been seen at the championships in Europe, a team spirit and an effort to excel for their Chief, as we call him, their coach and manager. The other teams lacked that most important of all things, a master mind to train and direct them.

Hoffman readily accepted this generous view, recognizing that "team spirit" enabled this group to do "what potentially stronger teams, the teams of 1936, 1937 and 1938 . . . were unable to do."[8] Even considering that most European powers were still recovering from the war, it was a victory that Hoffman savored for years, and provided the inspiration for a golden age of American weightlifting.

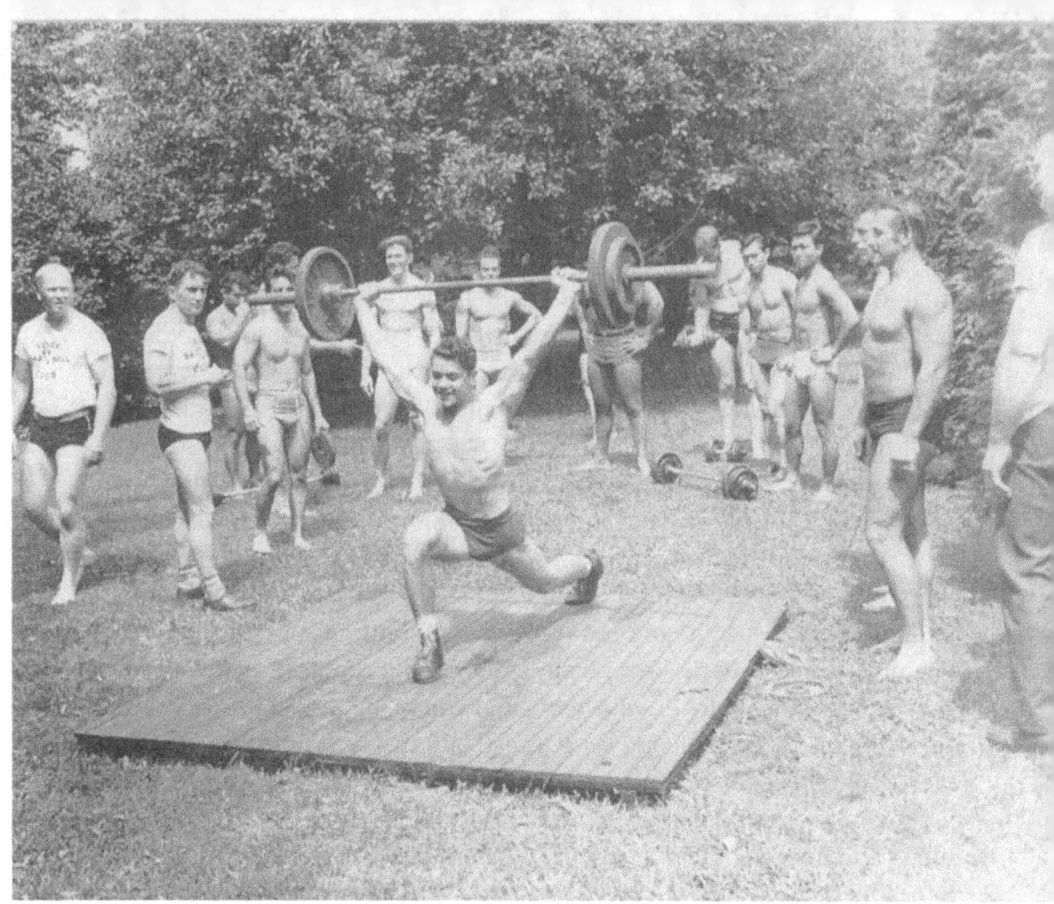

Postwar camaraderie. A young Dave Sheppard snatching on an outdoor platform at Bob's property in north York.

Success in 1946, however, brought mixed blessings. American lifting triumphs, Bob rightly complained, went virtually unnoticed, and what little coverage there was in the press was often erroneous. When Stanczyk broke four world records in early 1947, "there was not a line in the papers about it." This situation was rectified somewhat during the ensuing year by feature articles on weightlifting in several popular magazines. But the image they portrayed did not always please Hoffman. He objected to criticisms by foreign writers that American lifters were good only because he collected them, gave them jobs, and did not care whether they worked—just so they lifted weights. Hoffman retorted, "The job comes first in our organization and only those men who do a good job are here." Grimek confirmed that many visitors seemed "very surprised to see all the York men working." *Fortune* magazine referred to York as "mecca" for at least a half million Americans and to Hoffman as the "Unquestioned Czar of American lifting." In 1946 his annual

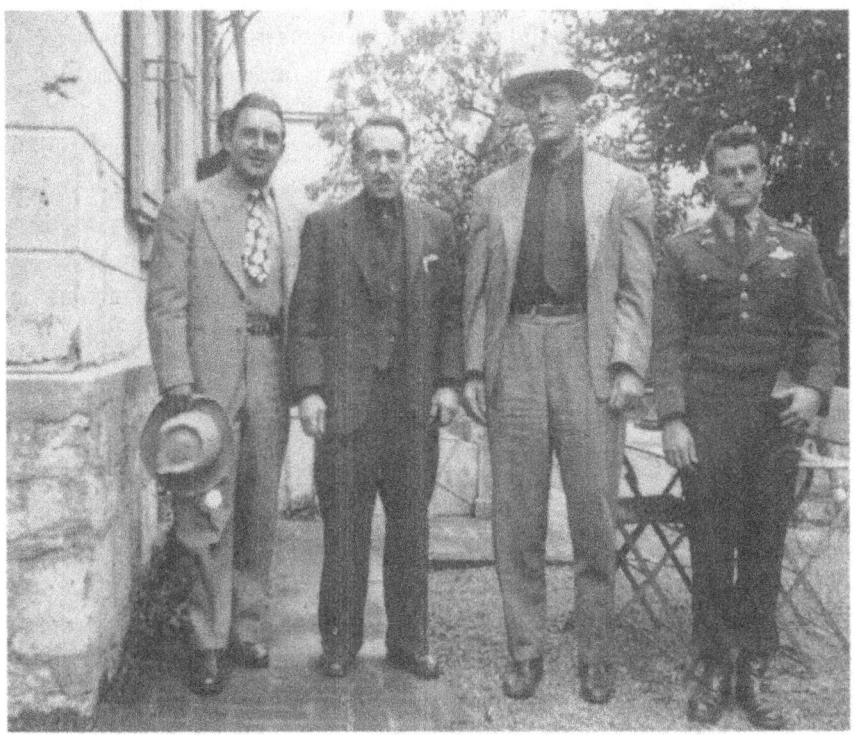

At the 1946 world championships in Paris, Terpak, Hoffman, and the team trainer, Sergeant Alvin Roy, met with Professor Edmund Desbonnet (left center), "Father of French Physical Culture."

salary was estimated at $50,000, and his lifter employees received between $35 and $200 weekly. He provided some with houses and

> set up fifteen of his former champions in businesses that include a restaurant, a taproom, a roadhouse, a curiosity swap shop, and a food market. And he has not been less generous to his two girl friends in York, each of whom has a house and a business; one operates a little taproom and the other a dress shop. About his private life Bob Hoffman is earnest and frank. "I'm strong," he says, "I have to have two girls. I've been going with both of them for eight years and I can't bring myself to break either's heart by giving up one or the other. . . . A strong man can take more than anyone else, but there are limits. He can smoke or drink or make love to the ladies. I don't smoke or drink." His two friends are both proficient weight lifters, and a pleasant evening spent in the

company of either often consists of competition lifting in Hoffman's parlor. "We could use the gym out in the garage . . . but somehow we always seem to work out in here on that thousand-dollar rug."[9]

Unfortunately, despite his success, Bob was regarded as a social pariah in York. It was easy for the unenlightened to label his collection of young lifters as freaks, foreigners, and misfits, and for community leaders and citizens to look askance at this relative newcomer who pursued improper relationships with local women and published a magazine featuring pictures of nearly naked men.

The Weider Challenge

Hoffman's most serious problem was the rise of rival promoters. Joe Weider was marketing many of the same kinds of fitness devices as York, albeit with an emphasis on bodybuilding. Like so many other iron-game luminaries, Weider arose from humble circumstances. That he was ever penniless and undernourished seems doubtful, but at age thirteen he was "a gangling wisp of a lad," according to Jowett, "standing 5 ft. 6 inches, and weighing but 110 lbs." Though "fleet of foot," he was weak and the "butt of all his mates who took a delight in asserting their superior strength." Too poor to buy weights or join a YMCA, Weider "made his first barbell from a rusty iron flywheel in a junkyard."[10] Rick Wayne portrays him in much the same vein, adding that he joined a weightlifting club at sixteen, totaled 725 pounds in the Olympic lifts at eighteen, and in 1940, at nineteen, published his first issue of *Your Physique*.

With the outbreak of World War II, Bob Hoffman's *Strength & Health*, the source of inspiration for Montreal's musclemen, became unavailable to Canadians. The magazine had been their only source of information on weightlifting. And there were no more contests. That left young Joe Weider with little incentive to practice his Olympic lifts. So he turned to bodybuilding and was soon fantasizing about a future in which that activity would enjoy the same recognition accorded Olympic weightlifting. . . . Weider assigned himself the task of publishing a magazine exclusively for bodybuilders.... From old editions of *Strength & Health*, the aspiring publisher copied names and addresses of about eight hundred Canadian musclemen listed as members of the Strength & Health League, and to each he mailed a penny postcard soliciting support for his dream publication.[11]

Not only did early issues of *Your Physique* borrow much from York, but Bob allegedly paid most of Weider's publishing costs (and supplied his own printer) in return for advertisements of York products. In 1946 a picture of Weider appeared in *Strength & Health* with an inscription stating that he had been "a York pupil for 2½ years and gained from 105 to 163 pounds" bodyweight. However much Weider might later minimize it, Hoffman's promotion techniques served as a model for his own fledgling efforts. There was also much that was innovative in Weider's initiatives. He presented a glitzier approach to fitness and physique by emphasizing appearance rather than use of muscles. "Charisma" and "glamour" are terms later applied by Vince Gironda to Weider's movement: "He glorifies mister bodybuilder." But even when competition from Weider became more intense after the war and a second magazine called *Muscle Power* appeared, York made a pretense of cordiality. It noted a "friendly feeling" at a 1946 Montreal strengthfest attended by the twenty-three-year-old Weider. And congratulations were extended when Joe married Diana Ross in Manhattan in January 1947.[12]

Clearly, however, concern was mounting over the growth and audacity of Weider, who offered not only a colorful format, but an abundance of authors. Some were prominent figures—Liederman, Jowett, Tilney, Cliff Byers, and Roger Eells—who were disaffected from York and sought continued affiliation and remuneration in the iron game. Alyce Stagg and Ed Yarick, who ran a physical-culture studio in Oakland, California, were torn both ways. In 1947 Alyce was considering whether to accept Weider's invitation to write for him. She believed that "Bob Hoffman and Joe Weider aren't too keen about each other" and "did not want to do anything that might spoil things with York and Ed." Later Ed expressed to Terpak indignation over the use Weider had made in *Your Physique* of some photos Alyce had sent him: "[Joe] sure made a mess of things saying I started Leo Stern, Jack LaLanne and John Tucker. The Tucker fellow I have never met. Typical Weider to do a trick of this kind at someone elses expense." Yarick also recalled that some years earlier he had furnished information for a piece on himself: "When the article

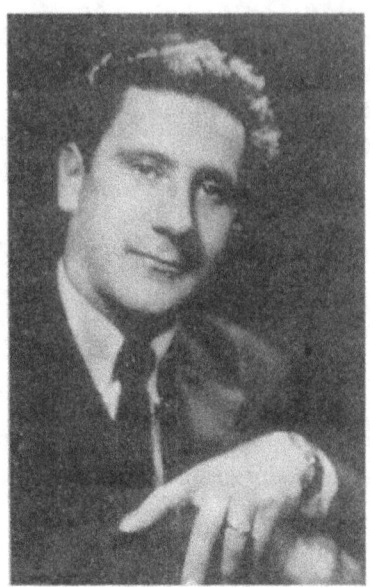

Bob's nemesis, Joe E. Weider. Weider's promotional activities in bodybuilding eventually surpassed those carried out by York in weightlifting.

appeared and it had been rewritten I sounded like a conceited ass. Every contact I have had with Weider has been a bad experience."[13] However culpable Weider may have been for misappropriating information, it could be argued that he was merely elaborating on a promotional tradition established by Macfadden, Jowett, Liederman, Atlas, and Hoffman. Virtue simply was not the most reliable road to success.

In the summer of 1945 Weider confronted York by promoting Dan Lurie's challenge to John Grimek for the title of "America's Most Muscular Man." Lurie contended that Grimek had repeatedly appropriated this appellation, though he had never won it. Since Lurie's professional status barred him from competing with amateurs, he challenged just Grimek, whom he also regarded as a professional. Such was not Grimek's view. In an insulting reply, he insisted on an open contest and attributed Lurie's "supercilious actions" to his "self-inflated ego." Lurie, accusing Grimek of trying to "darken my name and besmirch my character," charged that his opponent had evaded the challenge, and declared the matter closed. Hoffman, however, arranged a most-muscular contest in May 1946 at the Turners Hall in Philadelphia, sanctioned by the AAU. Grimek placed first, followed by Stanko, Sam Loprinzi, Kimon Voyages, and Dick Bachtell. Lurie showed up as a spectator. *Strength & Health* reported that when Hoffman, as emcee, taunted him to compete, Lurie protested that the contest was not being conducted fairly. Besides, he was a professional. A battle of words followed, Lurie ultimately agreeing to compete in a professional showdown against Sig

Klein and Walter Podolak, who volunteered from the audience. The results were Klein 48, Lurie 43, and Podolak 41. AAU official Wilbur Smith observed that Klein, though much older, proved "that his musculature is superior . . . even though Lurie allows himself to be exploited as America's Most Muscular Man. In this contest he was a second rater, or as the racing boys say, 'he also ran.' "[14]

A different view came from *Your Physique*, which implied that Lurie, despite his "magnificent physique," lost only because he had verbally abused the judges during his altercation with Hoffman. Also, there was no reason for calling Lurie a professional and Grimek an amateur, especially since what the audience "definitely wanted to see was Lurie and Grimek on stage together." That they did not compete on common ground was labeled the "Mother of all the little mysteries born of the Turner-Hoffman union in Philadelphia." But harshest criticism was reserved for the way the affair was conducted.

> Why can't strong man shows be put on with some semblance of professional theatre? We, the audience, are accustomed to showmanship. We have it in radio, the movies, the dramatic and musical comedy stage, and when we pay more than a buck for a seat we resent being steeped in corn. Why can't there be a Master of Ceremonies with a smooth line of talk and a brisk but easy manner to keep the show moving? Why can't there be good music to put a little spirit into the evening? When Turners tin can piano began to beat out the Star Spangled Banner we all knew what we were in for. When that ordeal was over Mr. Hoffman assured us the man at the piano was a very fine musician, but that he hadn't heard him since he played at his mother's funeral! I am still wondering if that was an apology, an attempt at a joke, or just a dull statement of fact.[15]

Herein lay an essential difference between the approaches of Weider and Hoffman and a reason why physique shows eventually separated from weightlifting. The former lent themselves more to show business, while the latter was more an athletic competition. Weider and Lurie may have been premature, overzealous, and even arrogant in their efforts to promote bodybuilding and challenge Hoffman's hegemony of the strength world, but theirs was the wave of the future.

Hoffman's concern was betrayed by repeated attempts to belittle Lurie and to reassure readers of York's supremacy. But Weider refused to buckle under and even claimed some spoils of victory from the many "new admirers" of Lurie who "went over to his camp through a love of fair play." Weider's real victory, however, lay in the fact that he had lured Hoffman to his own ground and thereby shared in the limelight of York's prestige. As underdog, Weider gained free publicity from this exchange. Further grounds for concern came from longtime associate Jack Elder in Texas. He observed that "all the boys here are turning into bodybuilders. Most of them are getting such nice, fat butts that I'm trying to get them to join the Navy and let me manage them. Just call me 'madam.'"[16] Hoffman realized that the multitude of returning servicemen, who were fostering the barbell boom as well as the baby boom, were turning more to bodybuilding than weightlifting. However much he favored the latter, he kept physique stars in the forefront of his promotional efforts. Pictures of Jules Bacon continued to accompany instructional articles and ads for York products, and Steve Stanko and John Grimek were given further prominence by winning Mr. Universe titles in 1947 and 1948, respectively.

At the moment, the future belonged to York. In 1946 the company sold fifty thousand weight sets and, with income from other enterprises, grossed a million dollars. Profits soared. "We are an organization," boasted Hoffman, "which employs from 140 to 168 men and women, has a payroll of from six to seven thousand five hundred weekly, we are doing a sizeable legitimate business." Bob sought an even greater following by combining his sales pitch with a high-minded patriotic appeal. Unlike organizations that were interested in "your dollars only," he professed a desire to "make America stronger and to lead the rest of the world." That Weider was based in a foreign country was rationale for Hoffman to portray it as anti-American and link it with the emerging Communist specter in eastern Europe. When *Your Physique*, by employing an alternative scoring method, credited the Soviet Union with victory at the 1946 world's championships, Bob accused Weider of "Pro Russian anti-American tendencies." And the term "comrade" was frequently bandied about in the columns of Venables and Paschall in reference to business rivals. Hoffman also invoked foreign metaphors for his outfit, but quite differently. "He said it like a prayer—like a Mohammedan would say 'Mecca,' or a Buddhist would say 'Nirvana,' 'York,

Pennsylvania!' "[17] Such words were attributed to 1946 Mr. America Alan Stephen when he first visited York. He later became a Weider star.

The International Challenge

It would be difficult to determine whether Hoffman regarded his greatest challenge as domestic or foreign. He portrayed Russia as "a strong nation where physical perfection and strength is more sought after than any other one quality." Against this popularity, supplemented by government assistance and rewards, there seemed to be "only the efforts of Bob Hoffman." "America's victory in weightlifting more than any other one thing depicts America's strength. In France we were told by pleased French officials that the American victory was worth more to the continued cause of world peace than the display of force by a fleet of battleships, by a thousand planes or by a dozen divisions of soldiers. For the world knows while America has sufficient interest in developing strength and muscles to excel the world that they are a strong virile race." However much he regretted lack of government support, his self-created image as a lone crusader gave Hoffman a special standing in the ruling councils of weightlifting. Though he did not always participate directly in decision making, those who did knew they had to reckon with him, especially in selecting athletes and coaches for international teams. York Barbell Club maintained a high profile, monopolizing the national championships for decades. Hoffman always said, "It's very important for our team to win the team championships." And Bob's goal was "to more completely dominate weightlifting than any other nation has ever dominated any sport."[18] Whether at home or abroad, success of his team was crucial for him to be regarded as the iron game's foremost promoter.

Further attention was drawn to York when Hoffman brought the 1947 world championships to Philadelphia, ninety miles east of York. There, with Russians and Egyptians absent, American lifters scored a 27-to-3 victory over everyone else and equaled or exceeded twelve world records. It was Hoffman's show. Staged in the capacious municipal auditorium (seating fifteen thousand), Hoffman provided $10,000 for expenses of foreign lifters and underwrote all other costs. Prior to the championships, lifters from across the country gathered in York, where they were quartered at Hoffman's expense. Most of the training took place at the York Barbell gym, until visitors made it so crowded that the team had to use his home. "There they had the use of the club gymnasium, the swimming pool, the extensive grounds," and "they were having a lot of fun going around together, palling around." Even Peary Rader, editor of *Iron Man*, commended Hoffman: "He spent a great deal of money and it is doubtful if enough tickets were sold to repay him. It was probably the smoothest run meet of international scope ever seen." In 1948 Hoffman raised American lifting to greater heights yet by achieving an Olympic victory in London, where his lifters easily beat the Egyptians. Again the American team gathered in York for final training. In Dorcas's newly remodeled King George Hotel, Bob provided accommodation even for those just trying out. With all the rooms occupied by weightlifters, and all eating, training, and playing together, a genuine team spirit developed. Hoffman expended $20,000 and even offered to provide barbells for the competition.[19] In the ensuing triumph, Americans won four of the six classes. The United States scored 30 points, as against 13 for Egypt and 11 for the rest of the world.

As in the 1946 and 1947 world championships, upwardly mobile immigrants and their attachment to Hoffman laid the basis for an Olympic victory. It was part of the American dream—the land of opportunity beckoned them to psychic as well as material fulfillment. The "league of nations" aspect of the American team was illustrated by the presence of "17 different nationalities." Hoffman was the patriarch for this aggregation—even to the extent that lifters performed certain lifts for him. At Philadelphia in 1947 Davis made his 308-pound world-record snatch at Hoffman's urging. "I'm going to make this one for you, Bob," said Pete George as he mounted the platform to try a 341-pound clean and jerk at the Olympics. And Spellman, who edged out George in the middleweight class, prior to his final lift said, "You've done a lot for me, Bob. . . . I'll make this one for you." Spellman claims that his "love for Bob Hoffman was so great, when I failed a lift I felt that I had let him down. He was my father image." Hoffman projected an all-American image for his lifters: "It gives me pleasure when one of our team not only makes world weightlifting history but obtains a better education, a better position, a nice car, a home, or a happy family."[20] It was evident that the unprecedented performances by the postwar generation of lifters corresponded with the widespread acceptance of Hoffman's ideology of success.

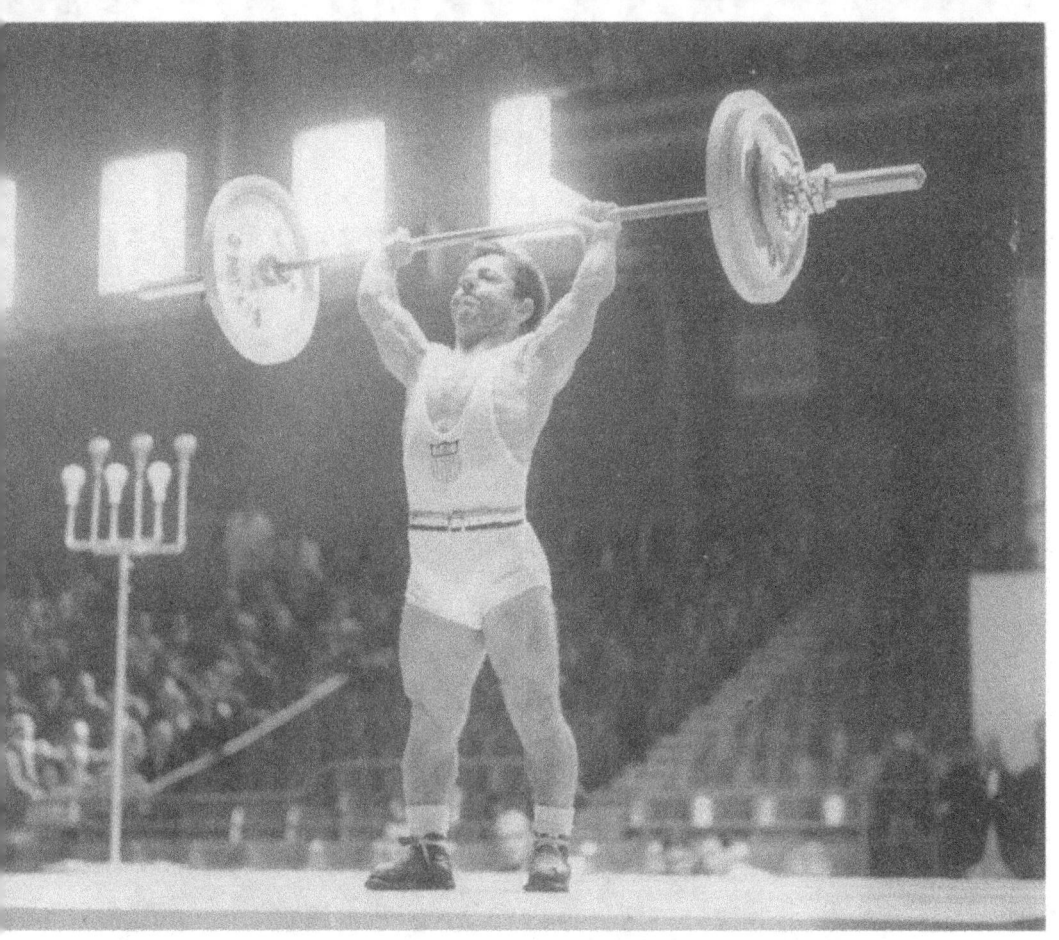

Joe DePietro, bantamweight gold medalist at the 1948 Olympics in London, shown pressing about 225 pounds.

The Olympic achievements of York's lifters could not be sustained at the 1949 world championships at The Hague. Though the Americans took a close second, Hoffman protested that the winning Egyptians were so heavily subsidized by their government as to be professionals and that the one-lifter-per-class rule militated against the heavier American team. By the following year he recouped his forces and added several more names to America's pantheon of heroes. A significant proportion again were ethnic Americans, including Tommy Kono, a Japanese-American from California; Norbert Schemansky, a Polish-American from Detroit; and James Bradford, an African-American from Washington, D.C. Kono, especially, fit the model of the striving ethnic American. The son of fruit-cannery workers in Sacramento, he suffered from asthma as a child and weighed only 105 pounds at age fourteen. When his family was shipped during World War II to a "relocation center" at Tule Lake, California, he found that desert air relieved his

THE "GOLDEN AGE" OF AMERICAN WEIGHTLIFTING

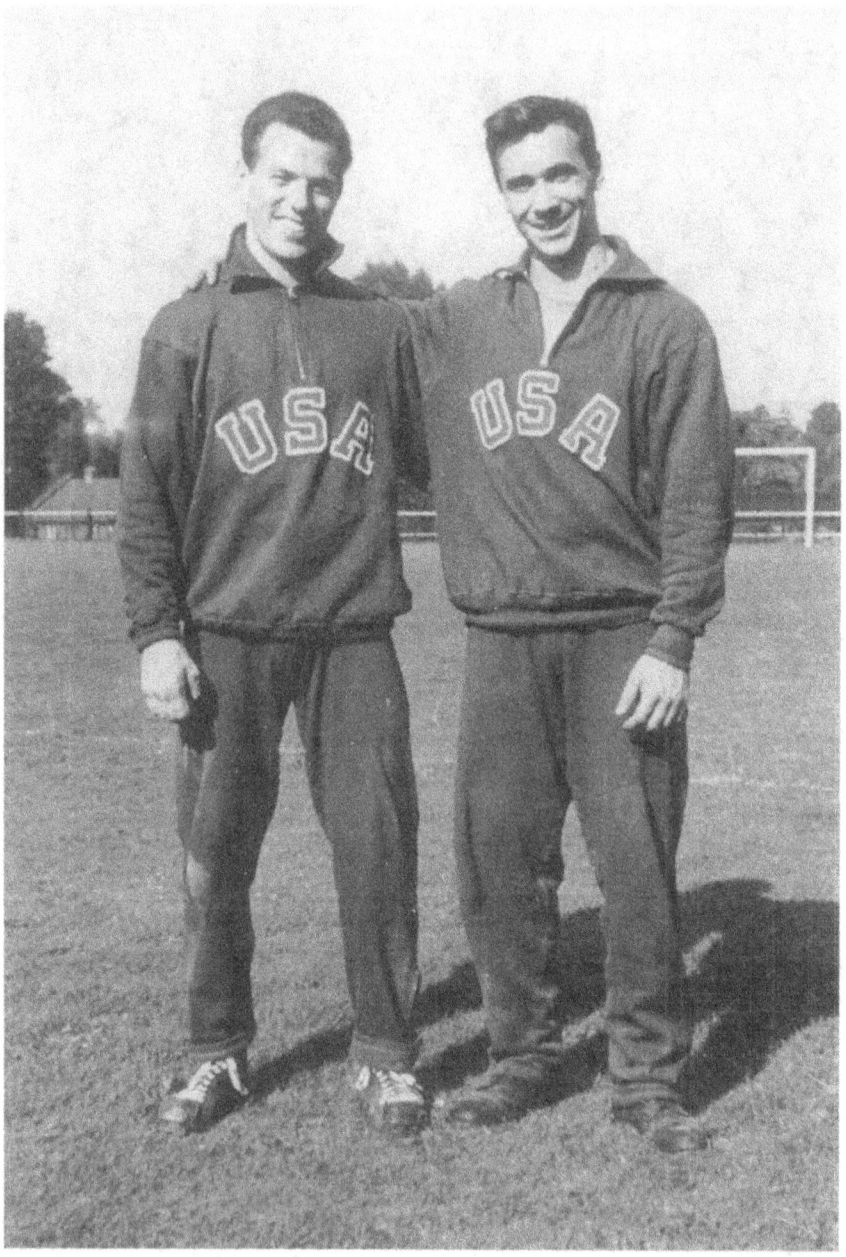

Frank Spellman and Pete George, two of York's top performers during America's golden age of weightlifting.

breathing and weightlifting strengthened him. Kono overcompensated and became America's brightest star in the 1950s. There were also a few traditional American types—Joe Pitman, Richard Greenawalt, and Dave Sheppard (another "boy wonder"), but they never reached the same degree of excellence.

By this time most of the older generation of York lifters had fallen by the wayside. Terpak, eleven times national and twice world champion, remained, but his powers were waning, and other lifters—Stanczyk, Spellman, and George—were beating him. As early as 1946 Terpak declared that he had "no intention of remaining in competition until I reach 40. . . . If I can represent my country in the Olympic Games in 1948 I shall be happy to retire immediately the Games come to an end." When that time came, Hoffman observed that Terpak, at thirty-six, bore "the weight of years upon his shoulders." Lifting as a lightweight to garner team points, Johnny could do no better than fourth. His clean and jerk of 297 was made "only after a terrific courageous effort," noted Hoffman. "It was the hardest lift I had ever seen him make."[21] It was the last time Terpak mounted the platform. Only the redoubtable John Davis seemed beyond reach of the newcomers.

New Bodybuilding Standards

Hoffman, of course, had long passed his competitive prime and no longer trained much, but to satisfy his craving to remain a champion, he continually conjured up opportunities for self-display. In the summer of 1946, applying his height advantage, he won a long-distance diving championship held in his backyard with seven current lifting and physique stars. Further reassurance of his virility was provided one evening when, in his words, "a group of us hiked over 25 miles to show we could do it." He claimed still to be able to work "hard for twelve hours at digging and making a garden, or digging a pool, picking, shoveling and wheel-barrowing all day." A bent press of 260 pounds at his fiftieth-birthday show in November 1948 culminated his efforts to defy aging. His achievement, however, was overshadowed by George's world record clean and jerk of 354. It was reported by Charles Smith, who, after learning that some of Bob's plates were aluminum, understated the former as much as he rejoiced in the latter. But the

THE "GOLDEN AGE" OF AMERICAN WEIGHTLIFTING

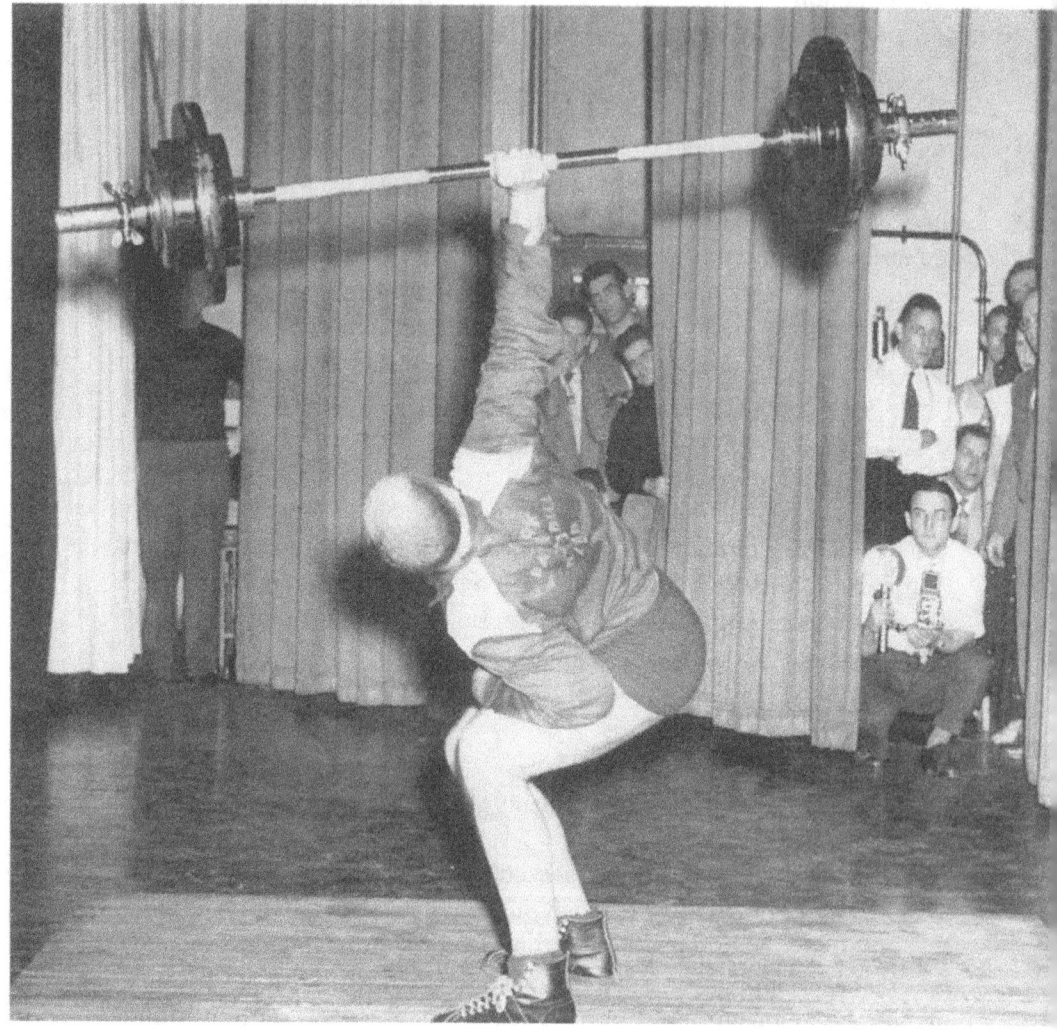

Bob performing a bent press (circa 1948) with a barbell purportedly weighing about 250 pounds. A shortened exhibition bar and aluminum plates reduced actual weight by about 100 pounds.

sensation of the evening was Melvin Wells, a black bodybuilder from Buffalo.

Melvin walked on the stage, the curtains parted, he took his jacket off—there was dead silence for thirty seconds, and then pandemonium broke loose. Never have I heard a roar like it before. It was a sheer cry of amazement, of almost disbelief one could be tempted to say. It seemed hardly possible that a man could be so big and yet so purely muscular.... You think Reeves, Ross, Pederson and Grimek are well built? Brother—you ain't seen nothing yet! Wait until you see Melvin.... His arms tape 18¼ inches cold. Pumped up they measure a full 19. Yet you can see every fiber. It almost seems he has no skin. His anterior deltoids run across his upper chest and meet there. The trapezius stand up from his back a full inch. The back development defies description. Standing beside Steve Stanko, I glanced around and Steve's eyes looked like they were on the end of stalks. "Man is he stacked up!" he kept repeating.

Notwithstanding being upstaged, Hoffman capitalized on Wells's physique by featuring him on the cover of *Strength & Health* and in an accompanying full-length article, the first such exposure of a black bodybuilder. And Bob was quick to point out that Wells, "one of the best of all times," had been following the York system since 1942.[22] It was obvious with the arrival of the likes of Wells, Steve Reeves, an ever-improving Clarence Ross, George Eiferman, Jack Delinger, and Reg Park from England that a new standard of excellence was emerging.

Grimek, of course, had been the undisputed king of bodybuilders for nearly ten years, but his days were numbered. Unlike most of the old gang, he departed in a blaze of glory. A surge of interest in physique was stimulated by such promoters as Vic Tanny, Bert Goodrich, Jack LaLanne, Walter Marcyan, Leo Stern, Alice and Ed Yarick, and Les and "Pudgy" Stockton. Their activism in the Golden State helped spark the Muscle Beach phenomenon that thrived in Santa Monica during the 1950s and early 1960s. Ross seemed to set the pace. In December 1947 he made his first appearance in the East at an "outlaw" show in Brooklyn staged by Dan Lurie for Weider. Though *Strength & Health* portrayed it otherwise as a "failure," Ross's final act was spectacular. "The audience realized from the instant he appeared upon the pedestal that they were observing a physical marvel in action.... Ross was the sensation of the show." In March 1948 at a Mr. U.S.A. contest in Los Angeles, Ross defeated a strong field that included two former Mr. Americas (Alan Stephan and Steve Reeves), Eric Pedersen, and Floyd Page. Ross "held the 5000 spectators spellbound." Grimek did not attend, but in the fall ventured to London, where he was hailed as an international celebrity

THE "GOLDEN AGE" OF AMERICAN WEIGHTLIFTING

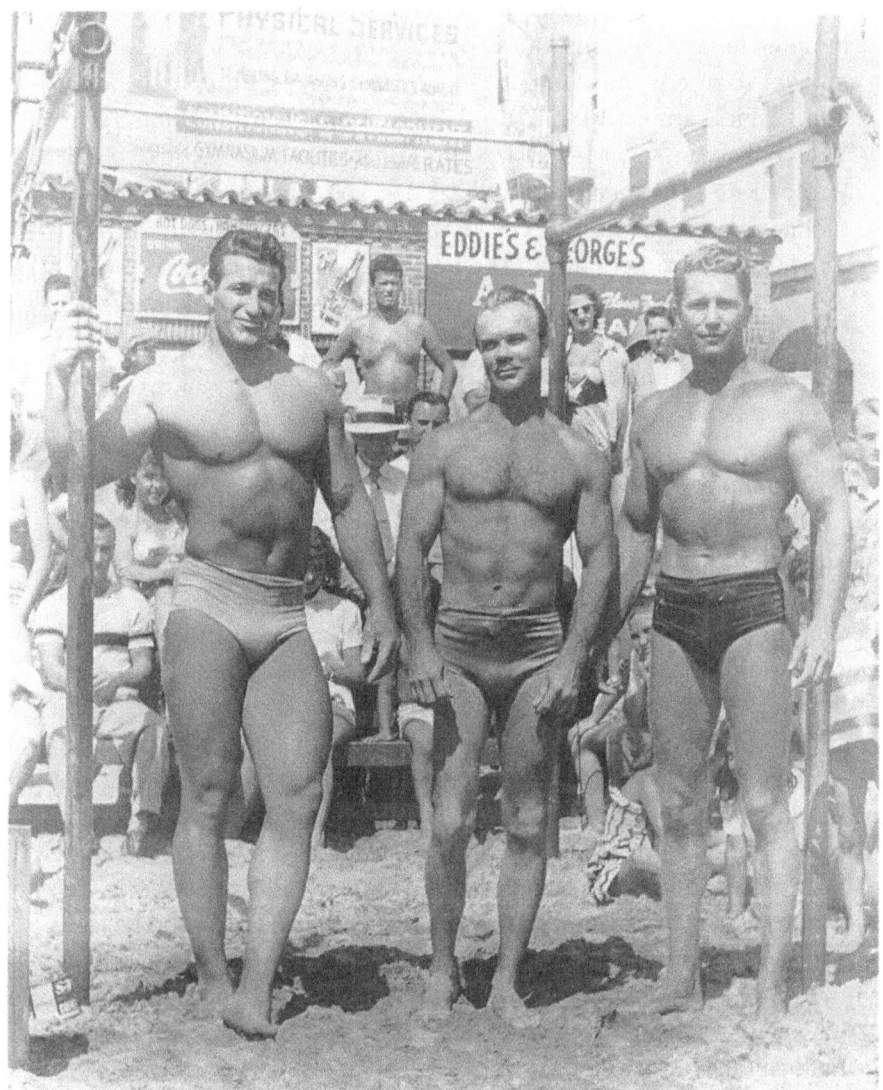

Winners of a chinning contest at Muscle Beach, July 1949—Kenny Achles, Bill Berger, and Bob McCune.

in winning the Mr. Universe contest. Reeves, relegated to second by the old master, was also swept away by the Grimek mystique. "I think that John Grimek is the greatest body-builder who ever lived." As Tanny put it, "[M]uscles will come and go but there will only be one Grimek."[23] Grimek had intended London to be his last competition. Therefore he greeted with dismay a challenge by Ross in *Your Physique*

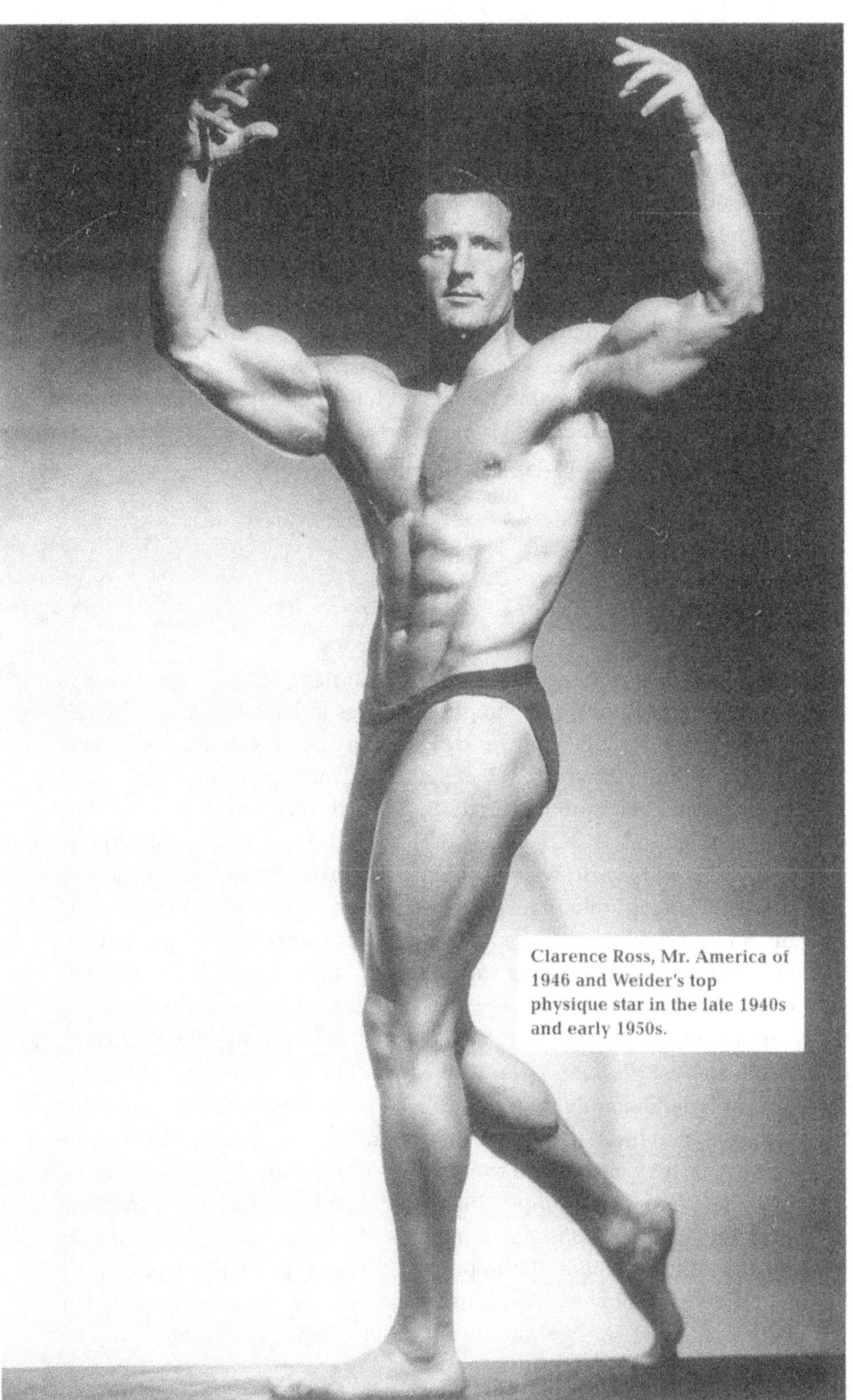

Clarence Ross, Mr. America of 1946 and Weider's top physique star in the late 1940s and early 1950s.

for a showdown at the 1949 Mr. U.S.A. contest hosted by Tanny and Goodrich in Los Angeles. But he must have realized that his status would never be immortalized if he did not contest the highly touted Ross. In the ensuing contest at a packed Shrine Auditorium, Grimek beat both Ross and Reeves. Ross quickly disappeared, but not before recognizing Grimek's supremacy. "Naturally I would have liked to have won and retained the title. However, I feel it's an honor to be second to John Grimek." The indefatigable Weider continued to try to draw Grimek out of retirement to "defend" his titles, but this final victory justified Paschall's observation that "J.C.G. is so far ahead of any other Mr. America or Mr. Anything else, that it is simply ridiculous for him to appear in a competition."[24] Grimek's loyalty to Bob over the next thirty-five years was an immense asset in sustaining York's reputation.

The IFBB

While Hoffman won this skirmish in the ongoing struggle for control of the iron game, it only encouraged boldness in his adversaries. Denied access to AAU levers of power by Hoffman and his cohorts, Joe Weider and his brother Ben in 1947 initiated a rival organization called the International Federation of Body Builders (IFBB). It was conceived by E. M. Orlick, a McGill University professor whose science-based articles had lent credibility to Weider publications. *Your Physique* boasted that the "shot" inaugurating the IFBB was "not only heard around the world" but had sparked "a rush for membership that is reaching the proportions of a torrential flood. Never was there any thing like it." The Weiders contended that bodybuilders were hampered by leaders who practiced "antiquated principles" and "discrimination," and hoped to rally dissidents against Hoffman. They also secured the endorsement of George Jowett to lend credibility to the IFBB. Phyllis Jowett confirms that her father helped the Weiders get started financially, and from 1945 to the mid-1950s they visited him every week or two with some lifters. Jowett became a figurehead for the IFBB, but he had a "great many problems with the Weiders." Joe continually used Jowett not only to lend the IFBB an air of tradition but to perpetuate the myth that his career as a "Trainer of Champions" began at thirteen, the age he first engaged "The Father of American Weightlifting" as his "father confessor."[25] Weider seemed determined to summon voices from the past to bolster his claim to the present.

Another angle pursued by Weider was employment of scientific authorities. Orlick's name, for example, was preceded by the title "Professor" and followed by a string of degrees—"B.A., B.Sc., M.A., Dip. M.S.P.E." Statistical articles by David Willoughby were a regular feature of Weider publications. In contrast to "unscientific" information purveyed by York writers, the statements of columnist George Weaver were supposedly "based upon the very best and latest of scientific facts." Dr. Tilney, Weider's Florida consultant, was depicted as a scientific superman. "Known far and wide as the 'miracle doctor,'" he allegedly held doctoral degrees in philosophy, divinity, natural law, naturopathy, chiropractics, and food science. Tilney was "the most forceful, dynamic and inspiring lecturer on 'The Science of Healthful Living' in the world" and author of hundreds of books, articles, and courses! Weider's most notable innovation was the creation in the late 1940s of the Weider Research Clinic at his new offices in Jersey City. It was little more than a name, but it lent an air of authority to his organization. Orlick confirms that "there was no clinic as such." When 1966 Mr. America Bob Gajda visited Weider offices, the door with the sign reading "'Research Clinic' led to a broom closet."[26]

Weider also, like Hoffman, promoted women, but he was more overt in exploiting the female form to attract his male clientele. Bob had paraded the likes of Rosetta, Gracie, Alda, Dorcas, and "Pudgy" before an admiring public to convey his conception of health, strength, and beauty. That his features did not convey greater sexuality and often included other females, especially athletes, suggests that there was more to Hoffman's appeal than ego gratification and commercialism. Weider, always the showman, stressed beauty more for its own sake. His photographs of women were sexier than Hoffman's, often with a cheesecake appeal. Most striking was Val Njord, a Swedish-born secretary from Los Angeles who won many local beauty pageants. Val served frequently as a cover girl. The November 1949 issue of *Your Physique* featured a pinup photo of her to keep servicemen "happy and contented." Her name also appeared as a byline on articles. Once she was described as "a perfect example of 'Beauty and Brains' with her lovely figure and brilliant mind."[27] The concept of sex and muscles was not new, but Weider employed it more fully. Along with a general improvement in his magazine's quality and a full line of fitness gear, Weider was making a strong pitch on many fronts.

Harry Paschall

Henceforth York's response to the Weider challenge took two forms. First, the 1948 AAU convention in New York, at Hoffman's behest, not only condemned the IFBB but promised disqualification for life to any athlete who participated in its "unsanctioned professional shows." Second, the scale and intensity of invective increased in York publications, where snide references to the triviality of bodybuilding culture ("Mr. Wavy Hair" and "Mr. Ingrown toe-nails") were employed to undercut Weider. The most acrid criticism came from Harry Paschall. When the IFBB appeared to make peace with the AAU by seeking sanction for its contests, Paschall twitted both parties. "A Year ago Weedy was hollering that the A.A.U. was unfair to bodybuilders, who should be highly paid for their efforts in achieving biceps with a larger circumference than their heads. Now we find him all snuggled up to the A.A.U., using the well known Red tactics of infiltration. . . . The plain facts are that the IFBB (Informal Brotherhood of Boobs) did not work out quite as well as Weedy expected, and now he is prospecting for gold on the other side of the street in the field of weightlifting." What struck hardest was Paschall's cartoon character Bosco, a superhero whose unlimited strength and integrity was contrasted with the effeminacy and vanity of "Weedy [Weider] Man," whose concern for the appearance of his "lats" and "pecs" was exceeded only by gratification derived from his puffed-up arms. *Strength & Health* featured a doggerel, sung to the tune of "Beautiful K-K-Katie":

> Wonderful Weedy . . . Wonderful Weedy . . .
> You're the only, only one that I adore;
> When the mule train goes over the mountain,
> It will carry "pecs" and "lats" galore!
>
> Wonderful Weedy . . . Wonderful Weedy . . .
> Let me sing your praises evermore;
> And when the moon shines over the cowshed,
> Don't let your "lats" get caught behind the door!

Also featured was a letter from George Walsh, a British physical culturist who accused Weider of unlawfully copying articles and photographs he had published. Walsh resented use of his work to support a viewpoint he disavowed. Weider's publication carried the "adulation of the male physique to hysterical heights," thereby "twisting the physical culture movement into dangerous channels." He prophesied that Weider's approach would lead to a demise of America's supremacy in this field.[28]

York Product Innovations

A more positive result of the Weider challenge was greater efficiency and innovation in Hoffman's organization. While most letters to York were complimentary, an increasing number were faultfinding. "Can it be Mr. Hoffman, that your organization is slipping?" wrote a customer in New York whose rubber expander had not arrived in six weeks. A patron from Philadelphia claimed he was defrauded. Having received neither the product nor replies to four letters after his money order was cashed, he angrily protested: "If your in such a *damn* hurry to get the suckers money let's give 'em an occasional break by filling the order. . . . Thank God we still got Weider Barbell Co." At the bottom of this letter Hoffman jotted, "More truth than comedy in this. We don't know how much business we lose this way." A *Strength & Health* reader in Texas complained of the "same old line of crap. No magazine again this month. What in the hell is the matter with you all up there anyway?" And a correspondent in the Dominican Republic pointed out that Weider was making a strong bid in the Caribbean.[29] It was obvious that the Weiders were making serious inroads into what had been exclusively Hoffman territory.

In self-defense Bob created some new product lines. In the winter of 1949–50 he made three trips to Florida to develop an aloe vera solution called Bob Hoffman's Sun Tan Lotion: "It has opened an entire life for me. It is pretty hard to feel better than what I thought was perfect, but I can find that there is a difference since I have been able to really soak up sunlight in large quantities." Articles, advertisements, and testimonials followed, describing the essential relation between sunlight and good health. Joe Barker, Bob's agent in Florida, reported that he had twenty-two retailers handling the lotion and that the solarium at the Hollywood Beach Hotel had successfully experimented with it. Further proof of its effectiveness was furnished by a trip to Guatemala, where several members of the York gang exposed themselves all day to the sun. "It

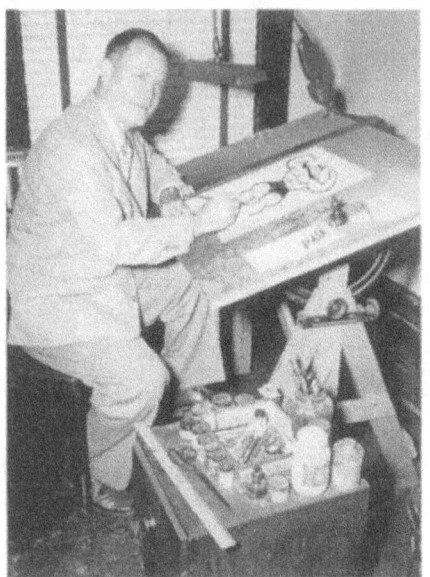
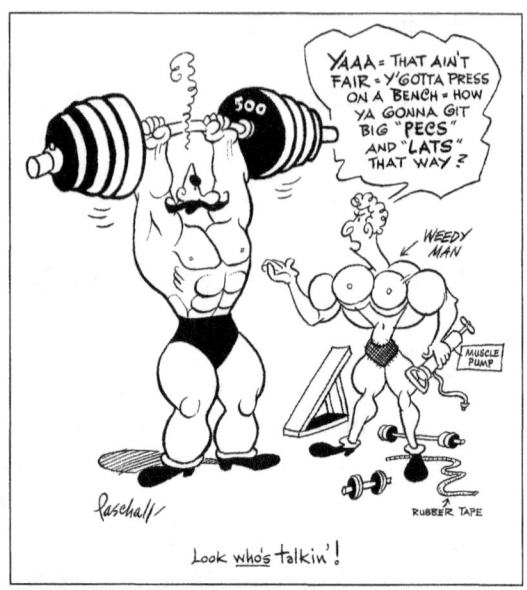

Harry Paschall, iron-game pioneer and editor of Strength & Health, **1955–57.**

Hoffman employed Paschall's Bosco cartoon to illustrate his philosophy of "useful muscles" and the superiority of York and the American way.

was so hot that the Indians kept under cover for 6 hours a day." Yet Bob, Johnny, and Dorcas "did not burn the slightest in these 12 hours of exposure." To Hoffman's four essentials to good health—exercise, nutrition, rest, and a tranquil mind—was now added fresh air and sunshine.[30] Hoffman's Athletic Rub was another product for which similar claims were made. For athletes it healed and improved performance, while others found it "a wonderful curative agent, an excellent pain killer" and inducer of sound sleep. "It's the best athletic Rub the world has ever seen." Unfortunately neither lotion nor rub was a major seller. "I naturally am disappointed that so wonderful a lotion sells so slowly," Bob wrote to Barker. "We are still going along getting about ten orders a day from fellows who use sun lamps. These are all from the north and all for big bottles.... We are not doing anything in a big way on the Rub, but the reports of users are fantastic." At the 1949 nationals in Cleveland, Stan Stanczyk was the "star of the show, not only for his lifting but for his promotion of York's latest product. Called "*Salesman Stan,* the Suntan Man," he set up business at the auditorium entrance, "hawking Hoffman's Sun-Tan Lotion with all the glib insouciance of a carnival pitchman."[31]

A better opportunity to move the company forward seemed to lie in new forms of apparatus. Owing in part to Weider, exercises to develop the pectoral and latissimus dorsi muscles, groups relatively unimportant to weightlifters, had grown increasingly popular. Hence such new devices as the bench with stirrups, the inclined bench, and the lat machine were needed. In 1950 Hoffman introduced his "5 in 1 Muscle Builder," which enabled trainees to perform bench presses, incline (or decline) presses, lateral raises, incline sit-ups, and lat pull-downs, all on a single adjustable apparatus. When not in use it could be used as a barbell storage rack.[32] York also produced a leg-press machine, squat racks, and a separate incline bench. Some of these new items were either clumsy, flimsy, or expensive, but they remained on the market virtually unaltered for decades.

To expand barbell sales, the mainstay of Hoffman's trade, it was necessary to move into the lucrative western market. "Weider Goes West!" was the catchphrase for a 1948 advertisement announcing that Weider weights were being manufactured and sold in California, thereby saving customers money and time. Weider's prices were already 15 percent below York's, and he stood to acquire an even greater advantage in the West unless Bob could establish a foundry there to cut freight costs. What brought the issue to the fore in 1949 was a 160,000-pound order from the army for West Coast delivery. Bob and Dorcas visited California in the spring and found labor costs much higher than in the East and extra charges for pattern making. Eventually, Bob negotiated a contract with Continental Foundry and Enameling in Tulare to manufacture weights at six and one-quarter cents per pound, but the company encountered too many problems in trying to manage production three thousand miles away. Another drawback to operations in Tulare was that the foundry's finances were in disarray, so much so that Continental was being foreclosed. Its creditor urged Hoffman to purchase it outright. That he did not, and resumed bulk shipments to California from York, was probably due to the fact that Bob's last major purchase, York Precision Company, had yet to turn a decent profit. Its products included fire extinguishers, medical sprays, and scalp-treatment machines. As he explained to Tanny, "[I]t has taken a lot of work with very little return."[33]

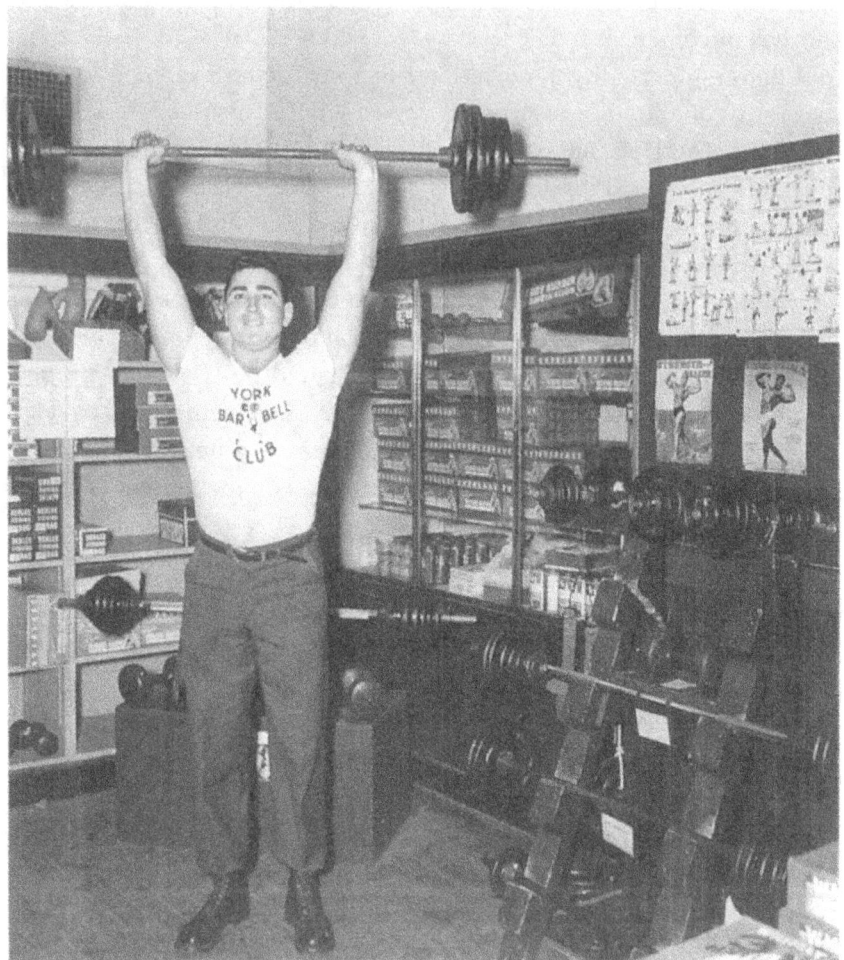

William Cirenza demonstrating York products at Macy's department store, New York City, December 1948.

Enhancing York's Image

Strength & Health too underwent changes to cope with increasing competition from Weider's publications and Peary Rader's *Iron Man*. Hoffman, piqued by Weider's claim of a larger sales volume, began to change the appearance of his magazine to resemble Weider's more colorful outlay, beginning with the August 1950 issue, featuring Mr. Universe Steve Reeves on the cover. More striking was the December issue, with a full-color cover of 1950 Mr. America John Farbotnik and his wife Joan and lots of "fancy work" inside. Hoffman admitted that he had "watched the added color in other magazines and the larger photos" and "wanted to keep up to or ahead of the rest." Also added were sixteen extra pages. What he did not reveal was that they were reduced in size and used poorer-quality paper, also attributes of his competition. These changes were a palpable admission of Weider's promotional wizardry, but Bob hoped that his customers would be less susceptible to his adversary's slick advertising. Ultimately the competition all centered on ego, and Weider could not resist observing that "the magazine which has spent so much space attacking us and running us down is actually copying us."[34] Although York initially served as a model and entrée for Weider, by the late 1940s Bob was drawing from his opponent to the point where it could be asked who was imitating whom.

Having to cater to the tastes of a new kind of physical-culture enthusiast for more specialized routines and muscles that looked good may have annoyed Hoffman. Yet his traditional training philosophy, centering on health, strength, and all-around physical development, continued to attract adherents worldwide. This was evident not only from product sales but from the many letters and visitors seeking advice and inspiration. After reading *Strength & Health* a fifteen-year-old lad from West Virginia ran away from home to meet Hoffman and become a weightlifter. Police in Spring Garden township picked him up at 3 A.M., and his parents were notified. Another youth from Staten Island wanted to assert his male identity by coming to live, work, and train with the York gang, thinking his life would be transformed. From distant Mozambique a novice bodybuilder wanted to know whether he could train the day after having sexual intercourse. All kinds of suggestions were received for new exercise devices and schemes. One from a man in Pennsylvania suggested the marketing of one-quarter-pound plates. A professor from Iowa visited York to see how high weightlifters could jump. He was surprised that they "jump considerably higher than the ordinary run of athletes"—further grist for Hoffman's promotional mill. A father from Kansas sought advice from Bob, unaware of his limited education, about what course of study his son should follow to become a physical educator. And a reader from New Jersey, after reading Bob's account of the 1947 world championships for the *tenth* time, referred to him as "far and above the greatest coach and athletic instructor the world has ever known . . . one of America's immortals."[35]

It is uncertain how much Hoffman desired national recognition, but in 1948 he was approached by a New York firm offering to "plaster the name of Bob Hoffman, as Olympic weightlifting coach, everywhere" for $1,500. And the proprietor of the York Airport offered bargain rates to introduce him to long-distance air travel. Both propositions were indications of his success as a small businessman and invitations to indulge in the riskier world of big business. Hoffman never crossed this threshold, but he must have relished the free publicity he got through AP news releases. Readers in Lufkin, Texas, were treated to a picture of Dorcas in high heels hoisting a 175-pound barbell overhead. Those in El Dorado, Arkansas, were informed that most of the cast-iron barbells used in this country were made in York and that Hoffman was the "spiritual leader" of weight men. Even the *Saturday Evening Post,* then in its heyday, described York as "the muscle center of America." This mythical portrayal alleged that it was "teeming with Tarzans": "Everything is weightlifting and strength exhibitions around York, and after you have been there a few days you are prepared to see people swinging on vines along Broad Street on their way to work. Living there, for instance, is Miss Dorcas Lehman . . . the world's strongest woman. She breaks chains with her chest for fun and lets a guy from Hawaii named Emerick Ishikawa jump on her stomach from a ten-foot-high stepladder, after which she gets up off the floor smiling." Coverage by the national media, however, was infrequent, and Hoffman was mostly confined to competing for visibility and support within the iron game. A York follower in Texas advised Bob just to keep up the "good work . . . and maybe if we ignore Weider he will go away."[36]

The Broad Street Gym

Bob reaffirmed his position as strength guru by showing that he supervised, in addition to his other regular employees, a real cadre of weightlifters and bodybuilders. Unlike Weider, who hid "behind a mailing address" and whose staff was "scattered from remote Canadian villages, to Florida, to California, where they engage in other vocations," Hoffman proudly declared that "you or the sheriff will find us . . . doing business where we have been since 1929." Paschall best captured the ambience of the training room visitors encountered on the second floor of 51 North Broad Street. The 40' × 60' chamber was divided by three large pillars and covered with weights, dumbbells, and other devices

> in such profusion, the stranger wonders if he has ventured into the torture room of the Spanish Inquisition by mistake. We suggest that you stop and seat yourself on the long visitor's bench just inside the entrance, or you may be struck by flying iron fragments. Usually there are a dozen or so visitors here—and you may run across someone from India or Iran, come halfway around the globe to see the Champs in action.
>
> Now look out over the big room, and pick out your favorite stars. The weightlifters will all be gathered around the old central platform with its deep grooves for the "wheels," cut by thousands of dropped bars. They line up and take turns, doing repetition presses, snatches, cleans, with the weight increasing until it approaches their limit. You will see lifts of over 300 pounds so often here that they are commonplace. Usually, too, you will see four or five of the big name physique stars training here, particularly if there is a contest in the offing. From this gym came nine out of ten of the Mr. Americas to date, and all of them . . . have trained here at one time or another.
>
> Glance carefully around the gym and note that every piece of training equipment you have ever heard of . . . is included as part of the apparatus of muscle and strength-building. But if you will look across the room, back against the wall under the windows right behind the main lifting platform, you will see the one piece of equipment that only York possesses, and which has built more champions than any other apparatus.
>
> This is a sturdy wooden bench, not much different than any other bench to outward inspection. Above it there is an old sign, "For Lifters Only," . . . to keep overenthusiastic visitors from robbing the weary athletes of a place to rest their bones. The real name of this bit of furniture is the "Dream Bench." Here Tony Terlazzo sat and thought and dreamed of becoming an Olympic Champion . . . and here too, the many York champions who followed him have made their lifts in their minds before they walked out on the platform to do them in reality. The seat is worn smooth and shiny,

for Terpak, Stanko, Grimek, Stanczyk, Terry, Davis, Bachtell, DePietro, Spellman, Schemansky, Mitchell, Hoffman, Pitman, Shandor, George and a myriad others have rested here between the series of consecutive lifts that have made them champions. Even Bosco has sat here! Surely no other bench the world over has been polished with the seats of such distinguished paragons of strength!

Only one so gifted with words as Paschall could sanctify a worn wooden bench. But there was something special about this place. Grimek recalls that some visitors were dismayed by the dilapidated appearance of the York gym. "But for those who came to train, the place grew on them."[37] This lifters' nest created by Hoffman was redolent of past and present camaraderie, which had catapulted American lifting to ever greater heights.

At the 1950 world championships in Paris, nationalism was more a factor than ever, for two reasons—the presence of the Soviet Union and America's involvement in a war against Communists in Korea. What gave the United States an 18–15–14 edge over the Egyptians and Russians was the unexpected win of Joe Pitman, "dark horse" of the lightweights. Again Bob financed the team, and his lifters functioned as a unit. They were almost always together—training, sightseeing, eating, and playing—with "an all for one, one for all attitude." Team physician Charles Moss called Hoffman "a second father to each of the team members. . . . I heard Joe Pitman say that he was going to win the championship for Bob." Stanczyk said, "Don't worry, Bob, the Russian is not going to beat me. I'm going to come [out] on top." America's victory in Paris dispelled any doubts that America's weightlifters were the best in the world. To Hoffman it proved not only that America was the "strongest nation," but that York men were the strongest Americans, for the victory was "won by Strength & Health boys, who now have grown to manhood."[38]

The Early-Fifties Slump

The Korean conflict necessitated preparations by York Barbell for material shortages and plant conversions for war contracts. "We have built up our plant in York rather extensively," stated Hoffman in early 1951.

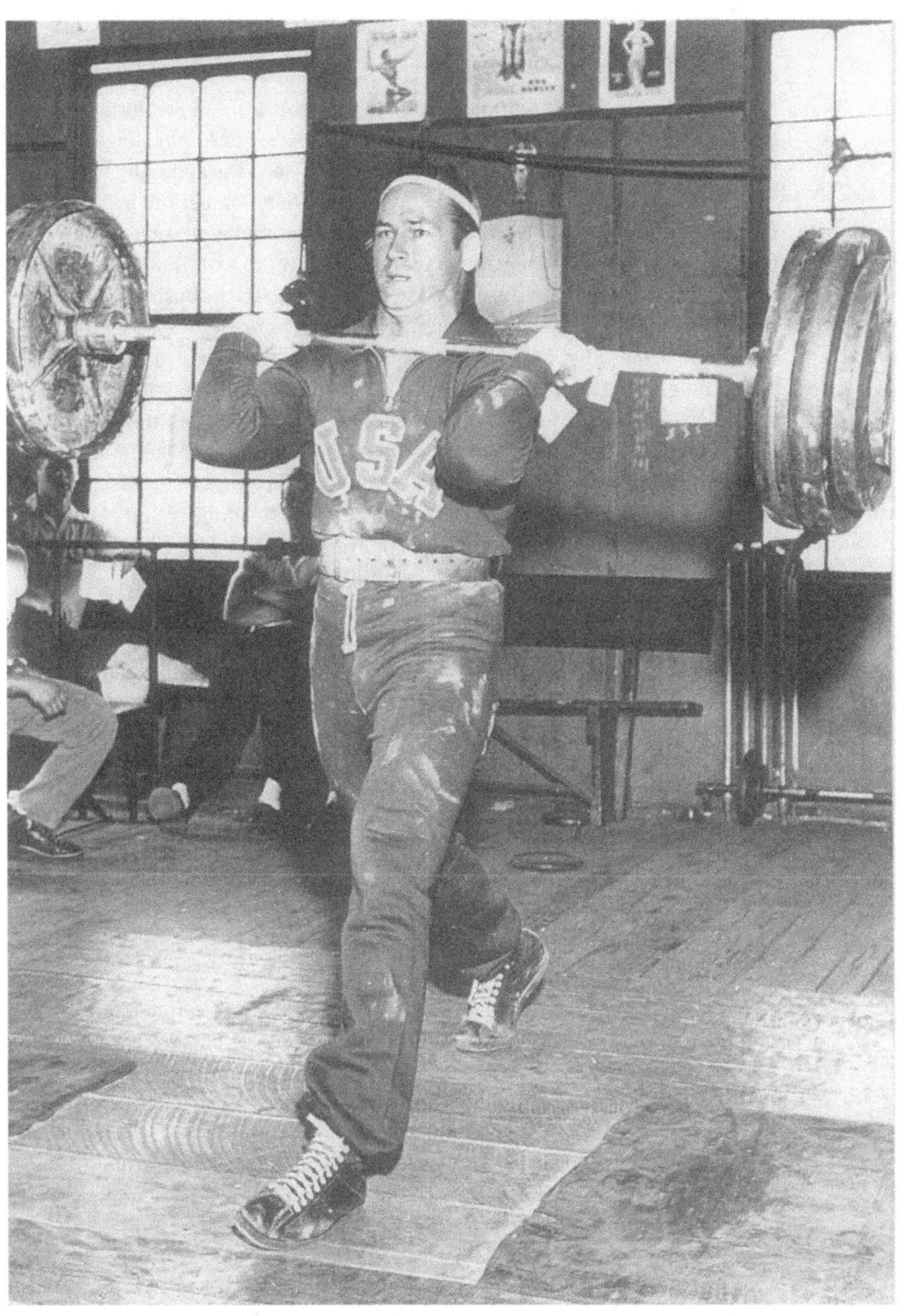

Stan Stanczyk recovering from a 320-pound clean at the old York gym at 51 Broad Street. Tommy Kono observes from the flanks.

"Some of our men are working 70 hours a week. All are working at least 50." Spellman and Pitman were working ten-hour days, five on Saturdays, with training being done after hours. Soon the company was producing parts for airplane motors, guided missiles, bombs, and instruments. Considerable sums were invested in new equipment, such as the twenty Swiss automatic machines that were accurate to 4/1,000,000 of an inch. Bob's claim that he put in a sixteen-hour day on the business and magazine might be exaggerated, but he did occasionally stay up with Spellman, who, after working the night shift on the Swiss machines, trained alone between three and five in the morning. Repeatedly he would fall asleep in the chair, but none could gainsay his devotion to the sport and his lifters. Such sacrifices give meaning to Hoffman's otherwise illogical statement that "we did not go in this business to make money"—for business was always a means to a higher end.[39] By keeping his company prosperous he could provide the wherewithal to enhance the prestige of American weightlifting and himself.

Sales figures for Hoffman products in the early 1950s, however, provided little reason for optimism. "The barbell business has not been very profitable for some time," Bob complained in 1952. While iron and steel costs had tripled and wages had doubled over the previous ten years, the price of his Big 12 Special had risen only 15 percent. Other York prices, including those for books and magazines, had also increased, but parcel postage was up by 25 percent. Company records show that sales were steadily declining through the end of 1951.

1946—$580,427	1949—$441,114	1952—$433,205
1947—$602,010	1950—$387,273	1953—$527,703
1948—$503,993	1951—$383,908	1954—$521,703

A nadir was reached in November 1950, when checks and money orders totaled $25,368, the lowest since August 1945. Profits from Bob's other enterprises varied. Accounts for *Strength & Health,* York Barbell Foundry, and Marietta Machine Shop show a deficit of $1,799 for 1948. A York Precision report from 1949 indicates a profit of $11,688. And a 1950 statement reveals a loss of $42.82 on Bob's real estate investments on south Duke Street. But reckonings of Hoffman's financial condition show that he did not lack resources, his net worth at the end of 1952 being estimated at $670,516. Bob also kept a large cash reserve in his safe at the House on the Hill.[40]

Years of Challenge and Achievement

Still, strong suspicions prevailed that he was not receiving all of the income he was entitled to. Ray Van Cleef, who edited *Strength & Health* for six years, confided to a friend in 1948 that he was frustrated and discouraged by the mismanagement at York. "I have learned little here, except how *not* to run a business." Jim Murray, who replaced Van Cleef in 1951, believed Mike Dietz was "taking money off the top" for himself and cheating on taxes for Bob. By such means Dietz could blackmail Hoffman. Far from expressing dismay over Mike's dealings or conspicuous wealth, Bob referred to him as a "financial wizard" and "champion cattle raiser" who "makes several times as much from his cattle as from the York Barbell enterprises." Fortunes were acquired "under the table" by collecting cash orders at the post office. From his gym across the street, Jules Bacon witnessed Bob and others making these pickups. In a year, Hoffman "got at least a quarter of a million dollars—never reported to the IRS." Jules could "not believe how a company could survive with everyone on the take and stealing." Jim Park, 1952 Mr. America and York employee for several years, confirms that the "business ran on checks, not cash." Charles Smith alleges that one of Bob's boys was fired for "dipping into the till" and another faked a theft to get money. When Bob was in Venezuela in the early fifties, $3,000 disappeared from his safe. When he returned, he blamed Dorcas, who promptly moved to Florida.[41] Increasing peculation by principals at York had a devastating effect on company morale and contrasted sharply with Hoffman's idealistic rhetoric.

What led erstwhile loyal members of the York gang to such desperate measures was a combination of low wages, poor management, and jealousy over Bob's generosity to favorites. But there was more. Bachtell confirms that the sense of community that had contributed so much to York's success "began to disappear in the late forties."[42] As aging athletes passed their prime, they engaged in various forms of compensatory behavior. Much of the malaise that set in during these years can be explained as a crisis of self-esteem, whereby York gang members had to justify continued personal worth in the face of palpable decline. Some, like Terpak, Grimek, Dietz, Bachtell, and Hoffman, coped with the challenge, while others fell by the wayside.

The most serious fall from grace was that of Gord Venables. Despite being Bob's highest-paid employee, Venables neglected his work and became an alcoholic. In 1946 Bob gave him a stern warning, likening him to "a hundred horse power machine which operates on about five horsepower." Gord's failure to reform, coupled with Hoffman's failure to confront the situation, was an example not lost on other employees. In 1950 Hoffman finally put Venables on probation. "You have continued to go from bad to worse. . . . either by accident or design you have done a great deal to hurt our business. Your failure to get the magazine out on time is the last straw. . . . I want you to stay away absolutely and entirely from 51 N. Broad St. for at least three months or until written notice from me. During this time we will pay you at the rate of fifty dollars per week. We will see if you straighten yourself out during this probation period or if you intend to skid right down to the bottom." Despite Bob's generosity, Venables did not improve, and it irked Murray and others that he was living rent-free while "pumping information to Weider" on activities at York. The June 1951 issue of *Your Physique* published an article by Venables entitled "The Best Bodybuilding System of All!" In heavily edited script, Venables explained that Weider's set system and specialization routines were responsible for advancements of modern physiques, including Grimek's. "At last, we have the truth," exclaimed Weider, "from the pen of a man who was there, and who saw the training sessions of their stars." Yet it took another year and more devastating blows from Weider (made possible by Venables) for Bob to evict Gord.[43] With nowhere else to go, Venables was soon writing for Weider and betraying more York secrets.

In 1953 Hoffman lost two more stalwarts. Frank Spellman, who had served him well as a lifter/employee, was being superseded on the lifting platform by Tommy Kono, Pete George, and Dave Sheppard. Soon Spellman gravitated into trouble with the law. Following extradition hearings, he and companion Clifford Dockey were brought back from California to face charges of looting $2,500 in equipment and supplies from the York Art Center, where Dockey had been employed. Testimony from Spellman's ex-wife Joyce, that the goods were used to set up an art studio in the attic of Frank's home, was critical to his conviction and six-month jail sentence. Bob's other loss was the death of longtime supporter Wilbur Smith of Pittsburgh. Originally from York, Smith had accompanied Hoffman on many trips, including the Olympics. His death at age sixty-six was a surprise to Hoffman, nearing fifty-five, and a reminder of his own mortality. This void was soon filled by Clarence Johnson, an accountant from Highland Park, Michigan, who like Smith would represent Hoffman's interests in the AAU. Cincinnati promoter Emmett Faris and Dietrich Wortmann passed away about the same time as Smith, evoking some nostalgic remarks from Paschall about their absence from the 1953 nationals. "Troubles run in threes."[44]

Bob's female relationships remained irregular. As with male comrades, he tended to discard female partners after their contributions to his company, cause, or ego were past. The farther back the relationship extended, however, the harder it was to sever emotional ties or cleanse himself of guilt. He continued to send Rosetta monthly checks and received letters from her combining fond memories with additional appeals to his generosity. There were also supplications from former in-laws, including Rosetta's mother, for money and housing. A letter from Gracie (Bard) Grabeel to Grimek about her plans for a trip to York in 1947 showed traces of nostalgia for the old gang. It is unlikely, however, that Hoffman ever saw her again. For years Bob had sustained relationships with both Alda and Dorcas and bestowed equal favors on each. And he continued to be drawn to other women wherever he went. When Dorcas disappeared from the scene, Bob picked up another girlfriend, a woman who worked at the Bon Ton in York and who, according to Murray, was "a total prostitute. She was arrested for performing oral sex in a parking lot." Bob entertained most of his friends at the House on the Hill, according to Park, who lived next door. He and his wife watched many women come and go. It is little wonder that when Murray informed Yorkers that he worked for Hoffman, their "eyebrows raised."[45]

The York-Weider Rift Deepens

When Murray came to York, he assumed naively that Bob's reputation, particularly from his prestige as Olympic coach, was good. He was soon disabused of this notion when Bob got into an altercation at the King George Hotel with a patron named James Anstine and knocked him to the front sidewalk. The victim suffered face lacerations, hemorrhaging of the right eyeball, loss of teeth, contusions and bruises to the head, and a fractured skull. Hoffman was convicted for assault and battery, and the judge had to guarantee protection for jurors against threats from him. Later Hoffman was sued for $21,000 by the defendant. Weider learned of these incidents and served them up to the readers of *Your Physique*. It was merely the latest of a long series of malicious acts, charges, and countercharges exchanged between Hoffman and Weider.

Their feud became vicious and personal. Most hurtful to Weider were aspersions cast on his manhood and integrity. Therefore he challenged Hoffman to a showdown whereby the two moguls of the strength world would vie for supremacy by means of a lifting and physique contest. Bob accepted Weider's challenge, but to compensate for his twenty-year age disadvantage, he proposed that a boxing match in skin-tight gloves also be included, and precede the other events![46] As with Berry and Grabeel in the past, Hoffman's resort to physical force revealed his frustration in dealing with an adversary who could not be subdued by other means.

The challenge never materialized. Joe, however, unexpectedly entered the 1951 Mr. Universe contest in London to show his own mettle. "I had to seek some other way of showing all bodybuilders that I was in good shape and practiced what I was constantly preaching," he explained. After placing only fifth out of six in the tall men's class (won by Reg Park), he rationalized that "the game itself" was more important than "winning for the sake of winning." However, the acerbic wit of Paschall cast Weider's performance in a different light.

> The highlight of Weedy's appearance was his tremendous struggle against a 200 lb. barbell, which he essayed to press in order to show his athletic ability. He failed three times to press the weight, during which there was some very audible caustic comment from the audience. Good Old Joe (no relation to Good Old Uncle Joe Stalin) was not to be stopped, however. Gritting both sets of teeth, he finally managed to struggle it overhead on a fourth try, and then did TWO (count 'em—2) deep knee bends with this tremendous weight on his manly shoulders. It looks like Joe forgot to read those Power Plus Routines in his own magazine.

The interminable feuding hurt all parties and undermined unity in the iron game. To Tony Terlazzo the "developing feud" between bodybuilders and weightlifters was evident by 1951. He regretted their looking on each other "with contempt." Grimek agreed, insisting that the two approaches were "closely related and one will achieve better results when both are included." That 1951 Mr. America Roy Hilligenn placed second as a mid-heavy lifter at the nationals seemed to support this view, but Paschall's stiletto stabs at "mirror athletes" and Hoffman's need for lifting talent for his teams gave York a weightlifting bias. Ken "Leo" Rosa recalls that "a lot of idealistic young bodybuilders, myself among them, had their bodybuilding dreams crushed, smashed, destroyed by the warfare going on between the Hoffman and Weider factions."[47]

Though seemingly poles apart, Jim Murray believes Hoffman and Weider were "very much alike." Weider wanted to be what Hoffman was, but "the AAU controlled lifting and the Mr. America contest, and Weider couldn't get in. Both wanted to be like the guys they trained. Hoffman and Weider were workaholics. Both had great ego needs." Murray believes it is "weak egos that need that kind of boosting" and that "in those days masculinity had a different meaning." Especially revealing is his observation that "what Hoffman and Weider said about each other was true—not what they said about themselves." As editor, Murray only printed about a third of what Bob wrote—the rest being mostly self-praise. Once Hoffman even compared himself to Jesus Christ. "He exaggerated everything he did and what other people did."[48]

Cold-War Triumphs and Tribulations

While Weider was luring bodybuilders into a separate camp, the Soviet Union, in its quest for supremacy, was compelling Hoffman to devote more attention to weightlifting. Though Russia had a larger population, many more registered lifters, state support, and a society more appreciative of strength, Hoffman believed the American system should and must triumph. His team's victory at Milan in 1951 over Egypt was one of the most convincing of Hoffman's career. In a study of world championships since 1937 and Olympic Games from 1920, British official Oscar State rated America the greatest weightlifting nation in the world by a wide margin: "Bob Hoffman can be well satisfied with the results of his efforts." To add even more to its standing, the United States beat the Russians again at the 1952 Helsinki Olympics. This was the climactic point in American weightlifting endeavors during the "golden age." No small reason for this success was that all gold medal winners at Milan and Helsinki—Kono, George, Stanczyk, Schemansky, and Davis—were hyphenated Americans unconsciously seeking cultural acceptance. That this was possible by feats of strength on behalf of their adopted land was the inspirational message conveyed by Hoffman: "This nation is a real melting pot, a real democracy."[49]

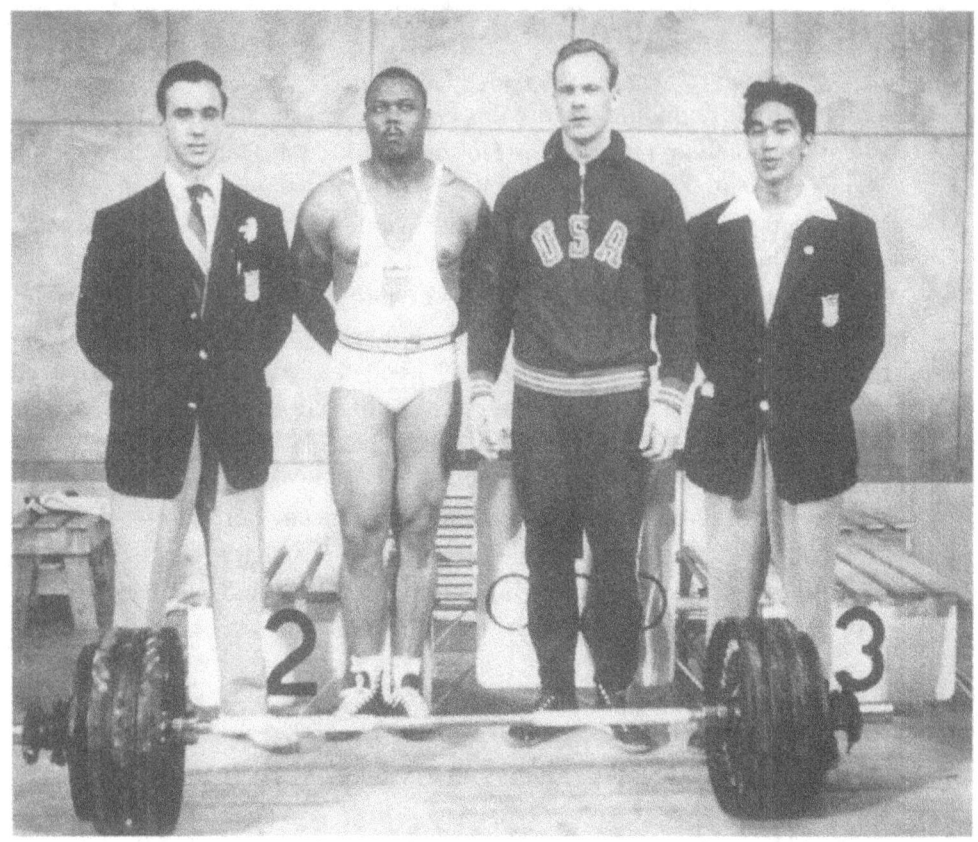

Gold medalists at Helsinki (1952)—America's greatest weightlifters of all time: Pete George, John Davis, Norbert Schemansky, and Tommy Kono.

The strength of the Russian team at Helsinki, however, indicated to Bob that American supremacy was in jeopardy. By this point he had spent nearly $300,000 of his company's profits to send lifters to championships and exhibitions, but it was hard for Hoffman's business-supported athletes to compete with Russians who were "wards of the state.... It is this professionalism," he said, "which makes it increasingly difficult to outperform the Soviet athletes." He noted with dismay the endless preparations made for state-subsidized lifters in the Soviet Union and recognized the need for greater American commitment. Hoffman could not understand why weightlifting, promoted so heavily in Russia, was virtually unrecognized by the United States government. Realizing the limitations of his own resources and the constraints of America's free enterprise system, Hoffman pleaded for "more weightlifters" and "more weightlifting contests." Weider publications played on these fears by publicizing Russian initiatives and denigrating

Hoffman's efforts as commercially motivated. Bob struck back, accusing Weider not only of not supporting American lifters but of promoting Canadian heavyweight Doug Hepburn and causing the ineligibility of promising middleweight Marvin Eder by using his photos in advertisements. It was a cruel coincidence that Hepburn's presence and Eder's absence at the 1953 world championships in Stockholm resulted in Russia's first-ever defeat of the United States, 25 to 22. But there were other factors too. The army effectively deprived the American team of heavyweight Jim Bradford, who had been serving in Korea and not training regularly. Also, unlike previous years, the team had not gathered in York for special training and was divided between two Stockholm hotels. "It was the greatest disappointment of my life," pronounced Hoffman.[50]

On further reflection Hoffman blamed the defeat on his countrymen's being "less ambitious, less athletically inclined, willing to take things easy" and "let the other fellow do it." America's weightlifting prestige, he alleged, was built and maintained by a handful of men, "and some of these are past their peak." Other reasons cited for America's lackluster performance included the increasing popularity of odd-lift (power) meets and physique contests. Hoffman "shuddered" at the sight of men lined up for odd-lift contests and believed, wrongly, that the best physiques were derived by performing the Olympic lifts. Hoffman was so attached to Olympic lifting that he could not imagine any upright American youth doing anything else. Victory in weightlifting was tantamount to victory over Communism and a validation of the American way of life.[51]

The Hi-Proteen Miracle

Ultimately Hoffman's ideology of success was bolstered by a new product called Hi-Proteen. He traced its origins to his fascination with the soybean as early as 1914, when he started patronizing Chinese restaurants. Then, in the 1930s he devoted several acres to soybeans on his farm. In 1938 he was introduced to a product similar to Hi-Proteen by a professional strength performer named Eddie Polo, but the soy base gave it an unpalatable taste. "For years" Hoffman searched for "the right product" and briefly sold a dietary supplement called Johnson's

Hi Protein Food. He introduced it in 1951 as a product capable of "sensational" results, with gains of "20 pounds in a month." But the taste was still not right. "So we took our problem to chemists, laboratories, and food processors and finally . . . developed the product which is now known as Hoffman's HI-proteen."[52] This "invention of the wheel" type of story no doubt satisfied Hoffman's need to validate himself as a patriarch and innovator.

Another, quite different tale is provided by Jim Murray, who explains that Hi-Proteen originated in Chicago with Erwin Johnson (Rheo Blair), who had a small gym for bodybuilders. He also liked to cook and became interested in dietary means of controlling subcutaneous fat—hence his interest in protein. Jim Park was a husky young trainee at his gym who was trying to limit his weight. When Park moved to York as a machinist after his 1952 Mr. America victory, he introduced Johnson's concoction to Hoffman. Bob marketed it long enough to measure public response, then changed its name and started selling his own product. "Next thing—Johnson's disappeared and Hoffman's replaced them. He got the ads going before the product was developed, complete with pictures of Grimek, etc. He ordered sweet chocolate from Hershey and was stirring his mixture with a canoe paddle in a soy bean flour container. He was sweating away while stirring and tasting, saying, 'yuk, no one will buy that,' and so mixed more." Murray was shocked by this lack of scientific process. Indeed the image of Hoffman sweating over a vat of Hi-Proteen mixture with paddle in hand is a far cry from "chemists, laboratories, and food processors." Hi-Proteen Fudge was developed later in much the same manner. Such dietary supplements contradicted Hoffman's erstwhile contention that "plain simple food" was best for aspiring champions. He admitted in 1951 that formerly he "was not convinced of the necessity for food concentrates and vitamin supplements." But his views "altered with the passing of time," as more evidence appeared on soil depletion. The exact nature of his evidence for "retrogression of the soil" was not revealed, but this revelation coincided nicely with his discovery of Hi-Proteen and York Vitamin-Mineral Food Supplement as a remedy.[53] And the fact that high-volume sales resulted from his own intuition, muscles, and canoe paddle must have been extremely gratifying.

Hoffman's new product appeared to be a panacea that would generate profits for his ailing company and give him a competitive edge. Soon Bob was producing articles on good nutrition, now the most important

Years of Challenge and Achievement

of his five essentials of good health. Undoubtedly the advancement of bodybuilding, perhaps more than weightlifting, was accelerated by the introduction of food supplements. "Muscles are being built at a pace never before attained," he exclaimed. Park, who followed his Mr. America victory with Mr. World and Mr. Universe titles, used the new Protamin tablet "generously and regularly" beforehand. "He took as many as 200 of these tablets daily, 50 each hour for four consecutive hours." Bob's favorite way of taking Hi-Proteen was in milk shakes, where he mixed it with milk, eggs, bananas, honey, and peanut butter. He claimed that Grimek, Stanko, Terpak, Bacon, and their families used Hi-Proteen regularly: "As for myself, I almost live on Hi-Proteen. Many days I take nothing else." Such was the anticipated volume of business that he formed a company, Better Nutritional Aids (BNA), and turned it over to Alda. Only Paschall, it seems, foresaw where this new emphasis on altering bodily makeup was leading. "They tell me that this year's 'Mr. America' is a vitamin and high protein guy," he wrote in 1952. "Maybe eventually we will come to a point where we can pile on the lumps by just inhaling iron pills instead of using them. That will be a sad day, brother, if it ever comes." But he stopped short of attacking Hoffman's formulas, resigning himself to Bob's rationalization that regular food "ain't what it used to be."[54]

In the meantime Hi-Proteen was becoming very profitable for York. Demand was widespread. In 1953 Tony Terlazzo told Terpak that sales generally were slow in January, but by midmonth he had sold out of Hi-Proteen. Likewise February sales were "not what they used to be," except for dietary supplements, which seemed in ever greater demand. When Terlazzo received thirty-eight boxes in April, he sold twelve the first day. Sales for George Yacos in Detroit were also brisk. He asked Terpak to "send as much Hi-proteen as you can." By 1954 Hoffman was soliciting distributors for his product. "It is customary to gain a pound of firm flesh to each pound of Hi-Proteen used," he claimed to a vendor in Nebraska. "Sales repeat, almost 100%" was his message to an agent in Dallas. To a dealer in Florida he claimed his product could supply the body "with all the elements it requires."[55] Not since his early days had Hoffman been so enthusiastic. It was Hi-Proteen that reversed the company's sales slump and instituted a steady rise in profits.

By no means the least important aspect of this new product was its potential for reversing America's sagging prospects in international lifting. Employing cold-war terminology, Bob referred to Hi-Proteen as "Our Secret Weapon." It was viewed as a magic elixir that would enable his lifters to gain muscular bodyweight and increase their totals. It also enabled him to train, transport, and provision his team without having to worry about money. The bitter experience of the 1953 world championships had shown him how vital Hi-Proteen was to victory. Tommy Kono was "lifting sluggishly." Then, before the clean and jerk, Bob said, " 'Tommy, you forgot your Hi-Proteen tablets.' He took a handfull and kept munching them. . . . When Tommy came out for the clean and jerk he was a new man. He asked for 325 to be sure, and then 347 to be doubly sure of winning. Having the field to himself after that he called for a record poundage of 369¼. He made it . . . for a new clean and jerk and official total record." Davis, on the other hand, was the only team member who did not use Hi-Proteen. "Certainly a little bit of added power would have brought him the title," Bob reasoned. It was his first loss ever, and deprived America of points needed for the team title. It was obvious to Hoffman that Hi-Proteen was vital to victory, which he uncharacteristically predicted, in 1954. His only hope was that "the Russians don't have Hi-Proteen."[56] Hoffman was a complete convert to Hi-Proteen as the "miracle food."

Even his team's 29–23 loss to the Russians at Vienna in 1954 did not cool his ardor. In an article entitled "Nutrition at the World Championships" he argued, speciously, that although Russia, with the world's best small men, outscored America in the lighter classes, the United States had the strongest big men: "Without immodesty we can say Hoffman's Hi-Proteen played an important part in this victory." In place of the team spirit that had prevailed in the past, a fetish was made now of Hi-Proteen. How misplaced such confidence was is indicated by an accompanying picture featuring the American "Hi-Proteen Kids," mid-heavyweights Dave Sheppard and Clyde Emrich, standing on the number two and three blocks, overshadowed by the great Russian champion Arkady Vorobiev on the winner's pedestal. Hoffman still could boast that America held more world records than Russia, 13–10, and could rationalize that "it is a greater honor to hold a world's record than to be a world's champion." But he was obviously feeling less secure. It was likely for that reason that in 1952 he adopted the title, first applied to William Curtis, of "Father of American Weightlifting." For good measure he publicly appropriated the tradition started by Calvert's Milo company "of making the best barbells . . . since 1902."[57] If Weider, by sleight of hand, could claim to have been a "Trainer of Champions" since 1936 at

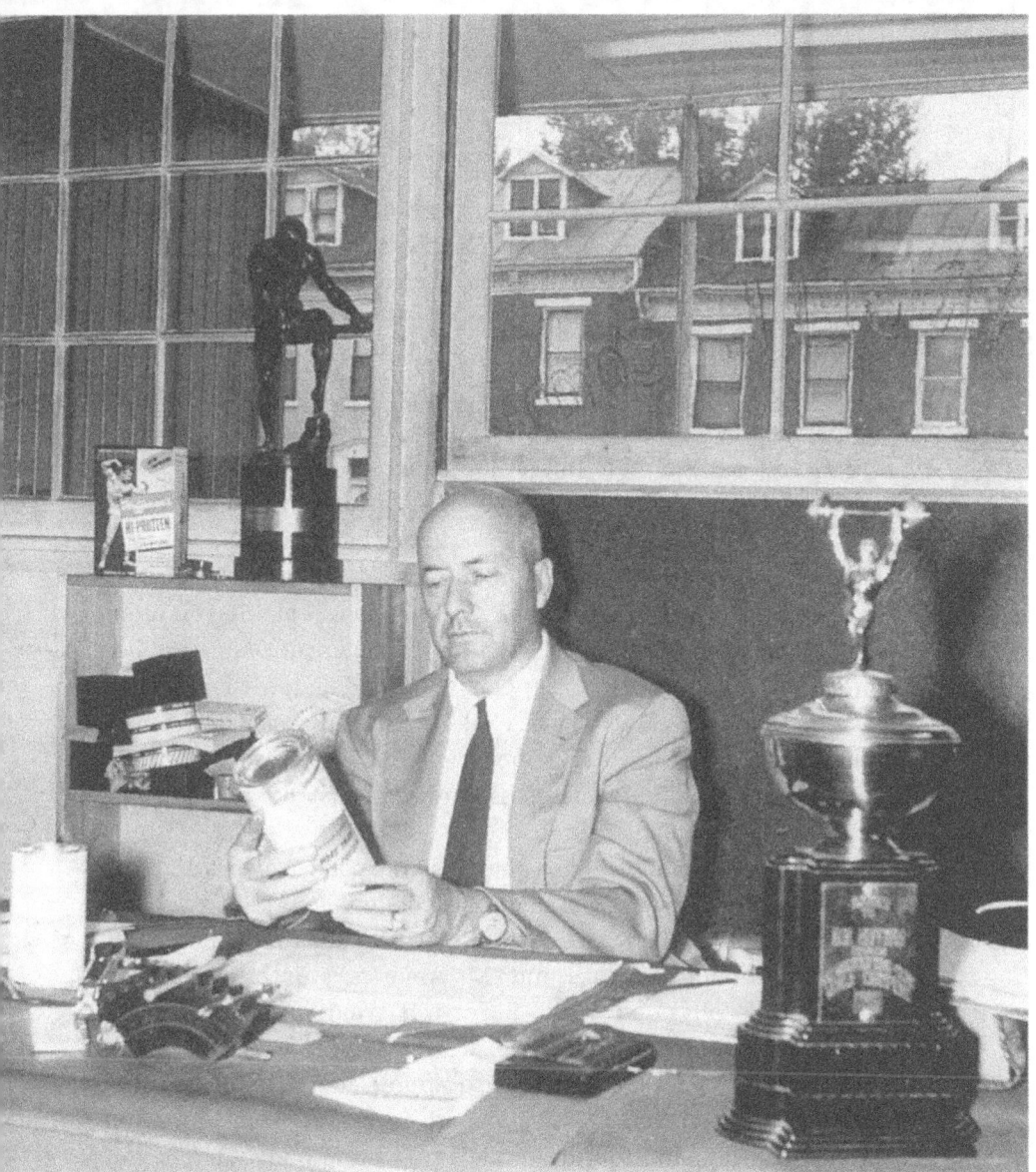

Bob admiring the product that made him a fortune, Super Hi-Proteen, at his Broad Street office in the late 1950s.

age thirteen, Hoffman was capable of staking out even more historical turf by "making" barbells since age four!

By the mid-1950s York had not only survived the challenges confronting it since the war but was thriving. It was a decade of struggle *and* achievement—a veritable "golden age." Business, owing largely to Hi-Proteen, was prospering again. *Strength & Health* carried an abundance of merchandise to supplement barbell training, which had become, mostly through Hoffman's efforts, an accepted means to improved health, strength, and appearance. The 1954 Mr. America, Dick DuBois, like his predecessors, was acclaimed to be a "York barbell man." In just one year BNA had expanded from one line of tablets to ten. There were "100 Ways to Use Hi-proteen," and a hundred outlets nationally where York products could be purchased. There is no way of knowing how successful Bob's rivals were, but the offerings displayed in *Muscle Builder,* Weider's new flagship publication, paled by comparison with those displayed in *Strength & Health.* In 1954 York won its twenty-second team title at the nationals in Los Angeles with fewer obvious immigrant types. Significantly, its only loss came in 1952 at the hands of a squad from Hawaii. Lifters from this tiny enclave of hyphenated Americans trounced Hoffman's team in the lighter classes, which should have served as an omen. Hi-Proteen was making his lifters stronger but also bigger. From 1953 to 1954 the American team, supplied with generous amounts of food supplements, made impressive gains in bodyweight and totals. Yet America still lost to the Russians at Vienna. Hoffman, oblivious of his team's top-heaviness, expressed pride in its lifting, vowed even greater progress, and set his sights on Munich.[58] The blush was still not off the rose.

Not only did Hoffman exercise near absolute control over weightlifting, but his influence was paramount in bodybuilding. Through the AAU, Hoffman controlled the structure by which aspiring young bodybuilders rose through the ranks, and "Mr. America" was the most sought after title in the physique world. But it was Weider, by stressing the body's appearance for its own sake, who catered more to the manly needs of aspiring youth. Hoffman also appreciated a good physique but always believed that muscles should be useful. Ironically, while his promotional apparatus and products catered to bodybuilders, Bob stubbornly adhered to Olympic lifting because it more fully satisfied his own psychic needs. It was the standard on which he had entered the iron game in the 1920s, the assumption on which he recruited his team in the 1930s, and the basis for his triumph over the Soviet Union in the 1940s. Big muscles alone hardly sufficed to fulfill his philosophical ideal of manliness. Using them was critical. And Hoffman was as much a moral crusader for strength and health as he was a businessman. Although he rarely attained the high ideals he prescribed for others, he embraced integrity, truth, and justice as peculiarly American virtues that were also his own. Hoffman's adherence to these traditions was best symbolized in 1954–55 by Paschall's Bosco, the "Hope of the Free World—

Years of Challenge and Achievement

the 101% American Red Blooded Boy." All who subscribed to the York way cheered for Bosco in his epic battles with the villainous Luke the Gook (Russia) and Latissimus Q. Superpex (Weider) for supremacy of the strength world—much as everyone did then for the Phantom, Hopalong Cassidy, or Superman.[59] In the 1950s such simplistic images were widely accepted as analogous to reality. Needless to say, the hero always won in the end.

6
ALL ROADS LEAD TO MUSCLETOWN USA

> We met the Shah personally and concluded that he is all man. He is the best tennis player in Iran, the best football player, he is a good revolver and rifle shot, a fine rider, a good golfer, an expert swimmer, a water skier, a weightlifter, and his picture in bathing costume showed that he is a Mr. America type.
>
> —Bob Hoffman, *Strength & Health*

By any measure of American success in the 1950s, Bob Hoffman had achieved greatness, more so than any previous physical culturist. Admittedly, Bernarr Macfadden in his prime had a larger following and exhibited more splendor, but Hoffman's more conservative approach was producing a more durable phenomenon. There was greater acceptance of muscle building, and York was the chief proponent of barbell use. What helped sustain sales of this commodity (which lacked built-in obsolescence) was expansion of its market to target average Americans after World War II. York also promoted weight training for athletes in all sports—an extension of Hoffman's all-around training philosophy. Most important, there was an increased emphasis on nutrition. Remembered chiefly as the era of Wheaties and Wonder Bread, the fifties was a period when Hoffman was able, with protein supplements, to stake the same kind of claim on the future as he had done earlier with barbells. At the same time, the unique cultural factors that had helped produce international weightlifting teams of the highest caliber were weakening. America was becoming healthier and more homogeneous, thus obviating the need to overcome physical deficiencies and the stigma of foreign birth. Weight training was accepted more as a matter of course, and Hoffman, still robust and striving harder than ever, was the acknowledged leader of America's strength empire.

Performance Enhancements

Bob was obsessed with factors influencing athletic performance. After losing to the Russians in 1953, he seemed stunned at first, then rationalized that "the Russians do nothing but lift. At Stockholm they were fresh from three months of special training at an athletic camp where they trained 14 times a week, twice each day." Obviously his adversaries had perfected York's socialization techniques by nationalizing their programs. Hoffman, constrained by America's amateur code, envied such practices. Modern training methods and better nutrition were other factors behind improved performances, but he placed most faith in the power of positive thinking. He believed "it was the desire, the will to win, more than anything else which made record breaking possible." This approach was institutionalized by Akron coach Larry Barnholdt. His philosophy of mind over matter was applied with spectacular success to Pete George and his younger brother Jim, who ascended to international heights in the mid-1950s. Barnholdt believed lifting was "mental, not physical," according to Jim. "If you haven't lifted it before you touch the weight, don't touch the weight."[1] That Hoffman did not promote this truism more fully may be attributed to its lack of commercial appeal or means for self-promotion.

Another development that influenced international lifting after World War II, and the recent Russian victory, was a change in pressing technique. Soviet lifter Gregory Novak perfected a looser style, starting a trend in which press poundages would surpass those hoisted in the snatch. In the 1946 world championships he pressed 309 pounds on his way to winning the light-heavy class. Hoffman called it "the greatest press ever made." His shoulder lay-back, wide grip, and elbows-back technique was soon imitated by other Soviets and became known as the "Russian press." York lifters did not immediately employ this new style. Instead, Hoffman staked his team's success at the 1954 world championships on Hi-Proteen. Bob administered this "secret weapon" to his lifters at a special training camp in York and hauled over a hundred pounds of it to Vienna. The Soviets, however, showed extraordinary strength. "None of the Russians finished lower than second," noted Murray, "and it was Vorobiev who fouled up the best-laid plans of mice, men and U.S. Coach Bob Hoffman."[2]

Dr. John Ziegler and Testosterone

Additional light on Soviet gains was provided by Dr. John Ziegler, who accompanied the U.S. team. On returning, Ziegler testified that members of the Soviet delegation thought he was "stimulating our boys with some kind of drug to make them lift better." A Russian physician kept asking: "What are you giving your boys?" He was especially curious about the chewing gum Ziegler kept giving the lifters, so Ziegler "gave him a piece which he immediately wrapped in a note." Eventually "it reached an MVD agent and was perhaps sent away for analysis, as were samples of my liniment and aspirin." Much later, Ziegler talked about how the Russian doctor, after "a few drinks," revealed that "some members of his team were using testosterone." Soviet athletes were not only "using straight testosterone" but "abusing the drugs heavily," even to the extent of "having to get catheterized!"[3] To what extent the Russians were using testosterone remains unknown. But if drugs were critical to improved Soviet performance at Vienna or their subsequent win in 1955 in Munich, then it was the Russians who had discovered a "secret weapon" for lifting success, while Hoffman's "secret weapon" merely brought him financial success.

Actually, Ziegler, who fancied himself as much a scientist as a physician, had already gained some insight into the effects of testosterone, as a result of his Marine service in the Pacific during World War II, where his 6' 4", 235-pound body was riddled by Japanese fire. After the removal of a collar bone and a lengthy convalescence, he entered the University of Maryland Medical School, intending to help others recuperate from similar disabilities. Ziegler was a complex personality—highly intelligent, original, eccentric, and often outrageous. After settling in Olney in 1954, he specialized in treating handicapped and seriously injured patients. With a romantic's love for the Civil War and the old West, he often dressed up as a westerner and had friends call him Tex or Montana Jack. Ziegler was also a "hell-raiser." One friend describes him as "a big man with big appetites and a keen sense of humor . . . a man's man." Not satisfied with regular patients, Ziegler sought out unusual physical specimens. His initial contacts with York occurred when he began working out at the York Barbell gym in nearby Silver Spring. There he encountered Grimek, who occasionally visited this client establishment. Grimek recalls that Ziegler, who "really wanted to be in research," was receiving testosterone from CIBA pharmaceutical company for experimental purposes. The company also provided him with books and records from Germany, where similar experiments had been carried out by the Nazis. Ziegler's first test was on an appendectomy patient. Then he treated a burn victim and even administered doses to himself. By the time Grimek met him, Ziegler was giving testosterone injections to fellow trainees in Silver Spring.[4] But they were not advanced enough for him to gauge any significant effects. It was therefore advantageous for Ziegler to acquire some of the strongest and best-built men in the world.

That the administration of drugs would have much impact on bodybuilders or enhance America's international lifting prestige occurred to no one at first. Grimek's interest, like Ziegler's, stemmed from his curiosity about how such potions might stimulate muscular growth and performance. As early as 1943 he had asked a doctor about methyl-testosterone. By the summer of 1954 Grimek was taking a variety of substances provided by Ziegler, including syndrox.

> Thanks for *keeping me awake* last night. I didn't really get the sting of Morpheus (goddess, that is) until around 4 A.M. but wait, I feel fresh and alert as if I slept from midnight. Must be this darn amber colored *vitamins!* But at times I think I detect a bit of alcohol by my discriminating palate! Boy, I can't wait until I make a long trip by car. . . . say, boy, I'm going to make Calif. in less than two days flat . . . unless I get flattened before. But seriously that darn stuff sure has an odd reaction on me. I took two tablespoons this morning. . . . I feel like I've gotten 1,000 mgs. of testosterone!

However much Ziegler might have suspected drugs to be critical in the Soviets' triumph over American lifters in Vienna, his experiments on York musclemen were hardly enlightening. He administered testosterone to Jim Park, featherweight champion Yas Kuzuhara, and Grimek, who recalled how Ziegler "tried to convince me that if I took these shots 2 or 3 times a week, I would get stronger and more muscular without training . . . but I saw no reaction. In fact I told him I was feeling lousy compared to what I feel normally. So he suggested I return to training. I did. But after 6 weeks I gave it up [the shots]. I got no results." Nor did Park fare any better. He received one dose, and its only effect was to give him an instant erection upon seeing *any* woman.[5] There is no evidence that Hoffman or anyone else at York saw any potential for the drug. Whether Ziegler became discouraged, feared side effects, or was too busy with regular patients cannot be ascertained, but he did no further research with muscle-enhancing drugs until 1959.

Clearly the pharmaceutical age of sport was on the horizon. What continued to fuel American weightlifting success, however, was not drugs but the traditional patterns of socialization Hoffman had fostered since the 1930s. Immigrant communities still provided most new recruits, including Charles Vinci (Italian), Isaac Berger (Israeli), Jim George (Bulgarian), and Yas Kuzuhara (Japanese). And Hoffman was still regarded as a father figure. Bantamweight Vinci said, "Don't worry, Bob, I'll beat him for you—I'll make 800!" after his loss to the Russian Stogov at Munich. Vinci and featherweight Berger mixed Hi-Proteen in the York plant, competed with each other in training, and were a popular duo with the ladies of Muscletown. "After I moved to York . . . I made my big gains," recalls Berger. "The team environment was great, the equipment was great, and that's where I got all of the kinks out." Prior to overseas competitions lifters from across the country—including Paul Anderson from Tennessee, Dave Sheppard from California, and Kono and Pete George from Hawaii—would descend upon weightlifting's world capital. Spirited workouts in the Broad Street gym fondly reminded Hoffman of "the good old days when everybody was a weight lifter." Occasionally team members teased the ponderous Anderson (whose training poundages exceeded 400) of "being big and slow." One day Kono "goaded him too far, and Andy offered to race Tommy up the steps to the second floor at 51 North Broad Street. So they lined up on the sidewalk outside and took off at the signal—they hit the stairs neck and neck, and it sounded from our office as if the roof was coming in. At the half-way mark there is a turn in the stairs and Paul hit this first, switched gears and roared up the final flight. Tommy couldn't pass him because nobody had room to pass."[6] But such camaraderie existed less than in earlier years when Hoffman himself was an active athlete. There were no longer references in Strength & Health to the "league of nations" aspect of America's teams. There was also less emphasis on patriotism. By the late 1950s York Barbell was no longer as much an agency for acculturating immigrant youth. With increased urbanization, improved public health, and better diets, Americans were getting bigger, stronger, and living longer. Correspondingly fewer of America's top lifters were recruited from that once sizable body of souls struggling to compensate for inadequacies.

Paul Anderson

Still, Hoffman could feel encouraged by America's prospects for victory. Vinci and Berger seemed destined to reclaim valuable team points formerly earned by DePietro, Bachtell, and Terry. Both displayed outstanding strength and form, but their impact was overshadowed by that of Paul Anderson, the most amazing phenomenon in American weightlifting history. A native of Toccoa, Georgia, he began lifting secretly while on football scholarship at Furman University. He specialized in the squat and later, living in east Tennessee, was discovered by Bob Peoples, the legendary deadlifter. At their first meeting, Peoples asked how much weight he needed for warm-ups in the squat. Knowing the unofficial world record was 575 pounds, Anderson requested 600: "My three friends laughed. A smile escaped Bob Peoples. He loaded the bar with 600 pounds but cautioned the others to stay close and spot me. With the bar across my shoulders, I dropped to a full-squat and rose steadily, never wavering. When I was erect for a second, I squatted fully again and stood. They could hardly believe it. I had done the deep knee bend *twice* with a weight which had never been used *once* in the same lift before. Peoples and my friends were speechless." The squat, however, was still not contested, and Anderson did not attract much recognition until he learned the Olympic lifts. Then he eclipsed the achievements of Davis, Hepburn, and Schemansky, and acquired as firm a claim to the title of "world's strongest man" as anyone has ever held. Paschall, who had witnessed most past masters of strength in this century, was so impressed that he regressed to the impressionistic level

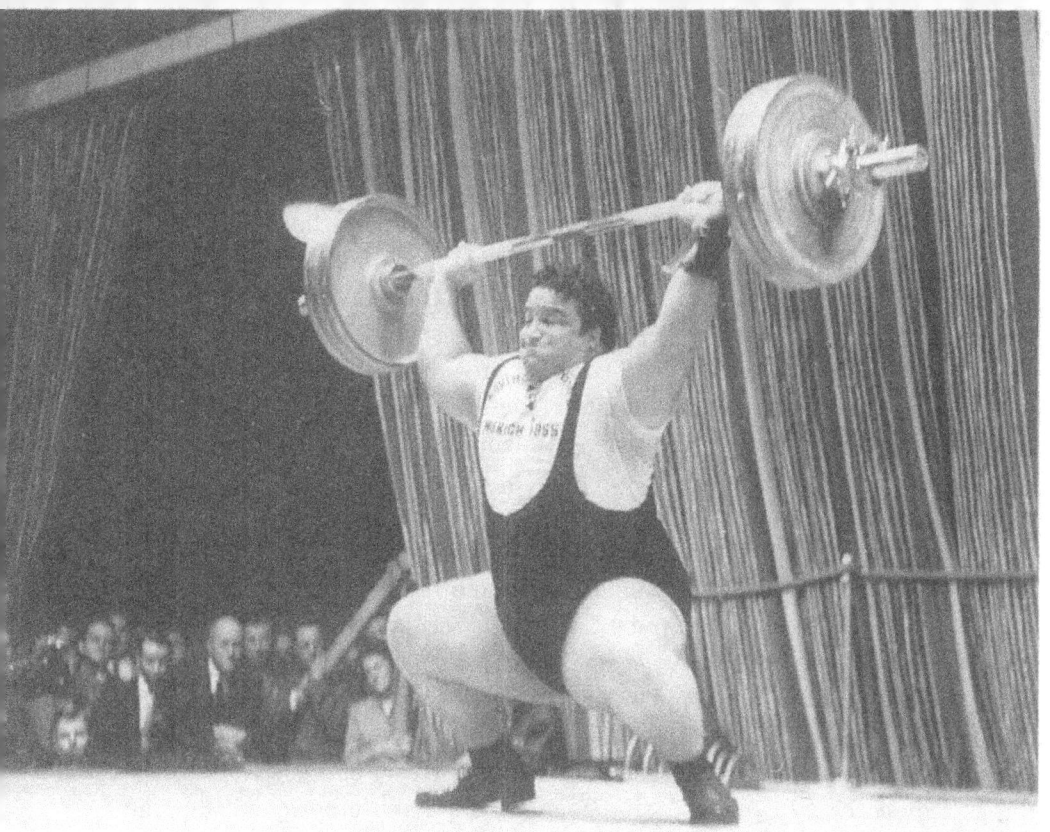

Heavyweight Paul Anderson came this close (note bent right arm) to making a 336-pound world-record snatch at the 1955 world championships in Munich. Anderson died in 1994.

of his youth. He sensed "an aura of physical power" in Anderson like nothing he had witnessed since 1911, when he "saw the great Arthur Saxon with Ringling's Circus.... The Strongest Man Who Ever Lived now walks the earth." A sports writer in 1956 called Paul a "fugitive from the 25th Century. In the natural development of the race, he had no justification for coming along for about 500 years." At age twenty-three and 5′ 10″, he "usually weigh[ed] around 350 pounds. His thighs measure[d] 36 inches around, the size of the average man's waist." By the end of his strength career Anderson, in addition to breaking many world weightlifting records, was credited with a 1,200-pound squat and a 6,270 back lift, the greatest weight ever raised by a human being.[7]

Anderson's size and strength represented a new standard, almost a quantum leap, in lifting. Henceforth most heavyweight champions would follow the Anderson model of bulk training and become superheavyweights, virtual giants of sport. Also, Anderson was not of immediate foreign extraction, had never been a ninety-eight-pound weakling, and was not deferential toward Hoffman. Nevertheless Bob appropriated him to serve his country and club. In 1955 the State Department subsidized a goodwill lifting mission to Russia, the first such visit to that country. At Moscow and Leningrad the Americans split wins with the Soviets, but the trip's sensation was the Georgia strong man who hoisted an unbelievable 402 press, 314 snatch, and 424-pound clean and jerk in Moscow. The capacity crowd of fifteen thousand dubbed him *Chudo Pirody* (A Wonder of Nature), and a flabbergasted Russian official exclaimed, "He's Mr. America." Later the team gave exhibitions in Egypt and Iran, where the shah, a lifting enthusiast, told Hoffman that he had been reading his magazine since he was ten. On returning home the team was greeted by Vice President Nixon, who praised the lifters as outstanding ambassadors and asked them to undertake an around-the-world journey. "All of this recognition came upon us with all the suddenness of an avalanche," remarked Hoffman. "I used to often remark to people in York that I was better known in Rangoon, in Manila, in Semerang, in Malaya than in my hometown. . . . It will be nice to finally meet these converts to our way of life." Their itinerary took them to Turkey, Iran, Lebanon, Iraq, Pakistan, Afghanistan, India, Burma, and Indonesia. Elaborate descriptions of their exploits appeared in *Strength & Health*, with pictures of Hoffman and team members in exotic places and attire. Despite government subventions, Hoffman estimated his share of traveling expenses for 1955–56 was still $36,000, mostly paid for by Hi-Proteen.[8] Whatever decline American lifting might have been undergoing by 1956, all roads to success still passed through York, and it was an Olympic year.

Hoffman believed the American and Russian teams were so evenly matched that the Melbourne games would be a team match between them. Anderson was "our only sure winner. In fact he [was] surer of winning an Olympic title than any man, from any country, in any sport." Yet the contest came down to Paul's final lift. While Vinci, Berger, and Kono handily defeated their Soviet rivals, an ailing Anderson won only by lighter bodyweight than the Argentine Humberto Selvetti. It was America's last great victory. Anderson turned professional, Vinci got married and fathered a child, Pete George became involved in his dental career, and Pitman and Stanczyk were past their prime. Bob's assessment in 1957 that "our chances . . . are not as bright as last year" was borne out by the Tehran world championships, where Russia won thirty-three points and the United States tied Iran for second with nine. Kono was America's only gold medalist. Similarly, when

All Roads Lead to Muscletown, USA

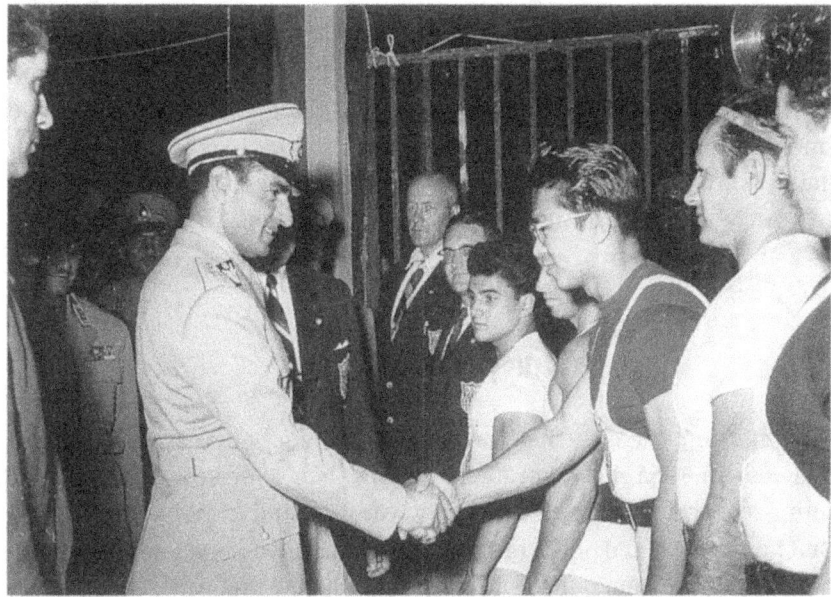

The shah of Iran greeting members of the York gang—Hoffman, Terpak, Chuck Vinci, Joe Pitman (partly hidden), Tommy Kono, Stan Stanczyk, and Dave Sheppard—during a goodwill visit in 1955.

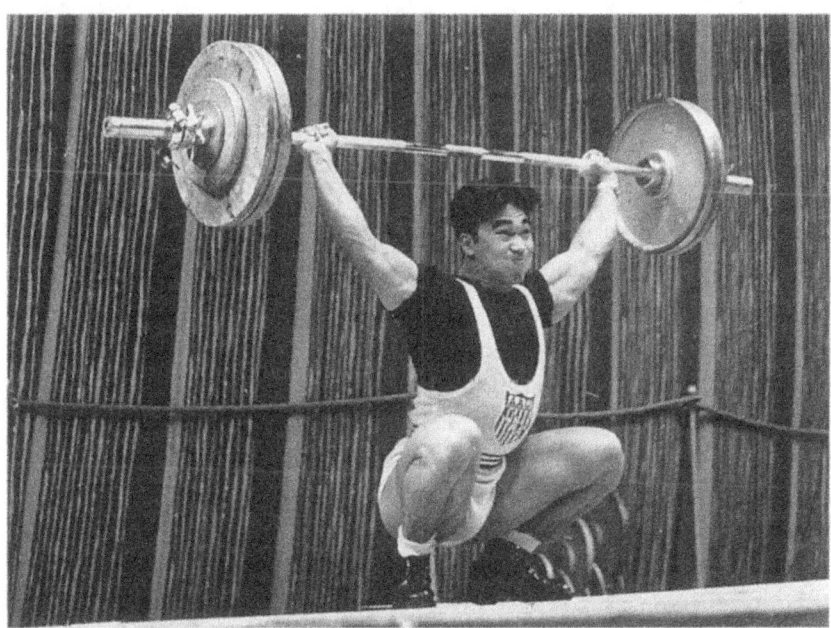

Light heavyweight Tommy Kono, widely regarded as the greatest weightlifter of all time, negotiates a clutch 281-pound snatch at Munich in 1955.

the Russians visited Chicago, Detroit, and New York for dual meets in May 1958, the outcome was a series of American defeats. Hoffman increasingly blamed his lifters. He chided Sheppard for drinking and smoking, Jim George for his attachment to cigars, and Stanczyk for doing bodybuilding. "If you want to beat the Russians, YOU MUST TRAIN LIKE THE RUSSIANS, AND WEIGHTLIFTING MUST BE FIRST IN YOUR LIFE."[9]

Struggling to Stay Ahead

Weightlifting, of course, had always been first for Bob. On returning from overseas in 1955, he reiterated, "[M]ore than ever now, I like weight lifting and weight lifters." So deeply was it related to his own self-worth that he simply could not tolerate losing. He blamed his lifters' loss at Munich in 1955 on poor officiating, then rationalized that America's heavier men had lifted more absolute poundages than anyone, and finally, by adding another five points for Kono's winning the accompanying Mr. Universe contest, argued that the United States had actually beaten the Soviet Union, 30 to 29! Jim George confirms that Bob was "always fiddling with scoring systems," and says, "I was persona non grata when I lost. When we won it was Bob—when we lost it was the team's fault." Mike Dietz thought the lifters were a useless appendage, recalls George, and others of the old gang never regarded the current champions as their equals. But Hoffman treated them like his sons. If a promising lifter wanted to train in York, Bob provided a job, temporary housing, and even some meals. For others who represented York but lived in distant areas, he sent equipment and food supplements. George admits that as a competitor he thought Bob "walked on water," and regarded him as a father figure: "There was no way I could have gone on competing without his help." Hoffman tolerated a lot of things if you performed. On international trips Hoffman, a strict teetotaler, gave lifters money he knew they were using for beer. An anecdote revealing how awkwardly Bob communicated values to his young charges is related by George. Vinci was drinking coffee in a restaurant, and Bob ordered him to stop: "Pretty soon you'll be out drinking and carousing with Dave and Jim." Vinci protested, "But I don't do those things. I don't drink at all." To which Bob responded, "See here, that's how they got started—by not drinking at all!"[10]

All Roads Lead to Muscletown, USA

Sexual promiscuity was the vice in which Bob indulged freely, and he was probably best able to understand lifters' needs in this area. He had no objection to the boys' relieving their frustrations as long as they abstained completely for five days before a contest. Hoffman's own relations with women followed a pattern set two decades earlier with his failed marriage. At home or abroad, he used women to bolster his sense of manliness. Rosetta and Alda agree that Bob's sexual appetite, like his ego, knew no bounds. "Bob Hoffman did what Bob Hoffman wanted to do," recalls Alda. "If he wanted to date someone else's wife, he would." Such behavior was perhaps encouraged by the likelihood that he was sterile. Still, he paid for at least four abortions. He also lavished expensive gifts and favors on his girlfriends. There is no evidence that Gracie and Dorcas ever again shared in Bob's largess after he broke off relations with them, but he showed continuous concern for Rosetta. He assisted with the mortgage on her house in Fruitland, Maryland, in 1956 and paid for an operation she had in 1960.[11] Though Bob never remarried, Alda was in essence his wife and the most direct recipient of his generosity. But it was earned through many years of toleration and sacrifice to the immense needs of Bob's ego.

Controlling men was equally important to Hoffman, as made manifest in his competitive attitude. Winning at anything, especially weightlifting, was a primary emotional need, but aging made it difficult. When he could no longer display athletic superiority, he equated his own aspirations with those of his lifters, derived vicarious satisfaction from their attainments, and sublimated his energies into a superhuman daily regimen, knowing no one could equal or question it. In 1954 he attended "47 weightlifting contests," not including international matches. "Our usual procedure . . . is to start from York early Saturday morning, perhaps drive as many as 400 miles in time to help with the competition, and then about 3 A.M. start back to York. This has gone on week after week, month after month and year after year." In 1956 he attended a meet every week. His weekday routine was no less rigorous, allowing an average of only five hours of sleep nightly. On a visit to eastern Europe in 1960 he claimed the title of World's Champion Polka Dancer for dancing the polka all night. His manhood also demanded that he be acclaimed Champion Chinese Food-Eater in the Free World. But Hoffman's most extravagant claim was that he possessed perfect health. Although he repeatedly stressed the need for *"proper food, correct exercise,* and *sufficient sleep,"* he never ate properly, exercised regularly, or slept sufficiently. His supercharged ego never allowed time. Yet he convinced himself and his public that he had superhuman health, simply by saying it enough times.[12]

Weight Training for Athletes

Few would deny, however, that his long campaign for acceptance of barbell training was now won and that it was largely through Bob's efforts that protein supplements were gaining popularity. A further innovation for which Hoffman could claim much credit was the application of weight training to other sports. It coincided with his long-held notion that barbells increased all-round development. In the early 1950s staunch reinforcement came from Jim Murray, who included a "weight trained athlete of the month" in *Strength & Health* and departed from the usual musclemen covers to display athletes from other sports. Hoffman propagated his views in speeches and writings on how weight training led to extraordinary improvements in other sports. His best pitch, also employed by the tobacco industry of that era, was to show nationally heralded athletes benefiting from his system. Among those cited were Jackie Jensen and Gil McDougald (baseball), Mal Whitfield and Herb Elliott (track), John Thomas (high jump), Harold Connolly (hammer throw), Don Bragg (pole vault), Al Oerter (discus), Alan Ameche and Billy Cannon (football), and Bob Mathias (decathlon). What Hoffman recommended for these athletes was what he prescribed for bodybuilding (or probably any other human endeavor)—the three Olympic lifts—thus striking a blow for American weightlifting: "An athlete like the Rev. Bob Richards has done more for weight-training than all the Mr. Americas and Mr. Universes combined."[13]

Richards figured prominently in Bob's book *Better Athletes Through Weight Training*, written after his return from the 1956 Olympics. Modeled on *How to Be Strong*, it was a self-promotional repetition of earlier themes. Flush from his world travels, Hoffman elevated his status to "Father of World Weight Lifting," boasting, "We started it all." His egocentric outlook required that even athletes from other countries, especially the Soviet Union, be portrayed as York followers. He believed that complete acceptance of weights by American athletes was the only way to beat the Russians. What he prescribed for every sport was the "all-around" system he had been advocating for thirty years, using original York courses, along with such recent additions as the Simplified System and the Daily Dozen, a concept originally devised by Walter Camp. Much of Bob's book consists of sketches of famous athletes, who are made to appear to be York disciples. This was the insinuation made regarding West Point cadet Pete Dawkins, a media hero of the late 1950s. He not only epitomized Hoffman's ideal of all-American virtues but seemed to owe his success to imitation of Hoffman's *personal* exercise routine. Dawkins was captain of the corps as well as the football team, seventh academically, and president of his class of 503.

> Fabulous as this record is, this isn't all, for he is a dashing, slashing, hard hitting determined runner with tremendous speed, he made 9 touchdowns in his first three games this year. But he also is a worthy artist, sings in the Cadet choir, plays half a dozen musical instruments, is the highest scoring defenseman in eastern collegiate hockey. . . . When asked how he does it, he shows them the barbell he keeps under his bed in his room. In his room he follows the Bob Hoffman system, doing his exercises between his study periods in his room, performing his exercises at odd times. Perform an exercise, put on one's shirt and tie, another exercise, the shoes, another exercise, the trousers, another exercise more of the clothes. Or while performing one's ablutions in the morning, an exercise, brush the teeth, another exercise, put the lather on the face, another exercise, shave half of the face, another exercise, shave the remainder of the face.

Dawkins was the kind of man Hoffman admired—a real Frank Merriwell, who used barbells to become a self-made man. Even before it was published, *Better Athletes* was advertised in *Strength & Health* as "already a classic in its field!"[14]

Murray and Paschall

Strength & Health remained the chief means by which Hoffman purveyed his ideas and products, but more astute writers came to bear influence over the magazine in the 1950s. Murray not only pushed weight training for athletes but introduced a greater degree of professionalism. Despite his positive outlook, Murray became discouraged by the inequities and hypocrisy he found in York, especially Bob's failure to live up to the high ideals he preached. He thought Hoffman led "an unsavory life" and that "someone was going to kill him. He was a real cheap skate when paying employees, but lavished gifts and money on his girl friends." His ego led him to "brag about having serviced several a day." Murray, though a key man in the organization, never made more than $85 per week and was hard put to support his family. He disliked Bob's exaggerated claims for his products and personal athletic feats, most notably his bent-press records: "I really resented Hoffman's phoniness. When I found out my idols had feet of clay, I was angry." But in retrospect Murray regards his experience at York as unique and enjoyable: "Hoffman did an awful lot more good than harm."[15]

"A real pro" is how Murray characterizes his successor, Harry Paschall, who had no problem with York's double standards. He probably believed that far from being the worst of his kind, Hoffman was a paragon of virtue in a sea of shysters and miscreants. What Paschall saw in his long association with Hoffman was a basic philosophical integrity behind the huckster. He shared Bob's view on all-around development and the premier status of weightlifting among sports, and agreed that one should be as strong as one looks. For Paschall, his appointment as editor in 1955 was "like a dream come true." Every day, "as the human behemoths rush in for their regular workout" at four o'clock, the fifty-seven-year-old veteran would don a sweat suit and relive his youth

> where the Great Men train. Here are the four platforms, beaten and bruised by the weights dropped by world-famous strong men, thousands upon thousands of pounds of barbell plates, dozens of benches of various types, overhead pulleys, squat racks, dumbells, abominable (the spelling is intentional) boards, and all the paraphernalia of the weight world. Sometimes four or five former Mr. Americas are training here, along with a dozen of the world's top lifters. If there is one place in all the world which is the true heart and center of weight training—certainly this is it.

Though now "owned body and soul by his publisher," Paschall vowed to be honest and forthright: "Nothing will be held back, and nothing will be twisted. I shall continue to call the shots just as I see them."[16]

Such independence probably did not bother Hoffman, since Paschall's views on most subjects resembled his own. Besides, with Bob's preoccupation with Hi-Proteen promotion and Paschall's journalistic ability, the magazine was in better hands. Unquestionably Hoffman had secured for his organization the most powerful pen in weightlifting.

The new impetus was most evident in York views on the relationship of bodybuilding to weightlifting and athletics. Paschall supported Bob's notion that bodybuilders should be athletes and that muscles should be useful. Repeatedly he heaped scorn on "boobybuilders," those who valued muscles for their own sake. He stressed a balanced approach, and soon the term "Sensible Physical Training" adorned the covers of *Strength & Health*. A distinction was clear, as right was from wrong, between those who followed the York way to health and fitness and those who followed any other course.

> A *boobybuilder* is usually a young man who has nothing better to do with his time than to spend four or five hours a day in a smelly gym doing bench presses and curls and squats and lat pulley exercises. He usually wears his hair long and frequently gilds the lily by having it waved. He is supremely concerned with big lats, big pex, big traps, big delts, and flapping triceps. His ideal is the V shape—preferably one like the emblem on the rear end of a Cadillac. He lives for his big moment, when he can strut and posture under the glare of a spot light before an audience of several hundred followers of his peculiar cult. Athletic fitness and muscular coordination and superb health are completely meaningless to him.

Hoffman lent substance to Paschall's crusade for integrity and all-American values. At the 1956 AAU meeting in Los Angeles he secured important rules changes for physique contests. Henceforth contestants had to display "athletic ability" in the three Olympic lifts, a category worth 25 percent of the judging. A further 50 percent was divided between general appearance and symmetry, with only 25 percent devoted to muscularity. Hoffman was hanged in effigy on Muscle Beach, and there were protests that it was unfair for bodybuilders to be judged on lifting ability. In response to complaints that the new rules were killing interest in local physique contests, Hoffman admitted that people seem "fascinated by muscles." But he failed to comprehend why promoters called their contests "Mr. This or That, and then . . . select[ed] only the most muscular man."[17] Undoubtedly 1955 Mr. America Steve Klisanin, an all-around athlete, most nearly approximated the high ideal set by Hoffman and Paschall.

In any case, Harry never survived to see his side triumph over the perceived evils of the day. In September 1957 he died in harness. He was twenty-one days late with the December issue and had been bothered with chest pains, which a doctor diagnosed as the flu. After pounding the typewriter till midnight, he rushed copy to the printer in Bethesda. On the return trip he drove slowly and erratically, holding up traffic until he pulled off the road near Olney. His body was found slumped over the steering wheel. That he died at age fifty-nine of a heart attack inevitably raised questions about the viability of the Strength and Health life style and whether Hoffman and his cohorts practiced what they preached. When Mark Berry, a heavy smoker, died of a heart attack the following year, Bob observed that men of iron are often brought down early by not obeying the rules of healthful living. The deaths of Paschall and Berry proved that "everyone does not die of cancer who smokes. All you have to do is to smoke regularly and you will die of a heart attack." Indeed "Harry smoked so much and lived such a high strung life, he did not live long enough to get cancer." He also endured a prolonged bout with the bottle. Terpak relates that Paschall "finally realized the seriousness of his condition after he drove drunk to a meet in Detroit, checked into a hotel, and the next morning couldn't remember where he had left his car or where he was."[18] But such unsavory facts could never be revealed to loyal consumers of Hoffman's products and philosophy of life.

Material Splendor

Despite his outward calm, the deaths of old friends brought to Hoffman an awareness of his own mortality. In an uncharacteristic lapse, he told Dave Matlin, southern California weightlifting chairman, that Berry "looked good" at the funeral and that he had "felt for a moment that it would be nice to go along"; but he had "too much to do." He quickly recovered his promoter's verve. When Wally Zagurski died of a heart attack in 1959 at age forty-eight, Hoffman persuaded himself that he still felt younger than he did at twenty. The need to affirm the myth of his immortality was further evident in several building projects. Though Hoffman dated many women, he had been living with Alda at Brookside for a decade. In 1956 Bob decided to satisfy her desire for a large stone house. It was to be their dream home, a handsome one-story bungalow (with bay window) constructed of Italian stone by the same masons who had built the House on the Hill—"a veritable paradise." A spacious basement became the nerve center for his strength empire. Formerly his work had been scattered in four locations. "Now I have everything together," he told Marshall Ackerman of *Prevention Magazine*. "Sort of luxurious, a 20 by 30 writing room and study . . . with all my books, and everything where I can find it. Terrazzo floor, insulated ceiling, beautiful cherry pannelling, just a few feet from my beautiful home gym. Life can be wonderful." Nearby Bob was planning a health-and-fitness laboratory to be known as the Hoffman Foundation. Among other enterprises, he hoped to experiment on organically grown food, including wheat germ, which he would grow locally and market nationally. In line with his "hands-on" approach, he purchased a shredder and was acquiring a farm adjacent to the foundation site.[19]

His other great project was a new Strength and Health Center on Ridge Avenue, only several blocks from the Broad Street gym. The need for a new complex to improve weightlifting's image and showcase Bob's achievements is illustrated by Terry Todd's story about his first visit to York. A tennis player at the University of Texas in the late 1950s, Todd, after attending the national collegiates at Annapolis in 1958, persuaded his teammates to take a side trip to the weightlifting capital of the world. Instead of a splendid modern facility, they found a drab warehouse, and Todd became the butt of numerous jokes. The new building, completed in 1959 for $150,000, coincided more with the radiant image of York projected in *Strength & Health*. Measuring 160' by 160', it included a large gym, hall of fame, snack bar, offices, and space for clinics, movies, and so forth. Hoffman wanted "to encourage promising lifters and coaches to come here to learn more about weightlifting." Above the entrance was the 1,600-pound Travis dumbbell, and the foyer featured a forty-foot black-velvet painting of the labors of Hercules by Eric Askew. The hall of fame included trophies accumulated by Bob and many team artifacts. He also commissioned a life-size statue of Grimek and a bronze bust of himself. The hall was "a big step forward" in promoting weightlifting and ensuring his own place in posterity.[20]

The Marietta Fire

A small setback to Hoffman's progress occurred on January 10, 1955, when the York Barbell Foundry at Marietta burned down. When informed of the mishap by a local broadcaster, Bob reacted in disbelief: "Foundries do not burn at 10 o'clock in the morning. They might catch fire while the 'heat is on,' the molten iron running from the cupola in the afternoon." In Dietz's Cadillac, Bob, Jules, and Mike sped to Marietta to witness the raging inferno. The foundry was a complete loss. Hoffman explains that the fire started in the machine shop, where "Jim 'Mr. Universe' Park was welding a piece of gym equipment.... A spark flew into a tank of thinner and paint, and the flames leaped so fast that the workers could not retrieve their coats." This line was used to avoid negligence charges over the loss of patterns being stored in the building by several firms. With no insurance to cover such losses, Bob cast the circumstances in the best possible light. The truth, according to Park, is that the fire started when he lit a cigarette and discarded the match in some nearby paint lacquer. Nevertheless Bob's story held up in court. Until a new foundry was built, the company scrambled to maintain production. Bacon was dispatched "through the ice and snow" to Canada to fetch duplicate patterns, enabling York to resume manufacture of plates within days. Meanwhile "our competitors had spent hundreds, perhaps thousands of dollars calling the stores selling York barbells, telling them that we were out of business." Hoffman reassured readers that arrangements had been made with neighboring firms: "ALL ORDERS WILL BE FILLED WITH OUR USUAL PROMPTNESS." He also rationalized that "any foundry can sell you weights, but they are so much iron and steel unless you follow the right methods."[21] That the York way was indubitably the right way, especially in contrast to the hated Weider system, was argued with even greater gusto.

Success and Its Pitfalls

Ironically, in January 1955, the month of York's greatest capital loss, the company registered its highest sales record ($55,830) since August 1946 ($59,557), during the postwar boom. In fact, it marked the beginning of an increase that did not abate till the early 1960s.

1953—$527,667	1957—$919,592	1961—$2,207,782
1954—$521,703	1958—$1,280,056	1962—$2,235,187
1955—$637,862	1959—$1,565,232	1963—$2,207,444
1956—$806,722	1960—$1,875,923	

This was truly a "golden age" for York Barbell, as it had been for Hoffman's lifting teams from 1946 to 1956. Such growth may be attributed to a wider variety of health-and-fitness items, particularly foods. Although Hi-Proteen was first marketed by York in the early fifties, it did not fully "kick in" to sales and profits till about 1955. Then business became so great that Hoffman could no longer mix "every pound" of it himself. Henceforth a functionary named Squirrely (Charles Leader) carried out this "secret process." Hoffman told one of his distributors that Hi-Proteen sales by the end of September 1957 had equaled the entire previous year's total. For February 1958 Hi-Proteen business was 3.7 times that of February 1957.[22] By the end of the decade Bob was amassing a fortune, just from items with a soy base.

Another reason for the company's success was imaginative marketing. Bob began running ads in such trade journals as *Let's Live, Prevention Magazine, Organic Gardening, Coach and Athlete, Athletic Journal, Amateur Athlete,* and *Ring,* often in return for writing health articles. But mail orders were accounting for proportionately fewer sales by the late 1950s. Increasingly, dietary supplements and equipment were handled by gyms, stores, and food distributors. *Strength & Health* regularly listed over five hundred vendors for Hi-Proteen. Also, Bob began attending health-food conventions to establish contacts. Weider followed suit with his own line of copycat items. Displays of Hi-Protein, Vitamin-Mineral tablets, and Enertol in *Muscle Power* and *Muscle Builder* closely mirrored York products with similar names, hoping to capture the undiscriminating buyer. His food supplements were often carried in the same stores as Hoffman's with considerable success.

How much money Hoffman could have made can only be conjectured. For scattered amid his papers are thousands of dollars in uncashed checks and money orders. Why would a man who often circled countless city blocks to find an unexpired parking meter fail to cash his remittances? Possibly Bob obtained the checks and money orders while fetching cash from the company's postal box and then mislaid them. Whether the orders were ever filled cannot be determined, but this oversight no doubt resulted in much time and expense wasted on handling customer complaints. Likewise it is doubtful whether cash orders were properly handled, though the division of labor in the York management probably made for easy concealment of these irregularities. Dietz had total control of finances and learned to cover for Bob's carelessness, while Terpak supervised sales and assisted Bob with other matters, including weightlifting trips and AAU politics. Rarely did they tread on each other's turf. Terpak insists that until the 1980s he knew virtually nothing about the financial end of the business, and Bob was consumed with public relations. He did tell Terpak and others, however, "I know Mike steals, but as long as he doesn't steal more than what I'm getting I'm not worried." "Dietz was a problem, and Bob knew it," concurs Clarence Johnson. "It was easier to ride along than correct it."[23]

That money, even a lot of it, could be made under such management seems remarkable. Alda attributed it to "some very wise investments" by Dietz. But aside from Bob's properties (which produced little income) and a long-term insurance annuity, there is little evidence of outside investment. It is also true that while prices on weights did not increase much, the profit margin on food supplements was enormous. And the company saved money on labor. For 1957, as sales neared the million-dollar mark, salaries were only $118,654, or roughly 13 percent of sales. For the banner year of 1958 they were 9 percent. Terpak blames Bob for the low wages but rationalizes that they were "not low for the area," largely agricultural and nonunionized. Bob justified his practice and minimized complaints by telling gang members that they would be remembered in his will.[24]

What must have angered employees and sapped morale was the belief that company executives were helping themselves to cash at the post office. Arguably Bob, as proprietor, had every right to draw upon his company's resources as he saw fit. Dietz, as treasurer, also had the right to collect income the company received, but he also had the responsibility of placing it in York Barbell bank accounts and keeping records on it. Bob, owing to other interests, kept such a loose rein on employees that he could not keep track of them. Once, in the mid-1950s, Bob brought in a certified public accountant to go through the books. The auditor told him that Mike was making more money than anyone else in the organization. That some of Dietz's privileges were also being assumed by George Shandor, "one of the key men in the office," became obvious by sudden changes in his lifestyle. Conspicuous consumption was evident in the *Strength & Health* documentation of his indulgence in cars and clothing. In 1957 he was "Our Man About Town" who "does more than anybody in the gym" to keep a trim waistline "or else spend a fortune on having the tailor let out his 14 suits." George owned a new two-tone Chrysler and in 1959 acquired a "sporty brand new Karmann Ghia." In 1960 he graduated to a Thunderbird convertible. Bacon observes that Shandor acquired a beautiful home, joined the country club, and became the best-dressed man in York. "He told everybody he was running a whorehouse and a gambling outfit up in the coal region." Then Bob began complaining that "the money wasn't coming in," and a trap was set for Shandor with marked money. He was fired and later died of a heart attack.[25] More than any other incident, Shandor's termination highlighted the boundary between those who occupied the exclusive inner circle at York and others who merely aspired to "old-gang" status.

The IRS Challenge

The factor that enabled Dietz to separate himself so easily from relative newcomers was not so much age but a permanent lien he held on Hoffman, which made him virtually unexpendable. He knew too much about York operations. Were he to be relieved of his duties, he could do far more damage than Venables had done. "In the old days," Jowett recalls, Hoffman was "always cheating on taxes. He told me so." Nevertheless, Bob struggled with the Internal Revenue Service for a decade over charges that he had failed to pay $176,058 in taxes from 1948 to 1950. By 1958, with penalties and interest, this figure had grown to $359,615. What drew IRS attention was his purchases of York Precision and York Light House, and the various properties and gifts he had purchased with capital not generated by sales. The government further argued, according to Elmer Morris, the company's lawyer, that "certain amounts of cash" were not deposited, that for three years money orders exceeded bank deposits by $21,000. Bob had also underestimated his payments to Rosetta and deducted as business expenses what were actually "expenditures for the personal benefit of

Dorcas, Alda and others." Morris concluded in 1957 that Hoffman's income over twenty years was "substantially in excess of that which he reported." He informed Bob that the IRS was willing to settle out of court for $93,805, just 25.7 percent of its initial claim. Deeming anything under 50 percent a "fair settlement," Morris urged him to accept.[26]

Hoffman, however, refused to pay more than $10,000. To undermine the government's case, he got his sister Eleanor to testify that he had sent his mother $100 monthly and that she bequeathed him $25,000. Bob also extracted supporting statements from Rosetta and his brother Chuck, though neither of them knew about these transactions. This did not matter, Bob told Chuck, because he would "have knowledge of it if either Eleanor or [he told Chuck] about it": "So I am telling you about it and will appreciate it if you will write the letter." Here, perhaps more than any other incident in his life, Bob displayed his willingness to take on any opponent, regardless of odds. Dick Smith remembers him as "one of the most tenacious individuals I've ever come across. He was a real fighter. Bob would not back down to anyone."[27] But his tenacity only drew him into deeper trouble. He was so intransigent that the case remained unresolved several more years, thus incurring greater interest charges and legal fees. Meanwhile, in 1959 the IRS assessed him a further $13,000 for deficiencies from 1954 to 1956. Hoffman grudgingly paid it, but not without venting his anger: "For some years your office has been persecuting me. . . . You have done all you can to damage my reputation, to damage our business. If I weren't a pretty strong minded fellow, a man who won 11 decorations in the first world war, I would have been ruined physically, and mentally. . . . Some day the real facts will come out. When this case is settled, it will be my turn to tell my story. And I don't think it will be a pretty one. . . . I'll be seeing you in court." Next, smarting over the interminable delays and expense, Hoffman turned on his lawyers. Feeling overcharged and not getting the support he needed, he switched from Morris and Vedder to Markowitz and Kagen. But when the latter presented him a $12,000 bill in 1960, he protested that he was being ruined: "I will appreciate a revision of this bill." Arthur Markowitz was so incensed by Bob's request that he did not reply for several weeks. Not only was he unwilling to revise the bill, but he refused to represent York Barbell until the matter was settled: "I cannot do justice in your case if I have to fight you as well as the Commissioner of Internal Revenue." Eventually the tax court in

Philadelphia decided that the IRS had overestimated by about $250,000 the amount Hoffman was in arrears.[28]

Mudslinging with Weider

More damaging than money lost in this suit, however, was the fuel it provided for attacks by his enemies. The inaugural issue of Weider's *Mr. America* in 1958 carried an exposé of "Bob Hoffman's strange finances," with unflattering caricatures and the list of IRS charges, framed in such a way as to appear true. Its thrust was that the man "held up as a model for young America" was defrauding the government and that "conviction could mean prison." Also, pains were taken to show that he wrote off the money he donated to weightlifting as a tax deduction and thus furthered his own business. The next month, an article entitled "Portrait of a 'Medicine Man'" depicted Hoffman as a bully and womanizer, ridiculed his products, and continued the attacks on his philanthropy. A third installment, "Hoffman's Calculated Scheme to Ruin Bodybuilding," showed how he "fixed" physique contests, degraded those interested in bodybuilding, and attempted to sacrifice physique to weightlifting.[29] Much of what Weider published was true, but the AAU revelations were hardly surprising. Tax deductions drive philanthropy, and Hoffman would have been a fool to have ignored them. Most athletes and officials would probably have agreed with Pete George's statement that Bob had done more to advance barbell use "than any other man in the world. . . . Sure, his business benefits from the promotion of the sport, but how far would the sport have gotten without his business?" Hoffman's rebuttal of Weider, however, assumed an unusually venomous tone. At age sixty and distant from his adversary, he could not assault Joe physically. So he punished Weider with words, such as "rat," "skunk," "jackal," and "hyena," in an editorial entitled "Birds of a Feather." Alleging libel for these remarks and others in a sarcastic piece entitled "Pal Joey!," Weider sued Hoffman for $800,000. Bob filed a counterclaim for malicious conspiracy and character defamation. In May 1962 a U.S. district court in Harrisburg found Hoffman not guilty and awarded him $30,000. This verdict did not stand, since York could not prove monetary loss. In early 1965, after years of stressful litigation and expenditure, a judgment was rendered in Hoffman's favor with a nominal award of $1. Bob was vindicated, but decades later the court record struck Terpak as "still good for belly laughs."[30]

For Hoffman, however, the suit was no laughing matter and must have tested his tranquil-mind rule to the limits. He at least received comfort from loyal York readers who doubted Weider's accusations. One from Detroit related how the police had raided that city's newsstands and seized copies of Weider's *Body Beautiful* and *Adonis*. He was annoyed by attacks on Hoffman's iron-game contributions: "No man in the world has done more for this cause than Bob and we all know it." From Hollywood a well-informed writer needled Bob for not taking stronger measures: "We who respect & admire you will forgive you any 'Hollywood dramatics' you might display in the way of retaliation. In killing Weider, any means will justify the end!" A longtime follower in Missouri, aware that Weider had copied Hoffman's marketing techniques and products, suggested he charge Joe for copyright infringement. In 1960 Englishman John Barrs explained how his friend Charles Coster was "having trouble with Joe Wonderful. It seems that Joe got into the nice little habit of paying 3 weeks wages every 4 weeks!!" Barrs sought a place for Coster on Bob's staff, insisting that he had "always wanted to work full-time for you. . . . Much of his stuff for Weider has been re-hashed before publication—presumably to give a fuller commercial Joe-boosting flavour!" Coster never joined York, but there was a major exodus from the Weider camp in the late 1950s, including Charlie Smith, Barton Horvath, and Earle Liederman. Bob's acquisition of Liederman, whose iron-game experience antedated his own, helped compensate for the loss of Paschall.[31]

Especially pleasing to Hoffman, in light of charges of his own sexual misconduct, was a 1960 exposé by the New York *Daily News* of an extramarital affair Weider was having with "blonde model" Betty Brosemer. Accompanied by photos revealing their physical assets, the front-page article explained how Weider and Brosemer were "allegedly found early Nov. 29 in a Montreal hotel room in a state of undress." Joe at first told detectives confronting him "that Betty was his wife," but the situation was quickly clarified "after the protesting muscle man followed the three sleuths to a neighboring room at the Queen Elizabeth Hotel and found himself confronted by the real Mrs. Weider." Accusing Joe of "cavorting with this model," Diana Weider sought $350 a week temporary alimony and $10,000 counsel from the "weightlifter of note," who earned $100,000 a year from his publishing empire.³² Never had Bob's sexual improprieties, though hardly secret, been so widely broadcast.

Faulty Business Practices

Weider and the IRS were by no means Hoffman's only problems. As York Barbell assumed a higher profile, he was beset with problems from government agencies, distributors, and the scientific community. In 1956 the Labor Department determined that York employees who performed weightlifting duties outside the workplace were entitled to extra compensation. In 1958 a health-food vendor in Tucson reported that customers were complaining that the taste of Hi Proteen Fudge Bars was ruined by York's omission of inside wrappers. A Tulsa distributor grumbled about not getting an extra 10 percent discount from York to offset a new Charles Atlas line. Bob pointed out that concessions were rarely made to any jobbers and that his advertising costs were $28,000 per year: "We are not going to be stampeded into giving the stuff away." In 1959 William Pierson, a scientist at the College of Osteopathic Physicians and Surgeons in Los Angeles, took Hoffman to task for his editorials on smoking. Pierson insisted there was no hard evidence that it caused cancer or was detrimental to athletic performance. He did "not condone smoking," but he did "object to published statements which imply scientific substantiation where in fact none exists." Finally, Bob had to address complaints that sediment had settled in suntan lotion that had been bottled ten years earlier.³³ Quality control was always a problem.

It was magnified by probes into Hoffman's products by nutrition scientists and the government. In 1957 a laboratory in Eugene, Oregon, refuted Bob's claim that his Super Hi-Proteen contained over 90 percent protein and no sugar or sodium. An analysis showed only 65 percent protein and some sodium. Hoffman first questioned the commercial motives of the inquiry, then explained that the salt came from natural salt in eggs and defended his statement on protein on grounds that several *ingredients* contained over 90 percent protein. Another challenge came from Robert Bates of Chicago, who discovered Hoffman's tablets contained only 22 percent protein instead of the 44 percent claimed. "This is not a crank letter," Bates assured him. As "a research chemist for 28 yrs.," he was "completely familiar with the laws governing food products" and "as familiar with the determination of protein as anyone in the country." In his response Bob addressed each of his adversary's points with a wealth of facts based on his (somewhat dated) knowledge of nutrition literature and decade of experience in health foods. Again, however, he was forced to admit to misleading labeling inasmuch as the 44 percent claim applied only to nonflavored Hi-Proteen. Bates even threatened to turn Hoffman over to authorities, but Delmar Myers of the Pennsylvania Department of Agriculture was already on his case for false labeling of Hi-Proteen Cookies and Energy Bars. Again, much less protein was found than stated. When the Bureau of Standards banned the sale of Hi-Proteen tablets, Macy's department store canceled its large account with York.[34] Finally, Hoffman changed the contents of his products and altered their labels.

More serious and equally untenable were the claims he made for the medicinal and ergogenic properties of York products. Nowhere was his promotional flair more evident than in his dealings with VioBin Corporation, supplier of the wheat-germ oil used in Hoffman's Germ Oil Concentrate. Its president, Ezra Levin, forbade Bob to use the phrase "VioBin Oil" in advertising. Levin feared repercussions from the Food and Drug Administration owing to Hoffman's extravagant claims for his product, including prevention and treatment of arteriosclerosis, improved athletic and sexual performance, and prevention of "119 unnatural and unpleasant physical conditions." These included such ailments as cirrhosis of the liver, gangrene, epilepsy, gas pains, shingles, alcoholism, stunted growth, insomnia, irregular menstruation, cataracts, diabetes, forgetfulness, paralysis, sore lips, and edema. Simultaneously, the FDA required Hoffman to alter portions of his Energol label that were false, misleading, or irrelevant, and the California Department of Health seized twenty-four York products statewide and quarantined them for several months. Again Hoffman complied with federal standards, but when he was at the Rome Olympics, the U.S. Marshal in Oklahoma seized more of his merchandise.[35] While Weider's epithet "medicine man" is hardly apt, Hoffman's promotional verve led to frequent clashes with officialdom.

Amazingly, consumer testimony often supported Hoffman's exaggerated claims. Allen Jones of San Mateo, California, reported "instant results" from Hi-Proteen tablets. "When one buys Hoffman's he is not buying a 'Pig-in-the-Poke,'" opined Charles Green of Mt. Kisco, New

York, of Bob's suntan lotion. "I know from the experience of 4 summers how good it is: you see I have tried out over 20 brands and I find but *one* safe + good—yours." Allyn Avant of Chevy Chase, Maryland, found Hoffman's Hi-Proteen Fudge "excellent. I can honestly say that it is everything you say it is." From eating Hi-Proteen, Edward Lord of Hannacroix, New York, gained fifteen pounds of muscular bodyweight and increased his lifts. It now seemed possible, even at thirty-seven, to gain another twenty pounds "and lift far more than [he] ever dreamed possible." Robert Beaudoin of Biddeford, Maine, gained bodyweight and confidence with Hi-Proteen after an illness. He appreciated Hoffman's "scientific" approach to bodybuilding. It was Hi-Proteen and Soy Bean Germ Oil Tablets, according to the Reverend M. D. Loar of Wilmore, Kentucky, that was keeping his ailing wife alive. Mrs. Robert Sciaroni of Morro Bay, California, attributed her husband's full recovery from a heart attack, stomach ulcer, and enlarged liver to Hoffman's Hi-Proteen: "I know it was the powder, because being on the diet, he couldn't have many foods . . . so he fairly lived on Super Hi-Proteen and now at 60 years old, he is in perfect Health." Phil Crow of Waller, Texas, wrote that he found Weider's protein "completely unsatisfactory. . . . Once a 'York man' always a 'York man.'"[36] Hoffman, the consummate salesman, had bestowed on these individuals the most important ingredient to recovery from any ailment—confidence. Notwithstanding the efforts of his detractors to reduce him to life-size proportions, Hoffman's idealism (and power of suggestion) prevailed.

Investment Opportunities

Another consequence of his increasing prominence was a vulnerability to the promotions of others who wished to share in Hoffman's newfound wealth. The usual pitch was that they could use his money to make him even more rich and famous. So in late 1959 he opened an account with Merrill Lynch, and in the early 1960s he was lured into the Florida and Arizona real estate markets. The most alluring investment opportunity, however, was proposed by Dr. Richard You, who had gained Bob's confidence by marketing York products and supplying the American team with some excellent Hawaiian lifters. You had also used York's name for the athletic club he sponsored, and regularly ingratiated himself to

Hoffman by sending large wads of newspaper clippings detailing the feats of his lifters and track stars. As Terpak recalls, "Every time Dr. You came around, he had some big and new ideas—'It will make you famous' was the usual line." You proposed to build a twelve-story medical-professional building in Honolulu. He needed to rent at least two-thirds of the building before construction started, and wanted Bob to lease one or more floors: "Once the building starts you are not obligated & may break your lease with me because I can easily lease the space once the building starts." Somewhat more attractive to Bob was the prospect of increasing his wealth by reinvesting in his own thriving enterprises, a notion whose emergence coincided with a 1958 visit by George Jowett. Regarded earlier as a pariah figure who had sold out to Weider, Jowett suddenly was featured in an old-timers setting in *Strength & Health*. Jowett suggested a direct-mail promotion using the list of pupils who subscribed to his courses. When Jowett heard of Bob's IRS problems, he explained how Weider escaped taxes by expanding into the sterling bloc: "Take my advice Bob, begin to cover up. Funnel your funds, particularly overseas sterling, into Bermuda, or Nassau." It is doubtful that Bob employed this scheme, but he did take up Jowett's direct-mailing offer. Other opportunities he explored included the marketing of a Bulgarian yogurt that would prevent cancer and the shipment of castings and health-food ingredients from east Asia.[37]

New Promotional Techniques

Hoffman also discussed promotional strategies with the Irwin Rosee Agency of New York. They hoped to duplicate Bonnie Pruden's highly successful fitness program by having Bob perform his Daily Dozen exercises on national television. Realizing the body of a man his age could not rival Pruden's slim figure and not wanting to pay $7,500 a year for Rosee's services, Hoffman fell back on his own more limited designs. During the previous year the York High School football team, using weights, Hi-Proteen, and Hoffman's Germ Oil Concentrate, had won its first state championship. Similarly, the basketball team had won twenty-three straight games. Bob beamed with pride and hoped to get "the girls who lead our band at the football games to exercise with the DAILY DOZEN." Another opportunity arose at the Colonial Days celebration in

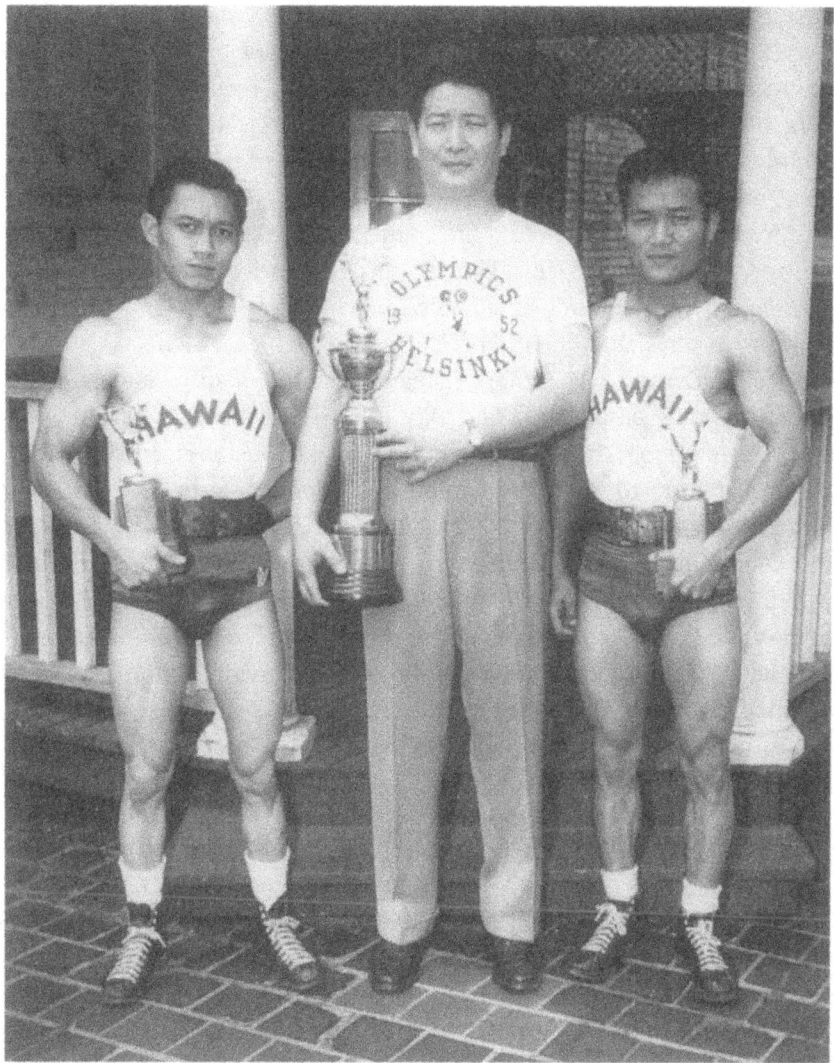

Dr. Richard You with bantamweight Richard Tom and featherweight Richard Tomita, both of whom were national champions and members of the 1948 and 1952 Olympic teams. You's Hawaiians upset York for the 1952 national team championship, Hoffman's only loss over a period of fifty years.

1958, which commemorated York's once being the nation's capital. The York gang grew beards, and Hoffman took charge of sports festivities. He broke chains with his chest and held an anvil on his stomach while Jules Bacon pounded it with a sledge hammer. "We had a great time, and it proved that I practice what I preach as well as the fact that a busy person can retain great strength by regularly practicing the DAILY DOZEN and taking Energol and Hi-Proteen every day." Even at age sixty he had to prove his manly prowess, so a picture of him in the *York Dispatch* had him hoisting "a 250-pound weight" overhead![38] But such local publicity stunts distracted him from projecting himself and his exercise philosophy in the national media.

It was largely by promoting the Daily Dozen that Hoffman developed civic pride and became a local benefactor. The York gang gave countless demonstrations at churches, schools, and clubs; and Bob donated $3,000 to improve physical education facilities at the York YMCA. As a result of these activities, city fathers realized that this man of means could help fund civic endeavors. The way to Bob's pocketbook was always through his ego. Thus, in recognition of the business and publicity he had brought to York, the Chamber of Commerce in 1957 honored him and his Olympians at a testimonial dinner attended by many of the community's best citizens. Also, a television film on York Barbell was broadcast locally. Hoffman was at last accruing the respect in his hometown that he had been denied in his leaner years. He responded in kind. Not only did he help stage Colonial Days but in 1958 hosted a thirty-kilometer run through the city. In 1959, the first time since 1932, the senior nationals were held in York, at the fairgrounds. Most symbolic perhaps of the reconciliation of company and community was the participation of four of the York gang—Dave Ashman, John Grimek, Jake Hitchins, and Vern Weaver—in a production of *Li'l Abner* at the American Legion Post. Bob's contribution of $1,000 to the York County Association for Retarded Children, though a tax deduction, indicated a willingness to share his largess with the city.[39]

His public spirit and eagerness to promote fitness extended to the AAU, where he became president of the Middle Atlantic District in 1958. Although it was an unpaid position and required frequent trips to Philadelphia, Hoffman enthusiastically assumed his duties, intending to create "the largest and most active district in the country." He told Asa Bushnell, secretary of the U.S. Olympic Association, that he was spending nearly all of his time "building a stronger and healthier America." When President Eisenhower appointed a council on physical fitness for youth, including the vice-president and five cabinet members, Hoffman supplied its chairman, Dr. Shane McCarthy, with long regular reports of his activities. With an eye to national recognition and political influence,

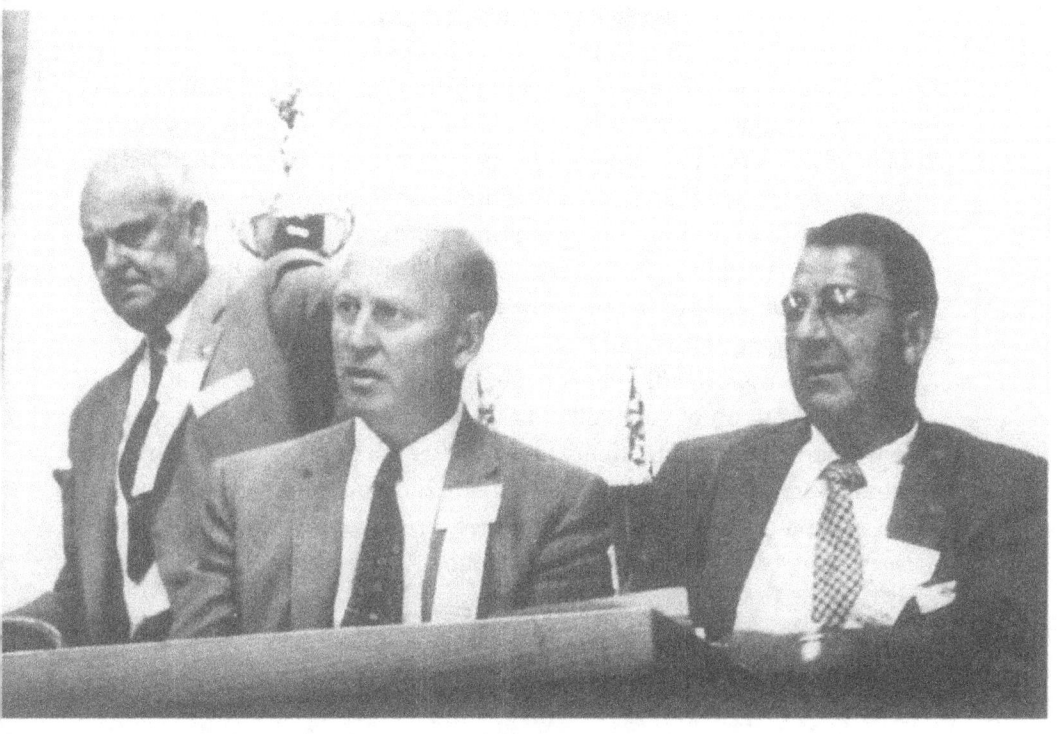

Clarence Johnson, a Michigan accountant, Ray Van Cleef, a San Jose gym owner, and David Matlin, a Los Angeles lawyer, were staunch allies of York in the AAU during the late 1950s.

he tried to secure McCarthy's adoption of the Daily Dozen and devised "The York Plan for Physical Fitness," with programs from "the capital of weightlifting" to serve as a national model. When the Democrats occupied the White House in 1960, Hoffman, though a Republican, was no less eager for recognition. He lent full support to the Kennedy program for physical fitness and professed to have a cure for the president's ailing back. An Associated Press photo taken during Hoffman's 1961 visit to Tokyo showed Bob stripped to the waist and hanging from a bar as he demonstrated to a group of curious Japanese an exercise he was recommending to the president. There is no evidence that Hoffman's ideas influenced those who controlled the nation's destiny, but he did secure election of his friend Clarence Johnson to the presidency of the IWF at the Rome Olympics.[40] In this sphere at least, he could exercise real power.

American Weightlifting Crises

As Hoffman entered his sixties, weightlifting remained his central passion. Unfortunately his lifters were no longer living up to expectations. Some of his brightest lights, no longer content to be company employees, were being lured by the more exuberant lifestyle of southern California. Isaac Berger and Dave Sheppard moved to Santa Monica, where they not only shared the camaraderie of the Muscle Beach crowd but engaged in some irresponsible acts. In June 1959 Berger was convicted of impairing the morals of minors, and Sheppard faced a charge of statutory rape. Hoffman admonished Berger to "come to life" and "make something of yourself" and castigated Sheppard, saying that if he would stop his dissipation, "he would be the greatest lifter who ever lived." Such sentiments must have made him sound like a Dutch uncle and a "square" to his youthful protégés. Frustration was evident in the assessment of his team Bob sent to Kono:

> Vinci went back to Cleveland. He would not do 5 cents worth of work for us. I asked him how come he would work in Cleveland and not for us. He said that he would get fired in Cleveland if he did not work. . . . His future is unknown. It was bad enough before, but with his wife, it makes it just twice as bad.
>
> Berger was exonerated in the trouble he was in, but still has a case hanging over him designed to keep him straight. Muscle Beach is still closed on account of the trouble they had with the lifters and the girls.

For Jim George he prescribed a regimen of "no drinking, no smoking, less girls," prior to the Rome Olympics. But it was obvious that Hoffman lacked the rapport with lifters of the late 1950s that he had had with earlier groups. He proudly called himself the "Father of American Weightlifting" and wanted to "help our country by showing what a fine group of young men we have."[41] But this generation was less willing to be patronized. Hoffman's old-fashioned values and fatherly gestures were viewed not so much as effusions of wisdom as old-fogyism.

In other ways as well, Hoffman's ideas were being overtaken by the early 1960s. Though more enthusiastic than ever, his outlook was ossified by his preoccupation with Olympic lifting, which was declining in popularity, and his failure to embrace the growing interest in physique and powerlifting. He called physique contests "cruel" because they were "killing weightlifting all over the world, except Russia, where they are getting a good laugh at all of us." The Soviets "put their efforts back of lifting, an event which brings them worldwide acclaim and respect, especially at the Olympics." That Hoffman did not admire bodybuilding, as he did Olympic lifting, accounts in part for Weider's success. In 1959 Joe staged his own Mr. America and Mr. Universe shows. In powerlifting, another of Hoffman's competitors, Peary Rader, assumed the initiative. Though professing to be an "Olympic enthusiast," Rader realized that "Olympic lifting in America today is a minor sport." For the public, bodybuilding had more attraction than the Olympic lifts, and physique training usually included the power lifts. While Hoffman would eventually host the first national powerlifting championships in York, he displayed little passion for the new sport. Even in Olympic lifting, Bob was out of touch with the trend toward squatting rather than splitting heavy snatches and cleans. Although the entire American team employed the squat style in winning at Melbourne, Hoffman remained partial to the split.[42]

While York Barbell was flourishing and Bob was gaining recognition as a patriarch, American fortunes continued to decline at the world championships at Stockholm in 1958 and Warsaw in 1959. Van Cleef rationalized that at Stockholm the United States was not expected to win—Russia's victory was as much a surprise as the Yankees' winning the American League pennant. But three American runners-up—Vinci, Jim George, and Ashman—"had the winning lifts overhead; had they held their lifts, we would have won our greatest victory over the Russians." After taking just one first, two seconds, and a third in Warsaw, Hoffman admitted that "we failed miserably." With other nations, such as Poland, joining the ranks of winners, he believed that in the future it would "take a miracle for us to beat the world." Failing to find any new secrets to success (Hi-Proteen being a short-lived panacea), Bob resorted to some old formulas. Pointing out that Communist nations had won eighteen of the twenty-one medals at the 1960 European championships in Milan, he raised the specter again of their possibly overtaking the West. The Communists "are out to prove that their system of living . . . is superior to that of the free world. . . . Only hard work will prevent us from being enslaved." There were still some ethnic-American lifters who looked on Hoffman as a father figure. At Warsaw, where he won his eighth consecutive world title, Kono, before attempting a 286-pound snatch that would place him well ahead of his Russian adversary, said: "I will snatch it, I must snatch it, I will make this for you, Bob." And he did. Furthermore, in an attempt to resurrect the team spirit of yore, fourteen lifters spent twelve days at York preparing for the 1960 Rome Olympics, and there was a strengthfest at Brookside Park prior to departure. The U.S. Olympic Committee even provided a partial subsidy.[43] Still, the Russians were victorious, 40 to 34, and Vinci was America's only winner. It was the last Olympic gold medal the United States would win in weightlifting.

After losing to the Russians in six consecutive world championships, and now, for the first time, in the Olympics, there was much consternation and soul-searching. At the National AAU Convention in Las Vegas in 1960, discussion centered on recent nutritional advances made by the Russians. Dr. You, a nutrition specialist, had attended a meeting on athletic medicine in Vienna after the Olympics and was amazed at advances made by the Russians in supplement use. Peary Rader remarked that "the Russians had that extra spark of vitality and drive that enabled them to come through and win, whereas our men lacked just a little of making their final lifts." Hoffman noted that "Communist lifters, who last year had been mediocre were now sensational lifters, transformed in both physique and strength." Bob continued to believe that Russian gains were due to improved diet. He observed that the solid muscle gained by Soviet heavyweight Yuri Vlasov since he had seen Vlasov at the European championships "was a marvel of the world, for with this 20 pounds he gained unusual strength too." He conceded that the Russians were "pretty smart people. Dr. Arkadi Vorobiev, who won his second Olympic title and sixth world championships in Rome, more than once in the past had learned about the contents of our Hi-Proteen and Energol. He realized that these products had something to do with the success of our great lifters and athletes. And so at Rome . . . the Russians had food supplements too. I hope they are not as good as ours, but something made these Russians perform sensationally." That this sudden improvement by the Soviets was due to steroids was beyond Hoffman's comprehension, such was his commitment to the efficacy of Hi-Proteen. But it was only too clear that the four hundred packages of Hi-Proteen he had sent with his lifters to Rome and other elaborate preparations for an American victory were to no avail.[44] The Russians had obviously discovered something better.

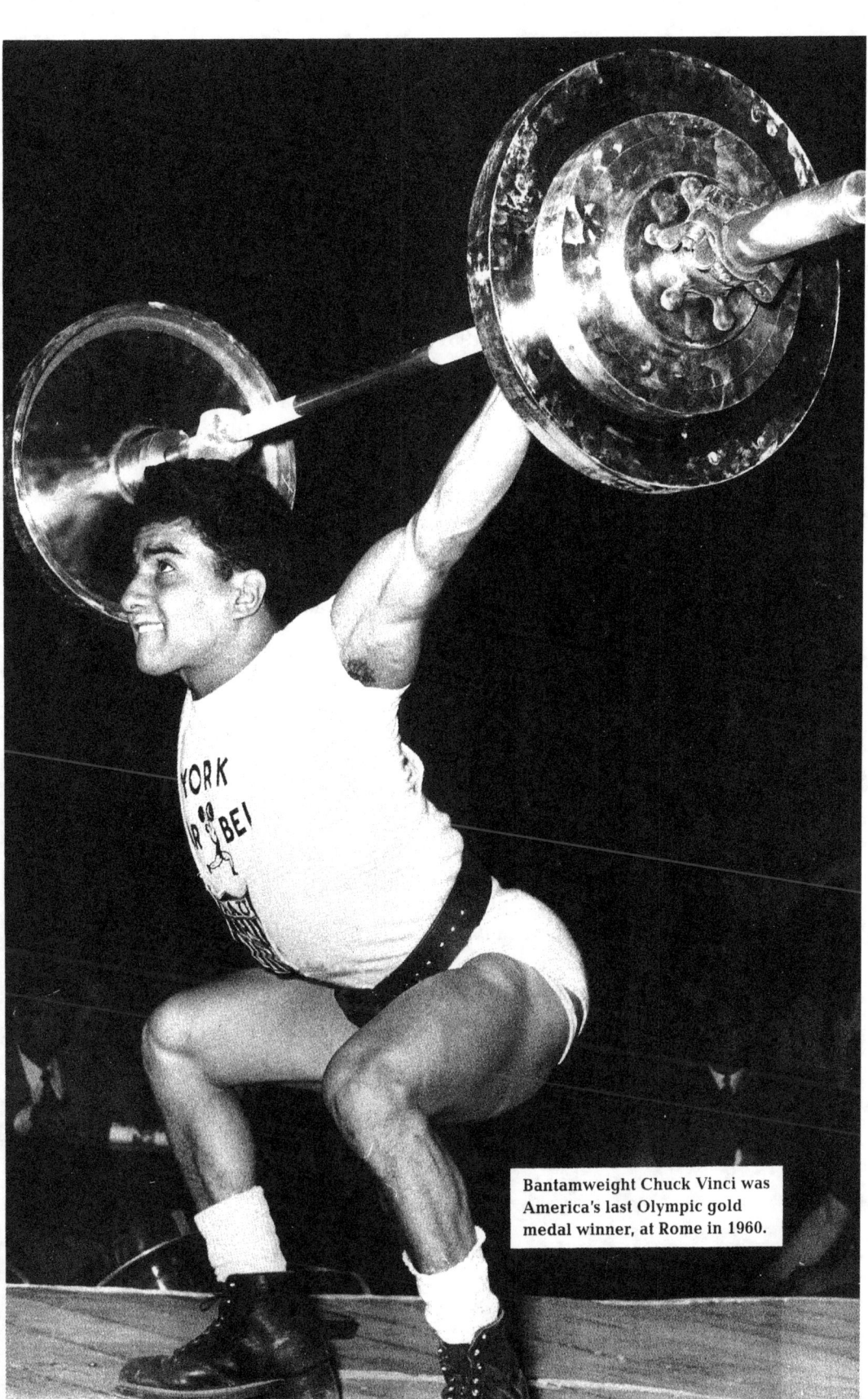

Bantamweight Chuck Vinci was America's last Olympic gold medal winner, at Rome in 1960.

THE "GOLDEN AGE" OF AMERICAN WEIGHTLIFTING

Still, Hoffman was immensely successful by the early 1960s. Hi-Proteen and other diet supplements had raised the company out of its financial doldrums and allowed him to amass a fortune. By dint of will, Bob survived a host of legal and bureaucratic hassles and rose above his own careless management practices. During this period he could also take pride in the widespread acceptance of weight training by athletes in other sports. After decades of propagating this notion, Bob observed to a friend in 1957 that "weight training for athletes is taking on like the Hula hoop for kids." York, however, was still beset by adversaries. One was the Soviet Union, which had clearly established dominance in weightlifting. Yet as late as 1959 the United States still held more world records than the Soviets, 14 to 11. Even after the loss in Rome, Hoffman consoled himself by calculating that if Berger and Kono had "made two or three snatches instead of just one each, they could have been gold medal winners, and the team score would have been 38 for the U.S. to 36 for the U.S.S.R."[45] Likewise, only by reading the past from a present perspective could Weider be characterized as outdistancing Hoffman. Though Weider was making gains, he was still in Hoffman's wake, even in bodybuilding. The spirit of "Muscletown" in this splendorous era was best captured by Harry Paschall, who observed in 1956: "Each new day is an adventure, for we never know who will next come through our door, nor from what far-flung country they may have traveled. These visitors represent every strata of life and every possible profession or calling. We meet ballplayers, wrestlers, boxers, track and field athletes, coaches, physical education men, professors, musicians, actors, entertainers, preachers, bartenders and hitch-hikers. All of these people have one thing in common . . . they have all been bitten by the virulent *barbell bug.*"[46] In the 1950s, all avenues to success and fame in the iron game led through York, as Bob realized his ambitions for power and glory. It was an era in which he probably came closest to fulfilling his manly aspirations.

7
THE "NEW" YORK GANG

> The vices of great men are usually on the same scale as their virtues.
>
> —Sam Keen, *Fire in the Belly*

For three decades Hoffman had been a father figure to American lifters, a tradition that went back to the inception of his oil-burner team. Some of the old York gang were still with him. By the 1960s Bob could be likened even to a grandfather figure. Unlike the first generation, many of his next group of champions, like Kono, George, and Schemansky, never resided in York, and administrators like Van Cleef, Murray, and Bob Hasse, never in full harmony with their elders, moved on. Hence no coherent transition group was displaced when the third generation (largely from Texas) descended on Muscletown in the 1960s. The new York gang was not only much younger but more innovative and ambitious, and eager to institute a new social order. A renewed camaraderie was evident during a Sunday visit to the Maryland State Prison by "two carloads of Yorkites" in July 1959. "Not since the tough but happy barnstorming days of the early 40's had York lifters put on a demonstration behind bars," Hasse noted.[1] The most distinguishing generational criterion, besides age, was education. Although most of the old gang were high school graduates, only Venables had attended college. For the new gang, college was the norm; some even held higher degrees. What they brought to York was a more scientific approach to training and fitness. Institutionalized in the Hoffman Foundation, this new spirit encouraged such innovations as functional isometric contraction, anabolic steroids, powerlifting, a journal for bodybuilders, and a new line of products designed to keep York in the forefront.

Bob's Books on Aging

Much of this progress, however, depended on Hoffman's continued vitality. More than ever conscious of his age, he published a book entitled *You Can Live Longer, 10–20–30 Years Longer*, which purportedly verified his claim to be the world's healthiest man. Here was "new hope, new scientific truths," for anyone affected by aging. Its message was that the elderly should follow his example by being active. Bob was inspired by York millionaire Mahlon Haines, an octogenarian who was "full of life and full of fun." He was a self-made man who epitomized Pennsylvania Dutch virtues of energy, enterprise, and hard work.

> I like him because he is the man I hope to be when I am 85, he likes me because I advocate the same habits of living he does. Mahlon Haines does not smoke, he will give anyone five dollars for a promise to stop smoking, he does not drink alcoholics, does not use tea or coffee, eats lightly and simply, natural foods when obtainable, and . . . follows the most important essential of health, exercise. In his case, surprisingly vigorous exercise.
> And I hope he won't mind me saying it, but he is a lover.

Hoffman's eulogy of Haines, however, was merely a segue to extol his own accomplishments. Even in his sixties, he needed to define his manliness in physical terms and portray an impression of perpetual youth. This manliness was characterized by his stamina in meeting the demands of a busy schedule. In 1960 he completed five books (along with six health-related articles per month), held "21 major jobs" in the AAU, attended eighty or ninety weightlifting meets, visited thirty-five countries for the State Department, was president of six corporations, and once a week danced "like a fiend" for the fun of it.² Hoffman appeared to be a sixty-two-year-old superman.

Underlying this hyperbole, however, was a fear of aging and a desire to delay the inevitable. In addition to information on nutrition, Bob provided advice on exercise and health. While much of it—avoidance of smoking, stimulants, and alcohol, and practicing the Daily Dozen—was sound, some of it, such as eating no breakfast and consuming almost nothing until evening, was questionable. But since *he* practiced this diet, it had to be right for everyone. In many respects, too, he fell short of the ideals he prescribed, flagrantly violating his rules for healthful living. He undertook the briefest exercise sessions and attributed miraculous results to them. It is unlikely that he had a balanced diet, given his neglect of fruit and his periods of eating little but Hi-Proteen. And he was addicted to junk foods, especially ice cream and candy. "Bob ate what he liked," recalls Terpak. "He loved chocolate. It was nothing for Bob to sit down and eat a pound box of candy." Hoffman's most serious shortcoming was sleeping too little. "Loss of sleep is quite harmful," he warned in *Old Age Is a Slow Starvation*. Yet he boasted of how his busy schedule never allowed him to sleep more than five hours a night. Such rules obviously applied only to mere mortals, not strong men! Whether he was too work-oriented to maintain a tranquil mind is arguable, but his frequent transgressions of sexual norms must have been unsettling. The latter half of his book on aging is devoted to diet, where the object of selling his products is obvious. "The shortage of protein," he stated, "is the greatest causative factor in aging."³ But much of his information, with extensive quotes from the 1959 Department of Agriculture yearbook, was derived from Arnold Lorand's *Old Age Deferred* and Elmer McCollum's *Food, Nutrition, and Health*, published in 1910 and 1925 respectively—hardly the latest scientific treatises.

Drawing from the same kinds of sources in his library, Hoffman in quick succession published the following paperback works: *The Protein Story*, *Protein-Building Blocks of Life*, and the *High Protein Recipe Book*. To make his writings credible, the covers featured the high-sounding titles he had appropriated for himself—"Father of American Weight Lifting," "Mr. Physical Fitness," "World Famous Authority on Nutrition," and "World's Healthiest Man." Also included were pictures of him with President Kennedy, former vice president Nixon, and the shah of Iran, which were intended to lend prestige by association. But over half of *Protein Story* and much of *Protein-Building Blocks* was copied word for word from *Protein Nutrition,* a 1958 publication of the New York Academy of Sciences. The recipe book was a collection of recipes, from beef stew to cookies, borrowed from standard cookbooks, with specified amounts of high protein added.[4] Hoffman thereby added another dimension to his marketing strategy.

Isometrics

A quite different innovation was functional isometric contraction. In what he called "The Most Important Article I Ever Wrote," Bob revealed his system to the world in the November 1961 issue of *Strength & Health,* and simultaneously released three accompanying models of isometric-isotonic apparatus priced at $29.95, $39.95, and $99.95. A book followed in 1962. As with earlier promotions of barbells and Hi-Proteen, he claimed to have been the first to discover the system and its benefits, stating that a prototype of the isometric power rack was mentioned in his 1938 *Guide to Weight Lifting Competition.* He dismissed earlier applications of the principle by educators at Springfield College in the 1920s and by E. A. Muller in Germany in the 1950s as "inconsequential," stating that its revelation came "like a bolt out of a clear sky" at a meeting in his office with Grimek and Terpak: "At that place at that moment an idea was born which was destined to revolutionize physical training." With isometrics "muscles may be worked to their limit for one supreme effort" and "do not become tired. New growth in cells and muscle tissues takes place at once." One "can train twice as often" and expect to "gain two to four times as fast." What Hoffman envisioned, reflective of his own abbreviated exercise periods, was "hope for American weightlifting." His favorite sales pitch became "One Minute a Day—The Functional Isometric Contraction Way." It was "the greatest system the world has ever seen."[5]

This portrayal was deceptive. Bob's enthusiasm for his new product far exceeded his understanding of it, and he failed to give credit to its real creator. Only once in his book *Functional Isometric Contraction* is Dr. John Ziegler cited. Since 1954 Ziegler had been associated with the York gang on an occasional basis, but in the months preceding the 1960 Olympics they became closer. Hoffman seemed pleased that men of science—medical doctors and educators with Ph.D.'s—were supporting a cause that could make him even more wealthy and famous. It was Grimek who, in January 1959, resurrected York's connection with Ziegler. Responding to his request for some magazine articles, Ziegler revealed that he was studying the "one a day maximum contraction of muscle" theory. He had collected "quite a bit of information," but had "not definitely proven anything. I am interested in following it up." How much Hoffman knew about the new technique is uncertain, but it was reminiscent of the Atlas system of "dynamic tension" he once condemned. Now it was being endorsed by various professors. One of them, C. H. McCloy of the State University of Iowa, is shown demonstrating these nonapparatus exercises in a 1959 issue of *Strength & Health*. "The results in terms of *strengthening* of the muscle," he argued, "may be very marked." With Bob's blessing, company assistant Dick Smith in late 1959 began making regular trips to Olney with Bill March, a budding young all-around athlete from York, who was to be trained by Ziegler. In addition to the isometrics, March was provided with "copious quantities of Hi-Proteen and Energol, vitamins, particularly Liver-Iron and Vitamin B12," and subjected to "positive-thinking" therapy that "verged on hypnotism." None of these aids appeared to affect him.[6]

Anabolic Steroids

Soon, however, another, even more potent training aid appeared. Anabolic steroids were developed in the 1930s, but their use in succeeding decades was limited to rehabilitating the weak and elderly.[7] That they could also be used to enhance athletic performance was a recent revelation, and it was fitting that Ziegler should be involved. Grimek recalls that "CIBA got in touch with him asking him if he wanted to try these steroids on athletes, since they knew he got involved with the lifters. He gave me one of those half-bushel baskets with the pills to try and get some of the lifters to try them. No one would." By the time Hoffman returned from the European championships in May, Ziegler suspected that "the Russians [were] giving their athletes 'something.'" He therefore asked Grimek to propose to Bob that steroids be administered to prospective members of the Olympic team. Hoffman, though interested, was cautious. The Olympics were "too close to give [steroids] to the men who will represent the USA," was Grimek's reply.

"Apparently, [Hoffman] doesn't think it will do that much good, and may even have detrimental effects." Meanwhile Grimek persuaded two fellow trainees—Jake Hitchens and Bill March—to take the drug. The former soon proved unsatisfactory. But March, after taking steroid tablets (ten milligrams per day) for a month, was "showing improvement and look[ed] better." In place of Hitchens, Grimek enlisted Tony Garcy, a twenty-year-old lightweight who had moved to York to train after winning the 1960 nationals. After only two months on steroids, he added nearly a hundred pounds to his lifts. Later, however, he attributed his miraculous progress to mental coaching he had received at York from Kono. "I was training hard at the time," Garcy recalled, "but the most important thing, I believe, was the fact that Tommy Kono was 'grooming' me mentally."[8] And what mental preparation seemed to be doing for Garcy, isometrics were finally starting to do for March. The lifting gains were obvious; that they came from steroids was not. By the time of the Olympics, Hoffman relented on his previous antisteroid stance. He administered steroids to certain American lifters in Rome, seemingly without knowledge of appropriate timing or doses.[9] A comparison of the Olympic performances of American lifters with their highest previous totals shows that four registered gains, two declined, and one stayed the same. The Soviets, handily beating them, displayed spectacular increases over previous outings. Admittedly there were many possible factors, including the added inspiration of the Olympics, but no one at York was prepared to ascribe any gains by American or foreign athletes to steroid usage.

Louis Riecke

At this juncture Ziegler developed a relationship with Louis Riecke of New Orleans, who had been a national-level lifter since 1947. Though he had won the junior nationals in 1955, he was never able to break into the top echelon of America's strongest men. With a B.S. in zoology and biochemistry and two years of medical school at Louisiana State University, Riecke established an immediate rapport with Ziegler. In October 1960 they met in the lobby of the Yorktowne Hotel, where Ziegler mysteriously mentioned a "discovery he had come across that would increase strength remarkably." Back home, Riecke pondered the gains made by March and Garcy under Ziegler's supervision and agreed to similar treatments. In November he spent several days at Olney to learn this new training routine. Riecke had been introduced to isometrics by Francis Drury at Louisiana State University (LSU) but had not been impressed by it. Now he was willing to give it a serious try, persuaded by Ziegler's pitch that "the way you improve is by lifting weights, the heaviest possible. What's the heaviest weight you can lift?—one you can't lift!" In Ziegler's garage Riecke experimented with various lifting positions on an apparatus called the power rack, a device evolved from a series of safety racks developed in the 1950s. His experiment called for a "single maximal contraction performed once a day in a group of eight exercises." Once a week he would test his gains by lifting limit poundages with a barbell. "To assure proper nutrition to the exerted muscles, the subject was given an anabolic daily," but Riecke had no idea how these pills would effect his performance. A different kind of experiment was undertaken by Hoffman. After administering steroids to his lifters in Rome, he took them himself for six weeks. A year later he told readers that he had conducted some "training experiments" with an emphasis on nutrition. As a result of "continued regular use" of Hoffman supplements, he had "gained at an amazing rate and soon developed noticeable muscles." Seven years later he admitted that he had taken "anabolics" and that they had increased his strength: "In five days I could curl and press more and I gained weight." Bob insisted that he never took them again and did not recommend their use.[10]

Isometrics Spin-Offs

During the next several months Riecke, using both isometrics and steroids, made phenomenal progress, posting a 925 total in Dallas in January 1961—thirty-five pounds above his official best and identical to the total of the bronze medalist in Rome. News of Riecke's gains aroused "more than a little curiosity" among his workout partners and friends, and Ziegler was badgered by York. On February 1 he informed Riecke that "Grimek & Hoffman have called me several times . . . asking if I have been working with you as *your* results in Dallas have been very well noticed all over the U.S.A. So far, I have made no admissions as per our agreement—but 'Ole Strong John' Grimek is getting wise with his 'come on Doc, you're up to something.' " Riecke also received a letter from Hasse congratulating him for his Dallas total. As Riecke wrote Ziegler, "I shall acknowledge his letter, of course, but shall neglect to make any mention of a question he asked. ('Are you taking Doc Ziegler's mysterious pink pills?')" Curiosity hounds were led still further off the scent by Riecke's statement in *Strength & Health* that his "recent sensational improvement" was due to "intensified *mental concentration*"— misleading perhaps, but not inaccurate. Privately Riecke was uncertain about any connection between his altered physical state and the pills. He told Ziegler, "[I am] amazed at this constant feeling of euphoria and energy I have. I don't know whether it is occasioned by the workout, the pills, or delight over my progress."[11]

In the meantime, March was receiving the same ergogenic aids as Riecke, the only difference being that he used a partial-movement (isotonic) routine. Since April 1960 his total had increased from 800 to 970, though he had advanced into the mid-heavy class. Hoffman was so happy with March's 950 at the national YMCA meet in Toledo, he told Kono in April 1961, that "I could stay awake driving all night for I knew what this would do to keep you, Bradford and Schemanski in the game for a long time, without . . . too much abuse of your muscles." Bob had seven more racks made for his champions across the country. "You are already the world's best presser," he told Kono, "and if this would help you, as it should, your records would be fantastic." Fearing "the Russians [were] using a similar system," Hoffman lent his revelations to America's best lifter an air of secrecy, but the secret was isometrics, not steroids: "There is the story about the acres of diamonds, looking all over the world for them when they were right on the farm. For nearly thirty years we have been writing and talking about making this machine, we have had the steps at the gym, and held weights overhead in a variety of ways, but it took us all this time to build this machine." Still, Riecke's even greater gains remained a mystery. Therefore Hoffman flew him to York on Memorial Day weekend to consult with him and Ziegler. As they sat in his living room, Riecke recalls, Hoffman asked what was responsible for his improvements. Ziegler looked at his protégé and said, "Tell him." Riecke then explained how he had been using isometrics over the previous six months and described the changes it had wrought. "We can't have this," was Bob's immediate response. "We have to sell weights."[12] Hoffman was at last enlightened.

The "New" York Gang

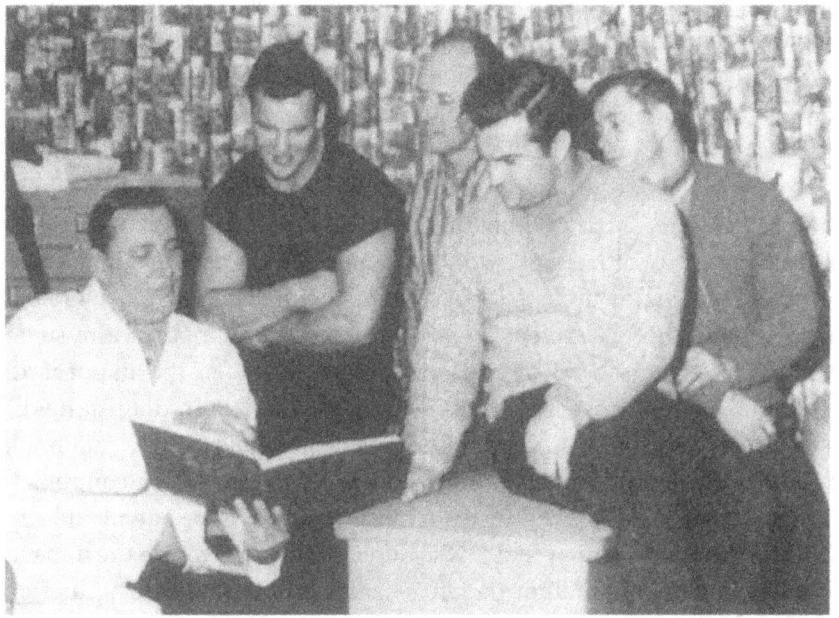

Dr. John Ziegler consulting with members of the "new" York gang—Bob Bednarski, Dick Smith, Homer Brannum, and Tony Garcy—at the Hoffman Foundation in the mid-1960s.

Whatever hopes Ziegler may have had for Riecke culminated in a showdown with Kono at the 1961 senior nationals in Los Angeles in June. After the press and snatch, the lifters were tied with subtotals of 600. In the clean and jerk Riecke made 365, while Kono made 380 and chose to save his last lift for whatever it might take to win. Riecke gambled that 380 would be enough for victory on lighter bodyweight. Despite all the components he had drawn from Ziegler's strength arsenal, he failed to negotiate it. But Hoffman was ecstatic. "Tommy was the champion, but Riecke was the sensation of the meet, for he lifted 105 pounds more than he did one year ago." Seeing was believing, and on the basis of such compelling evidence of its effectiveness, Hoffman decided to go public with isometrics. By the end of the summer he had assembled a line of static-contraction products for sale in *Strength & Health*. Soon *Sports Illustrated*, with testimony from Riecke, March, and Hoffman, was broadcasting the "no-sweat, no-pain" system of muscle building to a broader audience.[13]

Over the next year Ziegler plied his subjects with a variety of techniques to enhance the apparent benefits of isometrics. In addition to steroids, he used hypnotism, biorhythms, a medication that relieved fatigue by restoring potassium ions to muscle cells, and a machine called the isotron, which duplicated (via three watts of electricity) nerve impulses from the brain to skeletal muscles. March and Riecke differ in their assessments of the relative worth of the scientific notions conjured up by Ziegler. March regards the rack as "the most effective," while the pill also had much to do with his success. Riecke believes steroids had the greatest impact, followed by isometrics, the mental stimulation provided by Ziegler, and just "getting into the mainstream of American lifting." Both lifters also feel they benefited from hypnotism. But such estimations could be no more than conjecture, given the haphazard nature of Ziegler's research. Jim George, now an Akron dentist, holds a dim view of Ziegler's scientific approach: "Ziegler was a goddamn nut. He certainly was no researcher and worked in totally uncontrolled settings."[14] He administered such a large number of ergogenic aids in such an irregular manner that it was impossible to tell where the impact of one stopped and another began. Those who attribute conspiratorial designs to Ziegler, and by extension to Hoffman, must reckon with the fact that neither party was sure what was being discovered.

To most observers in the early 1960s it appeared that isometrics was the most active agent. Hoffman received abundant testimonials on its effectiveness. A real hotbed was LSU, where various individuals—Alvin Roy, Marty Broussard, and Francis Drury—were doing research. By 1962 Drury had three projects going on isometrics. One, with track and field athletes, was "getting unusually good results." At the University of Alabama, Paul "Bear" Bryant's trainer, Jim Goostree, expressed confidence in isometrics, and Norm Olson, a football and track coach at Florida State, reported "splendid results." In the 1961–62 season Olson's team posted a 10–0 record, including nine shutouts. His track team was state runner-up. Jim Rasmusson of Lansing, Michigan, found he was gaining more strength from the power rack than he formerly had from two-hour-a-day lifting workouts. He also sent a diagram for a collapsible model "to fit any automobile trunk" for Hoffman to market. Health-club operator Ken Stoller of Buffalo reported, "Isometric training is a great boon for my business and we have all noticed improvements training on the rack." In twenty-five years "as competitor, coach, and official," stated Eldon Dreher of Detroit, "I would unhesitatingly state nothing has approached your isometric-isotonic rack for assistance in physical improvement." Fourteen-year-old Gordon Stamp of Wayzata, Minnesota,

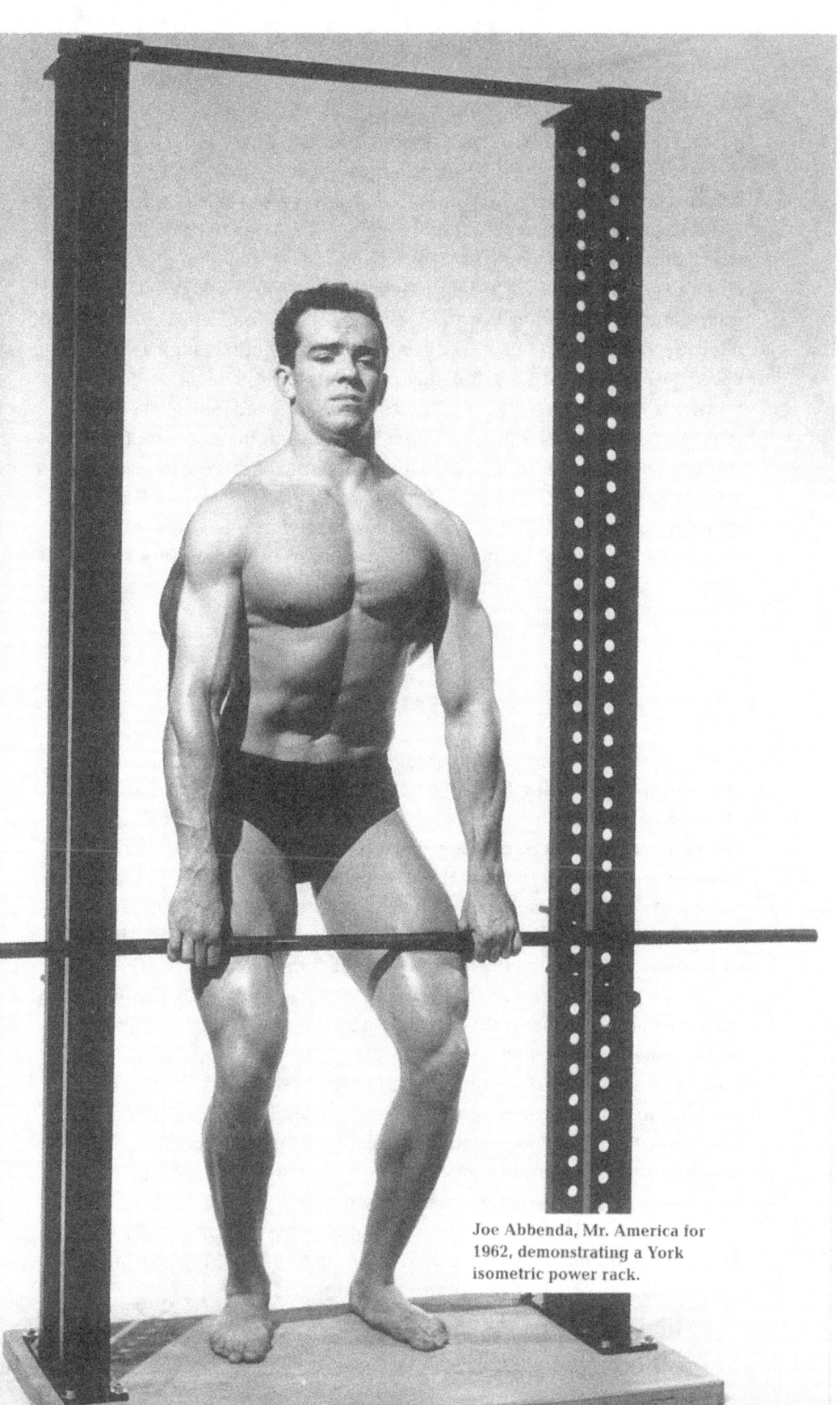

Joe Abbenda, Mr. America for 1962, demonstrating a York isometric power rack.

had never used barbells, but isometric contraction was "really working." He had "turned into one of the strongest boys in [his] school." After being stuck in the low three hundreds for several years, "old-timer" R. W. Partridge of Evanston, Illinois, reported a 9 percent bench-press gain after adopting isometrics. He even found reference to it in Victor Hugo's *Les Miserables:* "Certain convicts who were forever dreaming of escape ended by making a veritable science of force and skill combined. It is the science of muscles. An entire system of mysterious statics is daily practiced by prisoners." After making gains from isometrics, Robert Warner, a hammer thrower at Williams College, called himself "a walking testimonial." At first he was ridiculed for using the rack, but fellow students, administrators, and townspeople ("from barbers to ministers") were ultimately won over to it. Finally, Harvey Newton of St. David's, Pennsylvania, was a fifteen-year-old student who raised his total by ninety-five pounds on isometrics. It marked the beginning of a career that led to a directing role in American weightlifting two decades later.[15]

Science and Education

Isometrics and Ziegler were the most visible scientific influences at York in the post-Sputnik era. Doctors and educators were beckoned to Muscletown, where their academic attainments were flaunted to support the York way. For decades would-be strong men and fitness enthusiasts had visited Muscletown. Now there was a professional clientele, whose names and titles were dropped frequently in *Strength & Health*. An article by Pete George, D.D.S., on "The Psychology of Weightlifting" appeared in November 1961. Dr. S. E. Bilik, who "headed the Department of Physical Medicine at New York's famed Bellevue Hospital," authored an article in 1962. The July 1963 issue brought to light the work of Pat O'Shea, a physical educator at Oregon State University, and Dr. Frank Corbett, a graduate of Duke University Medical School, both lifting enthusiasts. An article entitled "Isometrics in the Home" by Dr. Richard Berger, a respected lifter and faculty member at Texas Tech, was featured in December 1963. In 1967 there was an article on "The Science of Health" by Francis Wm. Brown, who held degrees from MIT and Harvard and had taught at seven universities. Through Clarence Johnson, Hoffman became attached to Dr. Russell Wright, physician for the Detroit Tigers, who began to accompany American teams abroad as You and Ziegler had formerly done. York had come a long way since its reliance on Frederick Tilney. Even Hoffman was claiming that he had "attended a famous university" before World War I.[16]

In addition, more York lifters were pursuing higher education, some at Hoffman's expense. Scholarships were awarded to light-heavy Joe Puleo and mid-heavy Gary Glenney to attend York Junior College and to Garcy to attend Millersville State College. Pete and Jim George, with Bob's assistance, received multiple degrees from Ohio State University, and their classmate John Pulskamp, upon completion of his M.D., instituted the "Ask the Doctor" column in *Strength & Health* in 1964. Other physicians who were outstanding strength athletes included eye surgeon Craig Whitehead and John Gourgott, who placed third and fourth respectively at the 1963 Mr. America contest. And 1966 Mr. America Bob Gajda, influenced by his premedical training, introduced a training concept called Peripheral Heart Action (PHA), aimed at stimulating uniform development rather than focusing on specific body areas. Educational values were also embraced by such members of the old gang as Terpak, Bacon, Grimek, and John Terlazzo, who proudly sent their progeny off to college. The centerpiece of York's new emphasis on education and science was the Hoffman Foundation, originally housed in a wing of the Ridge Avenue headquarters, but in 1963 transferred to a separate facility built by Hoffman near his home in Dover. In addition to providing scholarships, the foundation distributed grants to professors working on isometrics and other projects, and tested food supplements. These tests were conducted in a laboratory under chemist Donald Nickol, who monitored quality and new-product development. Bob hoped eventually to host meetings of scientists and foster learning. In 1964 Terry Todd was brought in to coordinate these endeavors. Whether Hoffman was sincere in wanting to help retarded children or "those who suffer from cerebral palsy, muscular dystrophy, multiple sclerosis, polio and similar diseases" seems doubtful in retrospect.[17]

Planning for the Future

Directly related to Bob's foundation plans were a myriad of other enterprises and investments. "Next door" to his home he bought a sizable

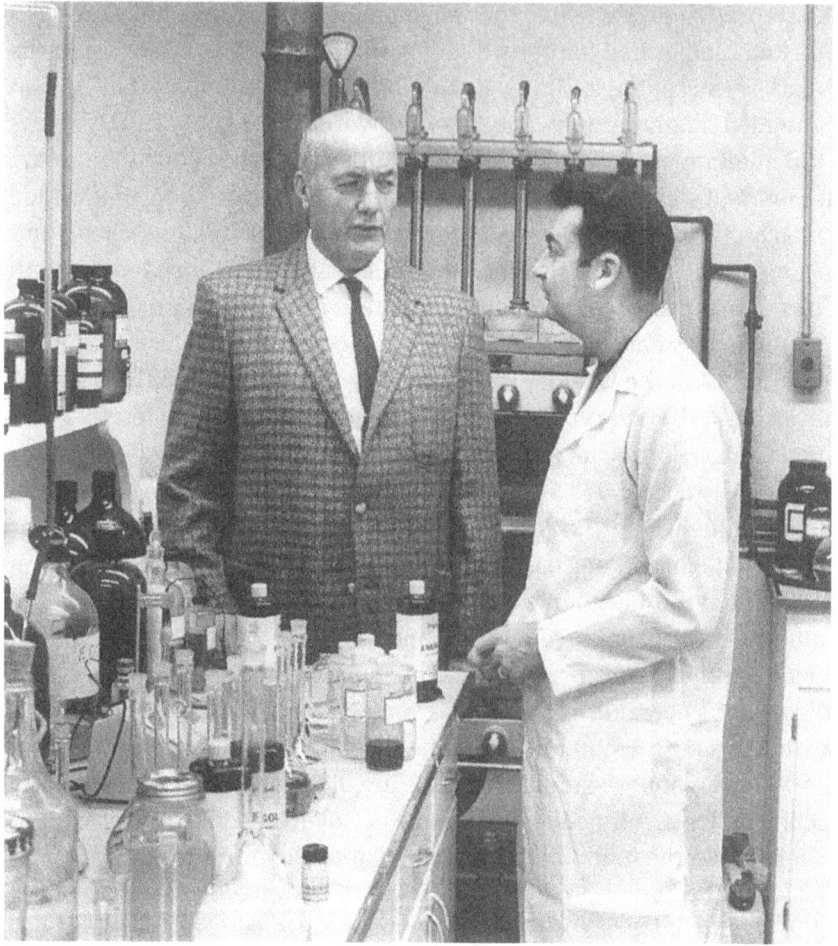

Hoffman with his chemist Don Nickol at the Hoffman Foundation laboratory. Although Bob used the foundation to provide scientific credibility for his products and methods, most of its work consisted of outside contracts, chiefly for water testing.

farm, enabling him to grow soybeans organically. In a new industrial park in north York he purchased a tract of land that would later become the center for all York Barbell operations. Seventy miles west, in Greencastle, he acquired, in 1963, half interest in Better Foods Foundation, producers of natural-food products. A few years later, after buying two additional city blocks, he opened a combination health-food outlet and bakery. "We believe that we have the largest health food store in the nation," he exclaimed. "It's fabulous!" And Hoffman could also boast of having the largest spring in Pennsylvania, at Boiling Spring, which produced 250 gallons of pure water a minute. Through Dr. Wright, he secured partial interest in a spring in northern California that produced hot water for bathing and cold water for drinking. In southern California he salvaged an ailing heath-food operation, much as he had done earlier with York Precision and York Light House, and established a Los Angeles outlet for his products under Tony Terlazzo. Even farther afield were arrangements he made after a visit to the East to import seaweed extract and other protein ingredients from Japan. Soon Bob was producing "Protein from the Sea" and a new "Oriental wonder food" called Forinake and importing juicers from Fuji Corporation in Tokyo.[18] He was still an opportunist and innovator.

Experience or Science?

Despite repeated references to scientific methods, the means by which Bob developed new products was not unlike the way he had conjured Hi-Proteen in a vat with his canoe paddle. At best he would peddle concoctions sent to him by his wholesale supplier in Philadelphia, Winston Day, confirming their efficacy on the basis of personal testimony. Whether gathering apples and hazelnuts in West Virginia at age ten or rowing for the "world famous" Vesper Boat Club on the Schuylkill River as an adult, personal experience counted for more than scientific evidence. Aside from the creative genius of Ziegler, whose method was flawed, Bob had no great faith in science: for athletes "we suggest that *improved performance* is what they seek when it comes to a weight-training program, not 'scientific proof of training methods.' " Typical of Hoffman's method of product development was the way he derived Hi-Proteen Honey Fudge. Inspiration came from John Terpak Jr. and his football companions at York's William Penn High in the late 1950s. The team used Hi-Proteen tablets—ten before the game and ten at halftime. Once, after Terpak made a ninety-six-yard run and was tackled on the one-yard line, he said afterward, "Dad, if I had had just one more Hi-Proteen tablet, I would have made it." Hoffman reasoned that not just one more tablet but the addition of honey and peanut butter could have made a difference. "So we came up with the Hi-Proteen Honey Fudge." By 1962 York offered fifty-seven packaged products, just like H. J. Heinz Company of Bob's native Pittsburgh.[19]

Hoffman realized that science, a two-edged sword, could support or refute the egoistic truths that underlay his endeavors. Any findings that questioned the viability of his products, techniques, or lifestyle had to be dismissed. The research of Karl Klein, a University of Texas professor who found that squats unduly stretched the knee ligaments, Hoffman identified as a threat. Klein's rationale for weight-trained athletes to perform half squats appeared in physical-education journals and reached the public through *Sports Illustrated*.[20] His formulations, based on *"scientific fact,* rather than personal observations," reinforced the prejudices of football coaches against squats. Rather than accept Klein's evidence at face value, Hoffman concluded it was wrong and announced a $1,200 grant for research "to prove that full knee bends are not harmful to the knees, do not stretch ligaments, and are a valuable form of physical training." Whether anyone did so is not known, but he rejected Klein's offer to cooperate in further testing at the foundation. In succeeding issues of his magazines, Bob marshaled three physicians who were sympathetic to his views (Corbett, Pulskamp, and Samuel Homola) but had done no independent research and three of the greatest figures in the iron game (Grimek, Sig Klein, and Paul Anderson) to condemn Klein's "scientific facts." Terry Todd is probably right in assuming that the characteristic these writers shared was that "none of them had read Klein's articles."[21]

A more stinging rebuke of York tenets came from Philip Rasch of the California College of Medicine, who tried to determine whether protein supplements, with weight training, increased strength and muscle mass. Contrary to Hoffman's claims, he found no differences between his two control groups (one taking a placebo). Rasch concluded that additional protein intake by male college students "does not increase the amount of body weight, muscular hypertrophy or strength" gained from weight training. "This article is not to your credit," was Hoffman's sharp retort. He criticized Rasch's research design—the short testing period, using tablets with only 20 percent protein, and employing just arm exercises. He also pointed out that hammer thrower Bob Backus gained fifty pounds in a year of training with Hi-Proteen, "more than he had gained in eight years without it." But such individual cases were "scientifically meaningless" to Rasch. He pointed out that the type and quantity of protein had been prescribed by Hoffman. The short time period was beyond Rasch's control, and he used arm exercises because he had no immersion tank large enough to accommodate legs or torsos. The cost of additional equipment for a larger study he estimated to be about $8,000. He suggested that Hoffman might be willing to underwrite it. Unsure of the results it would produce, Bob made no such offer. Nor did he take up the proposition of Gerald McCabe, a Chicago surgeon he met at the 1963 senior nationals. McCabe offered laboratory facilities to verify Hoffman's claims that Vitamin E and Energol lowered cholesterol: "I don't think a real objective study has been made and just because it makes you feel better that doesn't mean it works. You talked about cholesterol levels in the blood, but have samples really been taken, have laboratory studies been done?" Yet Hoffman, rather than obtain independent verification on product effectiveness, continued to elude the FDA and to protest when caught. That he had sympathy in high places is indicated by the reaction of Senator Edward Long, chairman of the Administrative Practice Subcommittee, when Bob had to remove his picture from labels because customers might think they too could win Olympic awards: "The thought arises as to whether Quaker Oats should be required to remove the picture of the Quaker from their package, or whether the FDA should mind its own business."[22] Long's implication was that consumers might believe they would start looking like the Quaker!

In light of his preference for experience over scientific data, Hoffman was receptive to testimonials from athletes. He also received enthusiastic endorsements from readers. Occasionally, however, he received one such as the following from the "poison pen" of Thomas Davis of Fontana, California:

> After having diligently practiced Functional *Isometric Contraction* Training for the better part of a year, I have come to the opinion that its usefulness is limited—very limited. . . . Your claim that you can double your strength in 5 months with this system if you are a beginner is utterly false or else my body is abnormal. . . . I've tried every conceivable position in each exercise & varying numbers of movements daily. I've rested & I've worked hard. The results total *zero* every time. . . . I've also come to the conclusion that if you tend to exaggerate in one thing, then you might have exaggerated in another matter, such as your health foods.

By this time Hoffman had concluded that his wonder system had not lived up to expectations. Not only had it not catapulted America back to the front rank of lifting powers, but it had proved unprofitable. Although many copies of his courses had been distributed, relatively few power racks had been sold. To such an extent had isometrics "weakened the financial structure of York Barbell" by 1963 that Hoffman curtailed further research on it and toned down his advertising. Ironically, isometrics, originally a promotional gimmick, has survived the test of time. As sociologist Jon Rieger notes, "[B]oth the power rack and isometrics have become centrally embedded in the strength sports right down through the present!"[23]

Health-Food Expansion

What kept York buoyant in the sixties was protein supplements. Hi-Proteen, a best seller in the 1950s, exceeded the million-dollar mark in 1960 and soon accounted for half of Hoffman's sales. In 1961 Bob gloated over an announcement by Balanced Foods, a major distributor in New York, that it was discontinuing its Weider and Atlas lines: "They came and they have gone. Hoffman's Hi-Proteen is the number one high protein product in the health food industry." That this was not an idle claim can be seen from steadily mounting sales figures in the 1960s, amounting to a near million-dollar increase in seven years.

1960—$1,875,923	1963—$2,207,444	1966—$2,582,917
1961—$2,207,782	1964—$2,503,425	1967—$2,856,388
1962—$2,235,187	1965—$2,704,014	

An interesting feature of these otherwise bright figures is the 1963 sales slump attributed to isometrics. What they do not show is income Bob received from his many other enterprises. Thomasville Inn, for instance, owned by Alda for tax purposes, netted about $12,000 in 1967, mostly from beer and liquor sales. Barbell sales remained brisk, and York successfully resisted a national trend toward composition (concrete, plastic, etc.) plates in the 1960s. Still, Hoffman had no recourse but to develop a larger stake in diet foods, where less manufacturing, shipping, and overhead left more room for profit. Net profits for 1965 were $161,993, noted Dietz, with facilities being "used to the peak of their capacity."[24]

The "New" York Gang

As his protein supplements grew popular, Hoffman sought promotional opportunities in various health-food organizations, thus adding another element to his hectic schedule. At the 1962 meeting of the National Health Federation in Columbus his lecture on strong and healthy children prompted one of the most remarkable tributes ever paid to Bob. Marie Elledge of the House of Natural Living in Springfield, Illinois, wrote: "Your great humility and humanitarian love which radiates as you so unselfishly serve for others, truly reveals that you have a deep spiritual understanding, such as manifested by Our Master." Never had Hoffman been credited with spiritual qualities or humility, or compared with Jesus Christ—all in one letter! Bob averaged four lecture/demonstrations per week, often assisted by Bill March. In a letter to Milton Low, president of the National Dietary Foods Association, he agreed to speak at his organization's 1963 meeting: "I could appear two or three times, for I sometimes talk for three hours and there are lots of angles to healthful living." At one of these gatherings, Terpak recalls, there was a forty-five-minute limit. When the emcee told him his time had expired, Hoffman stated, "I haven't finished my introduction."[25] He relished these occasions, not only to publicize his products or promote health and fitness, but to speak endlessly to a captive audience about his favorite subject—himself!

Any doubts Hoffman may have had about his mission were dispelled by letters from readers applauding York's stand for truth, justice, and the American way, at least as defined in the early sixties. In 1961 Dick Walter of Fort Wayne, Indiana, shared his regrets for following Weider's system. After building the "biggest set of 16 year old biceps in town," he acquired "the stretch marks and shrinkage scars to show for it" when he stopped training. Joseph Rexroad of Frederick, Maryland, reported that he had progressed with York programs and products until he read one of the competition's magazines: "I tried a few of the lifts using the weights that it suggested. . . . The next day I had to see a doctor who told me I would need an operation." In 1962 Arthur Abels of the Bronx noted that it was "too bad that you have so many 'rival bodybuilding' magazines which are published simply for the satisfaction . . . of homosexuals, the worst of which are Weedy's YOUNG PHYSIQUE and DEMI-GODS." Only *Iron Man* approximated York's quality. Particularly satisfying to Bob must have been a letter from Howard Corlman of Cheyenne, Wyoming, who analyzed flaws in a recent issue of Weider's *Mr. America:* "In most of his magazines we find testimonials by French-Canadians, Syrians, Turks, etc., BUT VERY, VERY FEW AMERICANS. Can it be that Joseph has to sell his gear abroad?? I know of no one who prefers his equipment . . . in fact, most are disappointed." Donald Miller of Chicopee, Massachusetts, was offended by Weider's concern for money over the welfare of his clientele: "All of this combined with slanted views on bodybuilding and weightlifting, fantasticly impossible self-defence courses and sexy pin-ups flocking around sexyer, he-man 'Weider built' muscle men almost made me sick."[26] While Hoffman's scandalous love life continued into old age, his magazines upheld the strictest standards of morality. Dozens of scantily clad bodies appeared in each issue, but they were never lewd. Wholesomeness, not sex, was used to sell his products and way of life.

The Texas Connection

Conditions at York, however, were far from idyllic and prompted important changes in the early 1960s. Bob Hasse had ably guided *Strength & Health* since Paschall's death. Unable to secure a decent wage, he departed in 1963, explaining to Murray: "I finally had my fill of Hoffman and his top partners in crime and walked out of that place the end of November. In spite of the fact that I have not yet found a new job, I have absolutely no regrets." Former marine fitness director George Otott and muscle-mag writer Gene Mozee were then offered the position and supposedly laughed at the salary. Eventually Bob appointed his friend Harry McLaughlin, sports editor for the Harrisburg *Patriot-News*. He was a "nice guy," observed Hasse, "but he [didn't] know beans about the game." Even Hoffman had to admit after five issues that he had turned *Strength & Health* into "a story or a picture magazine." To retrieve it Bob brought in Tommy Suggs, a young lifter who had studied business and law at the University of Texas. Art director Ray Degenhardt had been added the previous year. Together they put the magazine on schedule and returned it to "a more traditional format."[27] Suggs embodied all the attributes Bob most liked. Educated, strong, athletic, and good looking, he exuded the respectability of a good family man. It was Suggs who founded a Texas connection at York and formed the nucleus for an identifiable new gang in the 1960s.

Hoffman had always been in awe of Texans, and he seemed particularly susceptible to Suggs's youthful high spirits. The size of the state

The "New" York Gang

and the confident air of its inhabitants impressed him. They seemed bigger and better than other people, especially to Bob, who had always capitalized on his own size and self-confidence. The influx of Texans had started in the summer of 1958, when Garcy first came to York from El Paso to train with the champions. He returned during following summers and taught school in York from 1961 to 1968. Then came Suggs and Homer Brannum, a lightweight from Dallas. "It has been rumored that there is going to be a revolution in York about the time of the annual Strength and Health picnic," quipped "The Iron Grapevine" in 1964. "According to very reliable sources, the Texans are planning to take over Muscletown. Suspicion of this plot began when Texans started to filter into the ranks of the York Gym members. . . . Sid Henry and Terry Todd are due in a few days before the picnic to make final plans for the assault." Soon Henry, a heavyweight, joined the team on foreign trips, and Todd became managing editor with Suggs. The boys from Texas were "like peas in a pod since in York," and both settled in Dover near Bob. Suggs, in "hog heaven," bought an eighty-acre farm, and Todd moved into the Hoffman Foundation. Bob's pride in these two young educated Texans suffused an editorial on "dedication." In a fatherly way he described how the young men

> became dedicated to weightlifting, to weight training, to physical fitness and to all the precepts and ideals we stand for, by reading *Strength & Health* down in Texas, nearly 2,000 miles from York. Tommy Suggs brought his Texas-born wife, Kay, and his Texas-born children with him. Terry Todd brought his Texas wife, Ellen, who is a graduate of The University of Texas. Although she was born in Connecticut, she grew up in Texas and now speaks with a nice Texas accent instead of the harsher accent of New England. . . . So the buildings of the Bob Hoffman Foundation should soon be able to speak with a Texas drawl as well as in Pennsylvania Dutch. . . . To Tommy Suggs and Terry Todd, being here is a dream come true. . . . It is heartening to see the dedication and enthusiasm of . . . two young men who are just beginning to reap the rewards of a dedicated life.

Enthusiasm over their arrival was so palpable that their "first cover" on *Strength & Health* was envisioned to be a "picture of the Texas flag."[28] Admittedly Bob's expectations were high, but Suggs and Todd appeared to be made of the right stuff and enamoured with Muscletown. Hoffman felt new hope for carrying on his manly culture in perpetuity.

"The Magic Ingredient"

Partly through Suggs's efforts, the magazine assumed a classic appearance as chief medium for weightlifting worldwide. In a 1965 article, "The Magic Ingredient," Suggs tried to capture the York spirit that Hoffman spent a lifetime creating. He asked why lifters like Gary Cleveland, Berger, Puleo, and Garcy improved as if by magic when they came to York. After eliminating many factors—routine changes, form work, basic power movements, diet supplements, and sleeping habits—he concluded that there really was no secret training routine the champions withheld from the public: "The 'magic ingredient'—a combination of enthusiasm, competition, and good coaching that I like to call 'Yorkism'—is of the utmost importance to successful training."[29] To Suggs it was the camaraderie at York that fostered lifters of championship caliber, and he gloried at being part of it. The magazine, under his direction, became a major source of inspiration. An additional sixteen pages allowed not only more advertising but more articles and departments each month. These included a "Boys Club" section, "Lifter's Corner," "Success Stories," "Facts from the Foundation," "Tips on Good Eating," a "Self Improvement Contest," "Muscle Humor," and a "Behind the Scenes" column authored by Suggs. On the last page Pulskamp's "Ask the Doctor" replaced Grimek's "Your Training Problems," showing an upgrade in scientific emphasis.

John McCallum

The column that most characterized this era, however, started with Canadian John McCallum's "Weight Lifting for the Scuba Diver" in April 1963. Subsequent articles dealt with all aspects of training. Their conversational format captivated readers as probably no other series had ever done. Motivational effect was enhanced by artistry and display of muscles. McCallum's "Leg Specialization for Bulk," an adaptation of ideas promoted by J. C. Hise, Roger Eells, Mark Berry, and Peary Rader—but not Hoffman—was so inspiring that one reader called it "the best written and best composed article I have ever read." An undisputed classic in lifting lore is McCallum's description of how to perform the breathing squat:

> Take three huge breaths. All the air you can cram into your lungs. Hold the third breath and squat. Go down to parallel position and bounce back up as hard and fast as possible. Don't stay in the low position. Breathe out forcibly when you're almost erect. Take three more deep breaths. Hold the third breath and squat. Keep this up for twenty reps.
>
> You've got to work hard enough that the fifteenth squat feels like your limit. Then keep going and dig out the rest of the twenty. Each one of the last five reps should be doubtful.
>
> You've got to practically bleed on the squats. Work like you never worked before. When you finish the set you should be wiped right out. This is the hardest work you'll ever do but it's an absolute must for success.

For maximum effect this tortuous regimen had to be done with weights between three and four hundred pounds. In the next issue McCallum provided a recipe for his equally awesome 3,000-calorie "get-big-drink." A reader suggested McCallum write *all* the articles in *Strength & Health*: "Amid the mass of scientific, drab, fact riddled pieces which are informative, but at times boring, McCallum's work is quite a pleasing change." The ideas and style of McCallum, conveyed in a "Keys to Progress" series that ran from 1965 to 1972, are echoed decades later in Randall Strossen's "Ironmind" column in *Iron Man*. The popular "Iron Grapevine" section of this era has been reincarnated in the Todds' *Iron Game History*, replete with dumbbell trimmings.[30] A wellspring of nostalgia remains, striving to recapture the incandescence of Hoffman's promotional genius.

Terry Todd

Terry Todd's contributions at York focused more on academic concerns. As a doctoral candidate in education at the University of Texas, he was

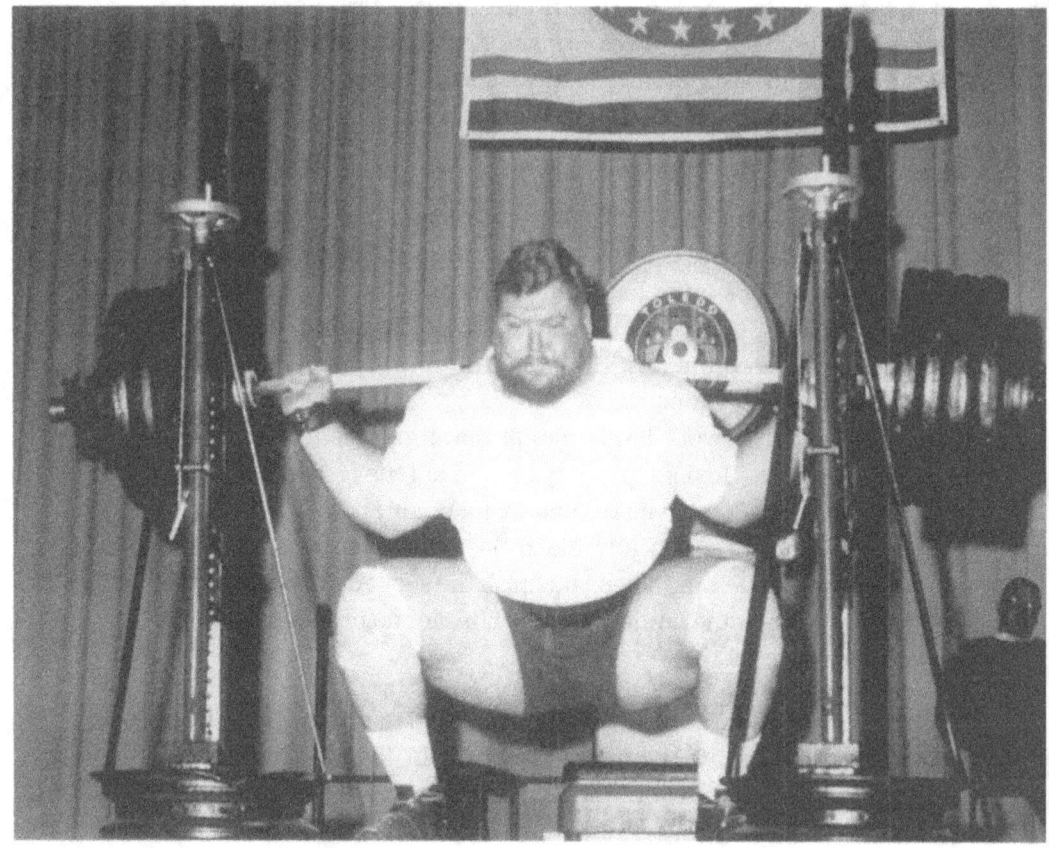

Terry Todd, squatting with 675 pounds, on his way to winning the first national powerlifting championships at York in September 1965.

writing a dissertation on the history of weightlifting. Knowing such a work would enhance his own image, Bob placed the resources of the foundation at Todd's disposal, including the vast quantity of literature he had collected. "We have done what we could to help," said Hoffman, by "building one of the . . . most extensive libraries [on physical culture] to be found in the world." He solicited further contributions of books from readers. Todd made a similar appeal, noting that he and his wife intended to build the "first reference library" that would preserve iron-game traditions "for centuries to come." Symbolic of this historical quest was a picture in *Strength & Health* of Ellen Todd browsing through Sandow's classic *System of Physical Training* with a copy of Hoffman's classic *How to Be Strong, Healthy, and Happy* at her side. Todd's other role at the foundation was to coordinate research projects, translate relevant foreign literature, exchange information with "other learned organizations," and arrange speakers. Dr. Craig Whitehead, another Texas link, represented the foundation by lecturing on medical aspects of physical fitness to sixty North American Aviation executives in 1965. Additionally, Todd collaborated with Ziegler on a monthly scientific column and planned to secure a grant from the Department of Health, Education, and Welfare.[31] Arguably Todd's most important impact at York was his instigation of powerlifting. He had made his mark as an Olympic lifter by winning the heavyweight class in the 1963 junior nationals. Then he won the first national power-lift tournament staged at York in September 1964. The next year, in a dramatic showdown with Gene Roberson, an Auburn University engineering student, Todd pulled out a victory with an awesome 740-pound deadlift. In a 1966 survey of best official Olympic and power lifts, he had the highest combined total of any lifter, making him the greatest of the "Supermen of the Iron Game." His final goal was to press four hundred pounds. Like Hoffman, Todd was a big man with big ideas. Only the incomparable Anderson, whose superiority Todd freely conceded, could lay greater claim to be the world's strongest man.[32]

Muscular Development

Todd helped define powerlifting's image in its formative period, when pictures of the ponderous Terry handling limit poundages caught the attention of *Strength & Health* and *Muscular Development* readers. The latter was launched in late 1963 as "the powerlifter's organ." In addition to news and meet results, it featured a "Powerlifter's Corner" edited by John Terlazzo. But it was also directed at the large bodybuilding clientele Hoffman had largely ignored. The first issue stated emphatically that it was "the bodybuilder's encyclopedia," its object to assist him in "developing a bigger and stronger looking body." Edited by Grimek, the new magazine was less family-oriented and carried articles on diet, exercise technique, inspiration, and pictures of bodybuilding champions. Its aim was chiefly to counter the influence of Weider, who, since the inauguration of his Mr. America and Mr. Universe contests (1959) and the Mr. Olympia title (1965), had made serious inroads on AAU-York control of Mr. contests. A 1965 editorial referred to the "heaping piles of drivel" published by Weider on "how to build 'Gladiator Pecs,' 'Cannonball Delts,' and 'Washboard Abs.' . . . Our *brains* feel 'Blitzed' and 'Bombed' after trying to wade through the refuse of half-truths, innuendos, false claims, and out and out bull."[33] Yet *Muscular Development*, with increased color splashes, more bold print, and the fantastic artwork of Gilbert III, imitated Weider's flamboyance. Through this magazine Hoffman hoped to stop the erosion in his control of bodybuilding and prevent it from happening in powerlifting.

However much Bob originally disdained this new sport, he soon experienced some attitude readjustment. That he could speak from both sides of his mouth is evident. He observed in 1963 that there were not enough Olympic lifters in America and that physique and odd-lift contests were "killing our chances of victory" in international competition, yet he professed not to be "against the power lifters" and insisted that York was doing its utmost to keep powerlifting in the AAU. He supported the efforts of weightlifting chairman David Matlin to establish a national championship and official set of records. Thinking that many odd-lift enthusiasts might be lured into Olympic lifting, he advocated the upright rowing motion and press behind the neck for inclusion in the power-lift program. He also hosted the first two national meets, in 1964 and 1965, hoping perhaps to become "Father of Powerlifting." Just as Hoffman had once collected the best weightlifters in the world and the greatest physique star in Grimek, he now took pride in having at York the "best power lifter in the nation." Todd he regarded as a "rarity—a mental as well as a physical giant."[34]

Harold Poole and Sergio Oliva

In bodybuilding Hoffman's reputation was adversely influenced by two emerging black stars, Harold Poole and Sergio Oliva. Their failure to capture the Mr. America title led to a decline of Bob's credibility among physique men. Poole was a strength athlete from Indianapolis whose exceptional development led him at sixteen to enter his first Mr. America contest in 1960. In 1961 he placed fourth, with *Strength & Health* noting that his "magnificent physique drew enthusiastic support from the packed audience. His improvement over last year, when he placed 18th, was remarkable." To Rick Wayne, Poole was "to black bodybuilding—what Joe Louis and Muhammed Ali had each in turn been to race and boxing." In 1962 Poole became the youngest man ever to win the most muscular award and graciously accepted the runner-up position overall to Joe Abbenda of Long Island. Clearly Poole was expecting to win in 1963. When he only repeated his most muscular title and finished second to York native Vern Weaver, an incident occurred. Hasse reported that he had

> improved in muscular development since last year, and his victory in the Most Muscular event was practically taken for granted the minute he began his posing routine. Harold accepted the huge Most Muscular trophy with obvious satisfaction, but his reaction to the announcement that he was placed second in Mr. America scoring gave proof positive that he is not yet ready for that honor. Confused and perhaps abetted by hooting and booing from a loudmouthed minority in the audience, the Indiana teenager foundered on stage, seemingly unable to make up his mind whether he should accept the runner-up trophy or not; when he did, amidst the uproar he continued to move about the stage. Not knowing what to expect next, the emcee . . . had the curtain drawn shut. Some minutes later the curtains parted again, and Weaver was announced as the winner. With apparent reluctance, Poole shook the victor's hand. A short time later the five top men were asked to pose as a group on the elevated posing platform. Poole, in tears, hesitated momentarily behind the other four, then walked off stage.

It hardly mattered that Weaver led Poole by five points or that the black judge on the panel, Rudy Sablo, rated Weaver higher; many observers knew that Poole had the better physique and believed he was placed lower because of his race. Two weeks later, at the Teen-Age Mr. America contest, when Poole was again relegated to second by "surprise winner" Jerry Daniels of Rossville, Georgia, he repeated his disappearing act, then smashed his trophy to bits off stage.[35]

Similarly Oliva, a dark-skinned Cuban weightlifter who had defected at the 1961 Pan-American Games, placed second to Daniels in the 1965 Mr. America contest and to Bob Gajda of Chicago the following year.

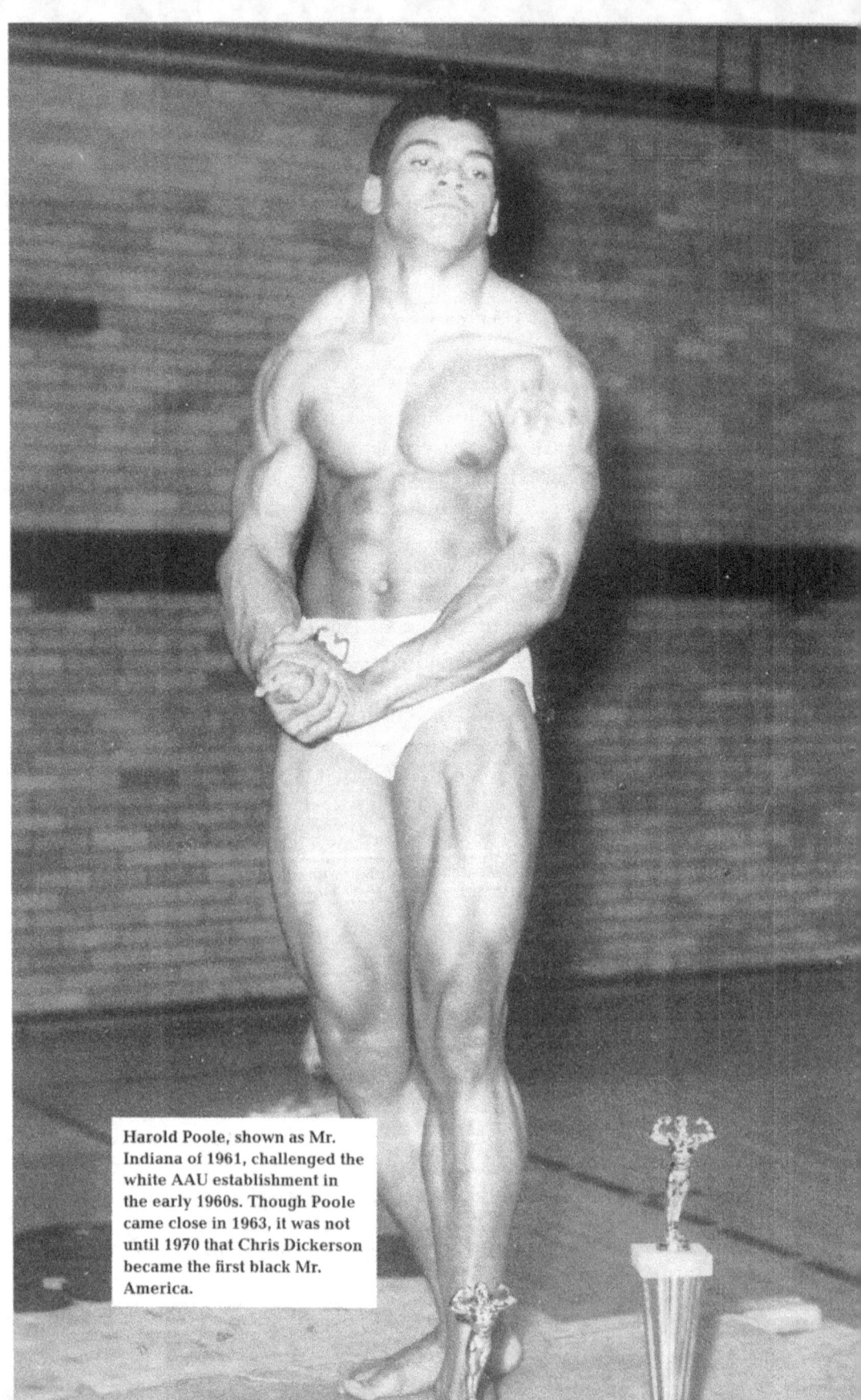

Harold Poole, shown as Mr. Indiana of 1961, challenged the white AAU establishment in the early 1960s. Though Poole came close in 1963, it was not until 1970 that Chris Dickerson became the first black Mr. America.

Oliva, though possessing arguably the best physique of the sixties, expressed no bitterness and even treated his denial as a joke: "The A.A.U. guys who don't know the Civil War is over, say Gajda is the winner when everybody in the house knew it was me." Although Hoffman was not directly responsible for Oliva's loss and could not be accused of racial bigotry, he did foster critical rules changes in the 1950s that stressed all-around athletic and personal attributes as well as muscularity. Even Oliva's judges, according to Wayne, "often apologized for playing by Bob Hoffman's rules."[36] Not surprisingly, both Poole and Oliva defected to Weider and captured top titles. Larry Scott, another superstar of the 1960s, had the all-American look favored by Hoffman but became a Weider man early. Even Hoffman felt constrained by the lack of any higher title than Mr. America within the AAU. Its international counterpart, the IWF, held a Mr. Universe contest at some world championships from 1947 to 1966, but it did not attract the best physiques. So, in order to provide a higher level of competition and combat Weider, Bob allied with Oscar Heidenstam's National Amateur Bodybuilders Association in London. Each year York would fly the AAU Mr. America to compete in the NABBA Mr. Universe in the fall. Although Grimek had won this title in 1948 and Ray Routledge and Joe Abbenda were worthy winners in the 1960s, Hoffman's entries were often beaten by British stars or the likes of Bill Pearl, Reg Park, or Arnold Schwarzenegger.

York Mainstays

What Bob really cared about was winning the senior nationals, the world championships, and the Olympics. His efforts were bolstered by such mainstays as Garcy, Puleo, March, and Schemansky. March displayed the most improvement at national championships from 1961 to 1965, with respective totals of 950, 975, 1,000, 1,010, and 1,020, while Puleo and Garcy each won five national titles and Schemansky three in helping Hoffman maintain his string of team victories. Schemansky, who turned forty in 1964, was dubbed "the professor" (from his stodgy appearance) or "the old master." After recovering from a back operation in the late 1950s, he was entering his third decade of competition. Hoffman had always provided him with financial assistance and training aids. In 1960, though still living in Detroit, Schemansky joined the

York gang. He won silver medals at the 1962 and 1963 world championships and bronze medals at the 1960 and 1964 Olympics, making him America's top international performer in the 1960s. He set twenty-five world records in his career. His 362 snatch, America's only world record in 1962, was heralded by many as the greatest lift ever made. A year later Hoffman referred to Schemansky, at 260 bodyweight, as having "the most powerfully athletic physique of all time." In 1964 he became the first American to total 1,200 pounds, with lifts of 400, 355, and 445. One of the last exponents of the split style, his flexibility and balance allowed him to drop to remarkably low positions, and his bull-like strength enabled him to come out of them. Though he respected Bob, Schemansky never felt any York team spirit. Blunt, outspoken, and brutally honest, he often quarreled with officialdom and experienced financial hardship because of his commitment. "I just about gave up everything," he recalls, "hoping something would come of it, and it never did."[37] National recognition outside the iron game was attained by relatively few competitors from this era, bodybuilder Steve Reeves (who starred as Hercules) and Olympian Harold Sakata (who played Odd Job in the James Bond thriller *Goldfinger*) being notable exceptions. Worldly gain otherwise seemed limited to clever promoters such as Hoffman and Weider, who could exploit the talents of others. Just being one of the strongest and most successful weightlifters of all time was not enough to open the doors to fame and fortune.

Also from Detroit, a hotbed of talent since the 1930s, was Joe Puleo. His first contact with York came when he witnessed the Russians versus the Americans in a meet staged by Hoffman in Detroit in 1958. He was amazed by Bob's capacity as emcee to recall perfectly lifts performed in previous meets. Puleo showed much promise as a middleweight in the 1960 senior nationals, where he placed fourth to Kono, Pete Talluto, and Gary Cleveland with an eight hundred total. He moved to Muscletown in early 1962 and received $30 a week for packaging Energol. He reaped the benefits of the abundant training facilities and camaraderie, as well as all-expenses-paid trips to meets and occasional bonuses. Puleo recalls receiving an envelope containing $50 at the 1962 seniors, and sometimes Bob would say at a critical point in competition, "There's a little extra incentive in this lift." Puleo became the first lifter to receive a Hoffman scholarship to attend York Junior College. He admits to being "a jitterbug kind of guy" who pursued the opposite sex much as Vinci and Berger had done. Terpak, a "no-nonsense kind of guy," advised

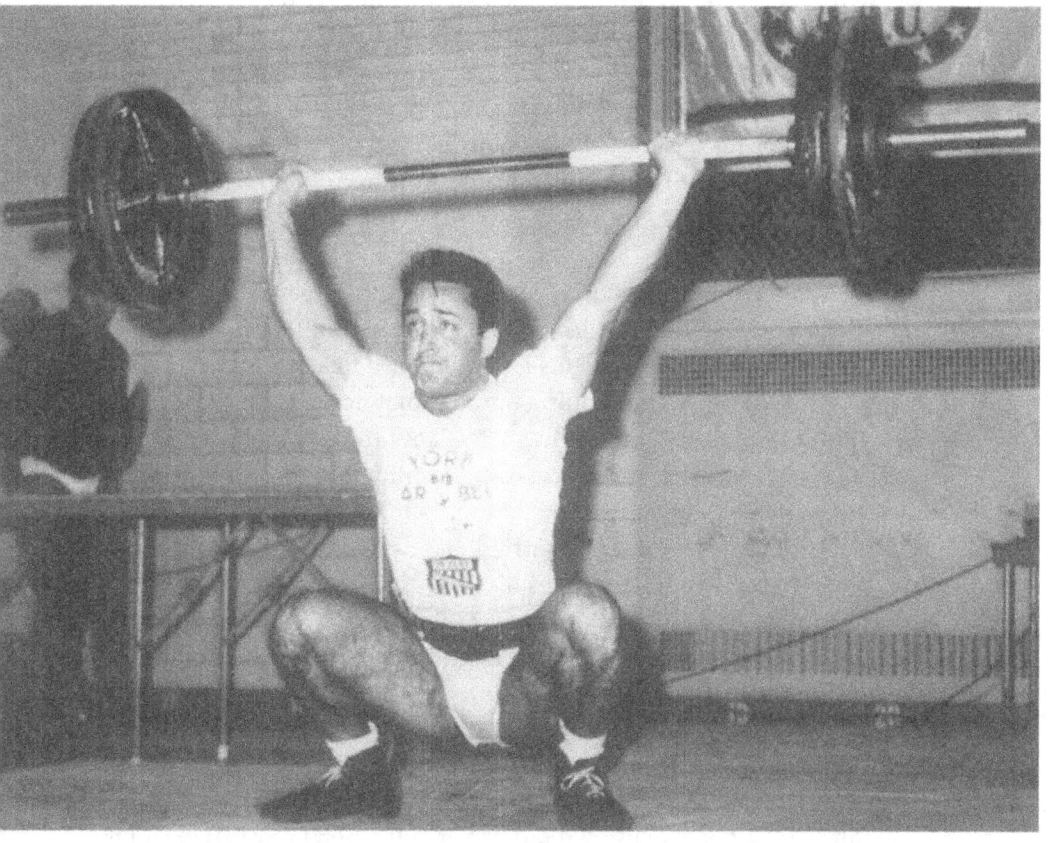

Joe Puleo, recruited from Detroit, was known for his quickness. He was one of many York lifters to benefit from Hoffman scholarships to further their education. Puleo eventually became a lawyer in Florida.

him to "leave these secretaries alone." Most evident to Puleo was a separation between lifters of his generation and the earlier gang, who had settled and raised families. For Puleo and others, like Schemansky, Sheppard, and Berger, York's conservatism and lack of social outlets was stifling. Puleo eventually concluded that "this place [would] drive you nuts."[38] Yet it was the place to be if you were a serious weightlifter in the 1960s.

Unlike some others of the new York gang, Tony Garcy related well to the older generation, including Grimek, Terpak, and John Terlazzo. And he was one of the few lifters who felt no ill feelings toward Dietz. Above all, Garcy respected Bob. Though he never regarded him as a father figure, he viewed Bob as a "dynamic force." A pensive person, Garcy was America's premier lightweight from 1960 to 1964. As a middleweight at the 1966 seniors, he held off challenges from Russ Knipp, who set a world-record press, and Canadian star Pierre St. Jean. "Garcy is more of a perfectionist than most any world lifter," observed Hoffman, "for he trained endlessly on form." When he totaled thirty-five pounds less the next year in losing to Knipp, Bob concluded that he was training too hard: "He lacked the vim and vitality that is so characteristic of Tony. . . . His 905 total was four pounds less than his lightweight total that he did at the Olympics three years ago. That's not the kind of progress we need. Tony is probably the hardest trainer in the York Barbell Gym. He trains long and hard nearly every day of the week. As if that wasn't enough, I am told that he does his squatting in the mornings before going to work."[39] What probably contributed most to Garcy's lifting demise was the disintegration of his marriage, which ruined his ability to concentrate. After retiring from the platform, he settled in Chicago and later remarried, but he always felt like one of the gang and harbors fond memories of York.

The most indigenous York lifter was Bill March, who began to train in nearby Dallastown with Vern Weaver and Dick Smith in the late 1950s. In 1959 Weaver and Dave Ashman were scheduled to give an exhibition with Hoffman at York Suburban High. When Ashman could not attend, March substituted. He impressed Bob so much that he was added to the team and given a job in the stockroom. For March, Hoffman was truly a substitute father, since his own father had left when he was two and his mother had died when he was thirteen: "I loved the man." The critical factor behind March's progress, in addition to Hoffman's support, was the cornucopia of training aids provided by Ziegler. And March was a willing patient: if Ziegler had told him to eat grass, he "would have done so to get strong." But he trusted Ziegler. Achieving gains on the power rack took so little time that March had to "make up training routines because nobody would believe [he] did it on thirty seconds a day." Mental preparation was the key. Bob exploited March's progress by including his pictures and stories in York promotional literature. What appealed to Hoffman was that March was homegrown, an international lifting and physique champion, and an all-around athlete who displayed "useful" muscles. March also was a gentleman. Always dressed in coat and tie, he was the idol of Gary Glenney, a York lifter in the late 1960s. "He always looked good," Glenney recalls. Once March even *gave* him his lifting belt. Ultimately, however, March was alienated from York

Barbell by Dietz, who, he contends, "hated weightlifters—or anyone who might get in there to get a piece of the pie." It was always a hassle to get the extra money he earned for exhibitions. "It was never Bob, it was always Mike," but this kind of treatment, unchecked by Hoffman, drove a wedge between oldsters with their hands on the controls and young men looking for a break in life.[40]

Terlazzo and Smitty

John Terlazzo, Tony's younger brother, was an outstanding lifter before getting wounded in World War II. Afterward he operated a gym in New York City for sixteen years. He came to Muscletown in 1960 to work in customer service and later helped launch *Muscular Development*. Then, using skills he had acquired in arranging contests and strength shows in New York, he organized various extravaganzas at York, including national championships and Mr. America contests, powerlifting meets, and Bob's annual picnics and birthday celebrations. The most unique was an "Isometric Birthday" in 1961 where guests gave Bob a trophy topped by a scale-model power rack and lifter. In retrospect, Terlazzo's "biggest mistake was saying salary was no object" when he came. Lack of money was always a problem. Terlazzo tried to increase his worth by doing his job well, but it never paid off. He would have been part of the old gang had he arrived twenty years earlier. Instead, though liked by everyone, he was never fully integrated with either generational clique at York and experienced "twenty years of headaches."

Dick Smith, affectionately known as "Smitty" or "Super Gopher," related well to both age groups. As a child in the 1930s, he started sneaking into the old Broad Street gym. He loved watching the strong men perform seemingly superhuman feats. Though he trained irregularly and never aspired to be a serious lifter, he continued to mingle with musclemen over the years. In 1955 he left his machine-shop job to become a handyman at York Barbell. He did so well that he graduated to trainer and eventually "chief technician" to Ziegler at the foundation and international coach. The longer he stayed, the more he learned, simply by observing. The elders trusted him, and the lifters loved and respected him. Bill Starr noted that in competition "having Smitty in our corner is worth ten pounds on each lift."[41] Like Terlazzo, Smitty never thrust himself into the limelight, but he was a catalyst for the socialization that made York special.

American Lifting Declines

Despite York's continuance as center of American and world weightlifting in the 1960s, the international performance of Bob's lifters declined steadily. A 1962 status report compiled by the German magazine *Athletik* showed only seven Americans ranked among the world's top seventy weightlifters, four being heavyweights. By contrast, Russia placed thirty-three lifters representing all divisions. With the retirement of Vinci in 1962 and Berger in 1964, Hoffman had virtually no one in the lighter classes. American lifters were getting bigger (on diets supplemented by Hi-Proteen and steroids), but they were not getting better internationally. As aging greats fell by the wayside, no one replaced them. The most serious blow was Kono's departure. From 1950 to 1963 he won eleven national championships, six world championships, and two Olympic gold medals. Always a linchpin for American teams, Kono, like Pete George, was a mental lifter who excelled in the clutch. He established seven Olympic, thirty-seven American, eight Pan-American, and twenty-six world records and is the only athlete ever to set world records in four weight classes. That the world was catching up with Kono was evident at the Rome Olympics, where he was upset by Russia's Alexander Kurinov. Then he placed third and second respectively at the 1961 and 1962 world championships. On the national level he was challenged by upstart Gary Cleveland and Riecke. To stave off defeat from a visiting Japanese team at the 1963 senior nationals in Harrisburg, Bob persuaded him to lift in what turned out to be one of weightlifting's great moments. All came down to Kono's final two attempts in the clean and jerk, in which he needed to tie Riecke and win on bodyweight. "He needed 375 to win," noted Hoffman.

> This did not seem possible, for he was out of condition. But what a competitor this man is. The yellow glow of the tiger showed in his eyes. He approached the bar, and three times he walked away from it. Then, with a double superhuman effort he cleaned the weight. It was too much for him. He simply could not jerk it.

The "New" York Gang

One more attempt. Tommy took more time to prepare for this lift than I had ever seen him take before. I was reminded of Pete George's ordeal at the 1948 Olympic Games, when the Olympic gold medal hinged on the 363 3/4 pounds this 18-year-old school boy weighing only 162 pounds had cleaned. Pete tried so hard to hold that jerk, but failed. Was that to be Kono's fate?

As he stood at the bar, I said to him, "Tommy, you can do it!" He cleaned the bar, and I shouted, "Now jerk it, step forward, bang your feet," and he did just that and was again the champion. Those who saw this lift saw the greatest effort of Kono's long championship career. It was a never-to-be-forgotten performance.[42]

Though he did not retire until 1965, Kono was never again a factor in international competition. Tommy never resided in York or lifted for the club, but he was very much a part of the York gang in the 1950s.

For a while it appeared that Gary Gubner, a world-class shot-putter from New York City, might resurrect American heavyweight fortunes against Russian behemoths Yuri Vlasov and Leonid Zhabotinski. When this new hope did not materialize fully, Bob fell back on an old hope from the 1950s, Paul Anderson, still the world's strongest man. In 1962 Anderson expressed interest in removing his professional status, maintaining that he had made little money as a strong man, boxer, wrestler, or Las Vegas showman. What he had earned had gone to his nonprofit youth home in Georgia. He wanted Bob "to see about getting my amateur standing back. If you will do this for me I will . . . beat the Russian for you. I will do 450-360-500." In 1964, with the Tokyo Olympics coming up, Hoffman tried to persuade the AAU to reinstate him. Despite Anderson's testimony and Bob's pleading, he was voted down by the board of directors, 106–40. Hoffman's plight was illustrated by the absence of Americans in a 1964 listing of world records. Even Schemansky's magnificent 362 snatch was surpassed by Zhabotinski. When Riecke broke the light-heavy record with a 325-pound snatch, he was treated like an Olympic champion. *Strength & Health* expressed hope that "Riecke's great lift will mark the start of another American assault on the world's records." But it was not to be. Only a handful more, including Berger's fine 336 clean and jerk in Tokyo, were forthcoming. Normally Bob's busy routine distracted him from this state of affairs, but he sometimes despaired: "After I saw the small list of entries for the District One [New England] Championships, I lay awake all night. I saw 4 o'clock come,

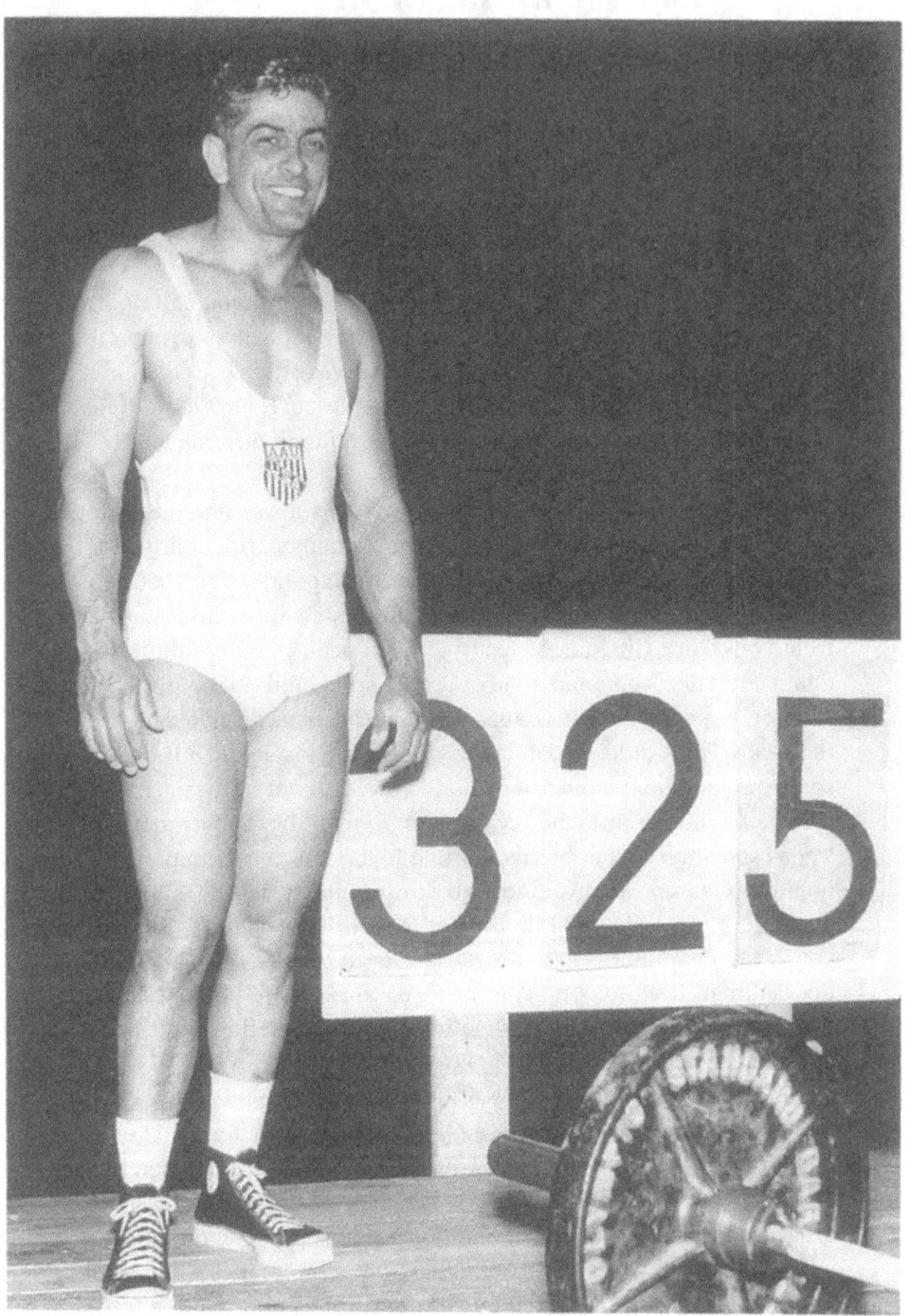

Louis Riecke beams following the completion of his 325-pound world-record snatch at the 1964 YMCA championships in Los Angeles. Riecke's hallmark was his black high-topped sneakers.

then 5 o'clock, 6 o'clock, 7 o'clock, and I finally dozed a bit before I got to start my day. People ask, 'Why do you concern yourself so much about lifting?' I reply, After you have spent 40 years trying to build up championship weightlifting teams, it hurts to see our country slipping back, back, and back in our favorite sport." Such a dismal outlook in 1965 justified Hoffman in saying, more than ever, that the international odds were stacked against him. It was "York Barbell against the Russian Government."[43]

Hoffman's Heart Fibrillations

This predicament clearly disturbed Hoffman's tranquillity. Whether it also undermined his health is debatable. A rumor circulated at the Tokyo Olympics that he was sick. "Not me," he protested. "I feel like a million." He was "fortunate to enjoy super health." However much he tried to minimize his condition, something was wrong. Demoralized at first, he sought help from Frank Corbett, one of his weightlifting doctors. Corbett arranged admission for him to the Lahey Clinic in Boston, where he was operated on for an enlarged thyroid gland in March 1965. Doctors' notes indicate the procedure was successful, but Bob's heart "continued to fibrillate throughout the operation." No one seemed to know what to do. An irregular heartbeat was not healthy, but it did not seem to be harming him, and there seemed no cause for alarm. Therefore Bob resumed his hyperactive schedule immediately after surgery, and even postponed his postoperative checkup. Bob expected the busy doctors at the clinic to adjust *their* schedules so he could fit them in between his convention commitments. In spite of his ordeal, Hoffman was heralded at the Natural Food Associates convention as never having missed an hour of work in fifty years. Myths of Hoffman's invincibility had to be sustained. And so the May 1965 issue of *Muscular Development* displayed an old picture of Bob with Al Stephen, the 1946 Mr. America. The caption read, "The years have been kind to both, thanks to weight training, and neither has changed very much."[44]

Yet the fibrillations continued, and Hoffman sought the advice of a heart specialist in Philadelphia as well as his surgeon in Boston. He noted that the latter said I could do anything I want to in a physical way. Not to get crazy but anything reasonable. Barbell training, running, Polka dancing as hard as I can.

Shock treatment would stop my fibrilation—but it does not always last. He thinks I would have a better chance for it to last than for others; should have it done at Laheys.

Does not know what caused the fibrilation.

Suggested keeping my weight down—more weight—more work for the heart. Told him that big horses live as long as small horses.

For the next year Bob, fearing the inconvenience of further medical treatments to his manly lifestyle and thinking he could will good health on his body, did nothing. Meanwhile his competitors learned of his problems and began to criticize his irregular ways and to speculate that he had had a heart attack. "He does not live like he tells you he lives," was the Weider line. "He frequents night clubs and you know what they do there." Hoffman insisted that he patronized them only for his "great love for dancing." To put rumors to rest, he published his Lahey cardiogram and quoted his doctor as saying, "As far as your heart is concerned you should live to be 102." All other tests, Hoffman claimed, "proved that at the age of 67 I have the actions, the responses and the organic, glandular and muscular condition of a man of 27." Further to dispel concerns, he went back to Corbett, who, after examining him in March 1966, pronounced him in excellent health. Corbett called Hoffman's publication of his electrocardiogram "a stroke of genius" that "should dispel all the gossip mongers. Since *all* your laboratory tests last week were so amazingly within normal limits I thought I would send a copy of them to you." Hoffman seemed satisfied from these results that he could conquer old age. But on his final visit to Lahey in May, he complained about chest pains. He betrayed concern privately by constantly checking his pulse and comparing it with others. Publicly he added running to his daily routine, aptly entitling an editorial "Run for Your Life." Readers now had to endure recapitulations of Hoffman's exploits on the roads and fields near Dover and in his basement, where he could do a mile in 1,800 steps (or thirty-six revolutions). By running five days a week he tried to convince himself and others that physically he was "truly one of the marvels of the world."[45]

That Hoffman could not dispel thoughts of aging was due in part to the passing of many of his contemporaries. The death of Ray Van Cleef in 1964 at age fifty-three was "the greatest shock of all." Van

Cleef had contributed to every issue of *Strength & Health* for over thirty years. "I see heart attacks happening all around me," Bob wrote in an editorial on heart disease just after his operation. When Tony Terlazzo and bodybuilder Vic Nicoletti (both in their early fifties) died on the same day in 1964, followed by Dave Hall, proprietor of Bur Barbell Company, the following month at age fifty-eight, Bob was moved to recall the high number of weightlifters who had recently died of heart failure. A preoccupation with his own mortality became evident in references to the future of his company and fortune. He emphasized youth and education.

> I am surrounding myself with worthy young men who should be with us for a long time to carry on our work. There are also many young physicians who show an increasing interest in the future of our enterprises such as Craig Whitehead, M.D., John Gourgott, M.D., Richard Wright, M.D. who is Dr. Russell Wright's son, and John Ziegler, M.D. . . . Also, the many young men who have been given scholarships through the Hoffman Foundation will help. As for the business itself, I am making arrangements to give the business to our retirement fund and to the Bob Hoffman Foundation. So there are many good reasons why we feel that our work will endure.[46]

A critical misconception of Hoffman's was that M.D.'s and Ph.D.'s were more perfect than other humans and that their professional expertise and judgment necessarily transferred to other realms. This flawed assumption was by no means limited to Bob, who clung to the self-made-man conceptions of his youth. The American public wanted to believe, in line with its ethos of upward social mobility, that those with educational attainments were less greedy, egotistical, or prone to financial miscalculation than others—that the noble professions of medicine and scholarship were worlds apart from those of money-grubbing businessmen.

Visions of Grandeur

At odds with such naiveté were the promotional activities of Richard You, who greatly admired Hoffman. According to Kono, "money meant nothing to Dr. You. Recognition was everything. Just like Hoffman, he

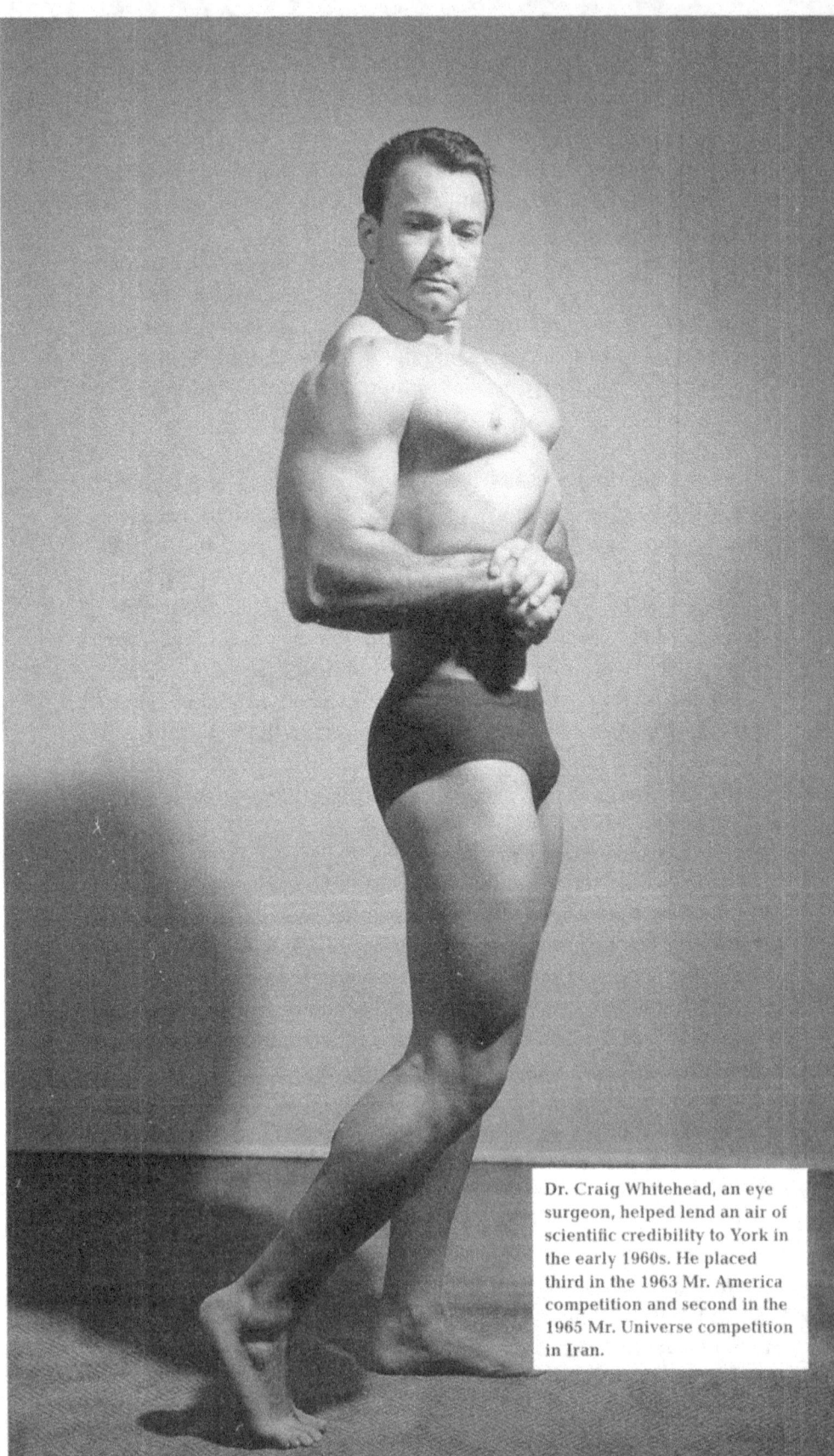

Dr. Craig Whitehead, an eye surgeon, helped lend an air of scientific credibility to York in the early 1960s. He placed third in the 1963 Mr. America competition and second in the 1965 Mr. Universe competition in Iran.

wanted his name in lights." Still trying to entice Bob to invest in Hawaii's tallest structure, You appealed directly to his ego by calling it the York International Building. It would contain a York Health Studio equipped with York barbells, a York Pharmacy to sell Hoffman supplements, a York Snack Bar, York Barber Shop, and even a York Laundry! Less commercial but no less egotistical and passionate about lifting was John Ziegler. After retiring from medical practice in 1963, he became involved in developing York products. In agreeing to head the Hoffman Foundation, Ziegler was motivated not so much by the prospect of making money as by the desire to become a renowned medical researcher. "It is *very very* possible," he told Hoffman in 1965, "that special training techniques and other *devices* along with greater physiological knowledge may enable man to achieve physical performances *now* considered SUPERHUMAN!" Such was the object of his treatments of Riecke and March. Now his goal seemed attainable through the isotron, which figured prominently in all subsequent transactions. For the services of this "top scientist," Hoffman gave Ziegler the title of medical director of research and paid him $100 to visit York one day per week. Ziegler successfully applied the isotron to athletes, handicapped patients, and Marine Corps volunteers. He boasted that eight minutes of electronic stimulation was equivalent to five hours of weight training. With his foot firmly planted in the Hoffman Foundation, Ziegler in September 1966 sprang his grand plan on Hoffman—a joint venture with Avon, a giant in the women's cosmetics field: "I have convinced my associates that you and York Barbell are leaders in your field. It is my opinion that AVON . . . would be a good organized market for a Female beauty model of the Isotron." Association with Avon could minimize research costs on new products, guarantee security from the FDA, increase York's market in related areas, and "guarantee a better future for us all."[47] That Ziegler's scheme never materialized may be attributed to its failure to satisfy Bob's need to be in charge.

What Hoffman cared about more than money (or even good health) was glory. But in his countless crusades for fitness and lifting superiority, his incessant bragging often detracted from any otherwise noble purpose and invited criticism. Such was the result of a 1964 editorial entitled "Dirty Water Is Plaguing Our Nation." Its stated purpose of drawing attention to the need for conserving the nation's pure-water resources seemed to some readers a thin disguise for the ulterior motive of stoking Hoffman's colossal ego. Glenn Bishop, a Michigan chiropractor, spoke out: "Your personal stories and vast accomplishments on this earth . . . have outworn their welcome in your magazine. It is as if you use S & H for your own personal soap box." Larry Fronheiser, a University of Dayton student, called Hoffman's articles "childish and poorly written, with such a conceited tone to them that I find it hard to believe that a man of your knowledge and fame would continually have to 'blow himself up.' . . . I hardly think Mr. Hoffman, that being 'a canoeist and an oarsman' is sufficient background for an expert on water pollution." It was obvious that Hoffman was lacking in those educational and scientific accomplishments he idealized for his organization. Even more wounding was a letter from "a long time friend" in 1967: "I read your BS about how strong, super healthy, and how far you can run. But the fact remains that you are not a young man. . . . You are known as the Father of American Weightlifting, but twenty years from now you will be father of nothing." Bob could respond only that he had run ten miles on his sixty-eighth birthday and that he planned to endow the Hoffman Foundation with "enough money to support American weightlifting forever."[48]

Exit Ziegler and Todd

Money, however, was not what was needed to sustain American lifting. Nor was another father figure on the horizon. Furthermore, Ziegler's miracle process, in which Hoffman had invested so much personal and corporate support—functional isometric contraction—had fallen far short of expectations. It had neither brought financial success nor restored American leadership. As Suggs explained, it suffered from becoming a "national fad," and "like all fads, isometrics was all too soon forgotten." By this time too there was general knowledge and accessibility of steroids. In 1964 *Muscular Development* expressed dismay that "readers constantly write to us asking where they can get the bodybuilding drugs (anabolics) such as Dianabol, Nilevar, Duranabol (nandrolone phenpropionate) and the new dehexy cream. Yes, they build muscles fast but we don't have them. We advise against their use. They are new and we don't know what effect they will have on their users five or ten years from now. Forget 'em and use the old weights and plenty of protein." Repeatedly York publications, acting on Ziegler's advice, condemned anabolics. Privately, however, an increasing number of lifters were using and abusing steroids. Ziegler was outraged: "What is it with these simple-minded shits? I'm the doctor!" Ziegler later recalled that "the York men went crazy about steroids. They figured if one pill was good, three or four would be better, and they were eating them like candy. I began seeing prostate trouble and a couple cases of atrophied testes." Unable to interest Hoffman in the isotron and fed up with drug-abusing lifters, Ziegler left York. In the January 1967 issue of *Strength & Health* he delivered a parting shot, a bold print "Warning" from the AMA sports medicine committee condemning the use of steroids by athletes.[49] Ziegler's attitude toward the monster he had created could not have been clearer.

The loss of Ziegler was preceded by another setback to Hoffman's plans for promoting education and science—the departure of Todd. Bob had high hopes for Terry, but other employees complained he was lazy, often did not show up for work, and relegated most of his duties at the magazine and foundation to Suggs and his wife, Ellen. Todd, however, attributes their alienation from him to the fact that he had become Bob's favorite. Suggs resented the large raise Terry received, placing Terry ahead of Suggs in the pecking order. Bob also put Ellen on the payroll, covered the Todds' housing and utility expenses, and provided tailor-made suits for Terry. "He treated me like a son," Todd recalls. "I was like one of Bob's mistresses. Bob let me get close to him." Terry even thought of succeeding him—after all, "he was sixty-five." But this situation proved intolerable to new gang and old gang alike. Soon Terry was demoted at *Strength & Health* and eased out of the foundation directorship in the fall of 1965 by Ziegler. According to Suggs, "Doc thought Terry was trying to take over more than he should."[50] Heretofore Todd and Ziegler had appeared to be collaborating, but a clash between two such assertive personalities was perhaps inevitable.

What was unexpected was Ziegler's diagnosis of Todd, aged twenty-seven, as having "hypertensive cardiovascular disease," an alleged victim of steroids. Smitty recalls that Todd's blood pressure was "going sky-high." At the 1965 Senior National Power Meet he had a hypoglycemia seizure. Smith says he quickly fetched a jar of honey, enabling Todd to make powerlifting history. "When Terry lifted, he strained so hard that his capillaries burst and there were traces of blood on his skin." Ziegler, arguing that he or York would be liable for any serious injury or collapse of Todd's health, notified AAU officials that he was not responsible for what his patient did. "Terry, I would recommend that you stop steroids dead, and get on a diet and a routine of regular exercise," was Ziegler's admonition, according to Terpak. "With Ziegler in control," Terpak saw no problem with steroids. It was only "when Doc lost control . . . that the situation got out of hand. Terry was abusing the steroids and getting them elsewhere." Todd denies he ever had high blood pressure, and claims that another doctor tested it at 125 over 70. His explanation for Ziegler's conduct is that Ziegler possibly thought his own position at York would be enhanced with Terry out. But "for Ziegler, a medical doctor, to falsify information is unforgivable."[51] To what extent personal ambition governed Ziegler's diagnosis will perhaps never be known. But Terry's vilification and ostracism for clutching the leader's mantle denotes a familiar pattern of conduct at York.

Soon Todd left for Texas to finish his doctoral studies. What he took from York, besides his expertise and youthful aspirations, is subject to speculation. Alda says he "stole a lot of weights" in addition to the two (one-hundred-pound) plates Bob gave him. Smitty recalls seeing him leaving with his Mercury "loaded down to the gunwales." Despite widespread suspicions, there is no evidence that Terry also took with him the strength collection he had accumulated at the Foundation. Todd completed his dissertation the following year, compiling a bibliographic survey from the collection of strength literature Hoffman had purchased from Ray Van Cleef's widow. Terry recalls that he took about eighty books with him. Bob had allowed him to borrow them and to continue writing for the magazine. But these arrangements were nixed when Terry received a letter requesting return of the items. He recalls doing so and calling Bob, who "apologized for this humiliating demand. . . . Bob said there was a lot of pressure on him. He was so apologetic that he almost cried. With me down here and all my enemies up there, there was no chance of continuing the relationship." The real basis for the Todd-McLean Collection, which Todd created at the University of Texas, was the Coulter collection, which he and his wife Jan purchased in the late 1970s.[52] Though scarcely realized by Hoffman and his cohorts, what was lost with the departure of Todd was much of York's link with posterity.

Bill Starr

Hoffman quickly rebounded from the loss of Todd and Ziegler by bringing in another lifter, at Suggs's behest, with Texas connections. Bill Starr was a native of Bel Air, Maryland, who had ended his stint in the air force at Sheppard Air Base in Wichita Falls. An engaging personality, Bill married a Texas girl and received a B.S. in sociology from Southern Methodist University. He also became an ordained minister. A sense of Christian caring led him to pursue a master's in social work at George Williams College in Chicago and to become youth director at the YMCA in Marion, Indiana. There he became interested in weightlifting and began visiting Muscletown. When Starr arrived in York as associate editor in 1966, with a flattop and a handsome family of three children, he projected the "all-American boy" image. Starr was energetic and innovative, and embodied Hoffman's emphasis on youth and education. The November 1966 issue of *Strength & Health* was dedicated to youth, featuring "America's strongest teenager," Phil Grippaldi, on the cover, pictures of the teenage nationals and Teenage Mr. America contest, a report on a European-style teenage training camp at York Junior College, and articles to inspire youth. A 1967 survey Starr conducted on reader preferences showed that 52 percent were bodybuilders, while 23 percent and 21 percent were weight trainers and weightlifters respectively. Remarkably, 47 percent were ten to nineteen, and only 9 percent were forty or older. McCallum's "Keys to Progress" was the most popular feature, while Vera Christensen's "To the Ladies" was least appreciated. That "Boys Club" should also be unpopular to largely young male patrons was unexpected. Others rated highly included the "Iron Grapevine" gossip column and the Mr. America instructional article. Curiously, readers showed the most apathy for historical pieces, such as "Old Timers" or Earle Leiderman's articles. Clearly, the relevant inspirational articles most wanted by York's clientele were exactly what Starr and Suggs were most eager to provide.[53]

A Lifting Hotbed

This dynamic duo also promoted a team spirit in the York gym, just as in days of yore. Lifters from New England, California, and Venezuela joined those from the middle Atlantic area in what seemed like a rebirth of American lifting. The old gang had always trained in the late afternoons, but soon noontime workouts were in vogue with the young enthusiasts converging on Muscletown. The York gym in 1967 was starting to "look like the entry list for the Senior Nationals." What made the experience unique was the "high level of competition in every workout," where every lifter "pushes himself to higher and higher performances." The team spirit generated at York carried over to the senior nationals at Columbus in June.

> All the lifters were in the same hotel. There is no way that you could be alone in your room for more than a few minutes. You were either down in the lobby, in another lifter's room, or had a group of lifters in your own room. Everyone was looking for friends that they hadn't seen for months. And this is when you realize that there must be a common denominator among lifters. The lifters ranged from high school students to Medical Doctors. But there was something that drew them to competition and . . . helped establish many a deep and long lasting friendship. It is . . . something that goes with being a competitor—you become a part of a certain fraternity when you meet and compete with other lifters.[54]

It seemed that Starr and Suggs had regenerated the socialization that Hoffman had ignited so successfully in the early 1930s and had rekindled at other times in his career. This quality, more than any other, allowed York to remain the Mecca for American and world weightlifting.

So infectious was the spirit generated at York that it spread to Chicago, where Bob Gajda, seized with Olympic-lifting fervor, began to recruit lifters at the Duncan YMCA, dubbed the "York of the Midwest." Such standouts as Winston Binney, Mike Karchut, Fred Schutz, and Chuck Nootens from the upper Midwest were joined by easterners Knipp and Grippaldi, who, according to Schutz, "[wouldn't] let you out of the gym until [you'd] had a good workout." Duncan and other teams, including the Los Angeles YMCA under Bob Hise and the air force team spearheaded by Homer Brannum, began challenging York. Most observers at the 1967 nationals "felt that it had the highest grade of competition in recent years." A statistical breakdown of senior national results for the top three places from 1960 to 1968 shows an 8.9 percent overall poundage gain. How much steroids and other scientific advances contributed to these increases cannot be determined, but gains in the heavier classes were much greater. From the Rome Olympics in 1960 to Tokyo in 1964 the total poundage increased for all classes by 1.6 percent, while from Tokyo to the Mexico City Olympics in 1968 the rate of increase jumped to 7.3 percent. Hoffman could have felt pleased with these improvements. But data show that international lifting was also increasing. From Rome to Tokyo, world gains were 6.7 percent, while for the second segment they were 2.2 percent, the two together equaling the American eight-year gain of 8.9 percent. The principal difference was that international gains were spread more evenly over all weight classes. But American teams were not out of the running—and there was cause for hope among America's teenagers. A poll taken by Starr in 1967 on the progress of eight of the fourteen youths who had attended the teenage training camp at York a year earlier revealed that each lifter had added an average of seventy-three pounds to his total. With such prospects on the horizon, inspired by young Bob Bednarski, American hopes were high.[55]

Bob Bednarski

A sure sign that weightlifting in the United States was on the move was the practice, reinstituted by the Texas contingent, of traveling throughout the country to lift, conduct clinics, or simply show the York flag. Starr recalls that they borrowed Alda's car for their first trip and eventually procured a van from Hoffman. Starr's trip with Suggs and Bednarski to the 1967 Cincinnati Open became a romantic adventure: "The weather that Saturday consisted of a mixture of wind, snow, and ice. But [we] decided to brave the elements and packed the York Barbell's Volkswagen for the trip. We carefully packed an assortment of suitcases, gym bags, the latest issue of *Strength & Health,* and a few cases of Chocolate Covered Hi-Proteen Fudge. Everything fit fine except that when we finished there wasn't any room for people."

Bednarski was the team goat, chided for his incessant chatter and his juvenile manner. For light reading he brought along a paperback entitled *The Real Life Adventures of Hoot Gibson.* But there was nothing frivolous about Bednarski's lifting. Under the tutelage of Joe Mills of Woonsocket, Rhode Island, his youthful strength had been harnessed. In 1965 he attracted attention by sudden increases in his lifts with relatively slight bodyweight gains. "Recent reports from New England verge on the unbelievable" was the reaction to news that he had made lifts of 355, 335, and 410, weighing only 210. Hoffman admitted he was "moving up fast" but doubted he was ready to take on Gubner and Schemansky.

THE "GOLDEN AGE" OF AMERICAN WEIGHTLIFTING

Yet at the 1966 senior nationals (at 234 bodyweight) he totaled 1,130, set an American clean-and-jerk record of 446, trounced Schemansky by 85 pounds, and placed second to Gubner, who outweighed him by 60. At the 1966 world championships in East Berlin he garnered America's only medal when he placed second to Zhabotinski with a 1,183 total. Dubbed "the ninth wonder" by his training mates, Hoffman proclaimed him to be "the greatest young weightlifter" in the sport's history. By this time he had moved to York and was employed at the company. He was recognized in a balloting of *Strength & Health* readers as "Weightlifter of the Year" for 1966 and was featured on the April 1967 cover and in an article tracing his meteoric rise. Bednarski was "the brightest light in the American weightlifting scene," wrote Starr, and he soon became an iron-game celebrity. On their trip to Cincinnati, there were so many fans backstage to watch "the ninth wonder" that he "couldn't concentrate on his lifting." Starr and Suggs served as bodyguards. "I think we would have had better luck protecting Elvis Presley at a 'rock 'n' roll' convention," quipped Suggs.[56] For Hoffman, Bednarski was America's greatest hope. He was capable of deluding himself into thinking that reclaiming the heavyweight title would herald a new era of American supremacy.

Clearly the new York gang—youthful, educated, and scientifically oriented—was making its mark. The influx of rising stars from Texas and elsewhere was having a leavening effect. Equipped with this new spirit, York, despite the loss of Ziegler and Todd, seemed capable of dealing with changing trends in sport science in the 1960s. As Garcy observed, it was "a period of tremendous experimentation" that led in many directions. But Hoffman's beliefs remained rooted in an earlier era, and to cope with these innovations and lend an air of scientific dignity to his undertakings, he embraced a body of illusions. As already noted, once Bob was convinced of isometrics' marketability, he jumped to the conclusion that it would restore America to the forefront of international competition and bring further fortune and fame to himself. By the same token, he rejected steroids and most other ergogenic aids, none of which coincided with his traditional values. Furthermore, he expected that the younger gang would abide by rules set by *his* generation. Arguably Bob's greatest illusion was the belief that he continued to be in perfect health, though he violated many rules for healthful living and began to be plagued with some ailments of old age. Still trying to prove his manliness, he clung to the paradoxical notion that, for him, "leading a

The "New" York Gang

good life makes it possible . . . to experience . . . irregularities and still remain at . . . peak physically." In all probability he truly thought he had the body of a twenty-year-old. "Because *he said* it was so, it was so," states Clarence Johnson. "Because he said it so often, it was so. And he came to believe it himself." So egocentric and self-persuasive was Hoffman, according to Starr, that "after he told a story a time or two, he started to believe it."[57] How little his outlook had altered was illustrated by the giant sign in front of the factory he opened in 1967 on Interstate 83 just north of York. Its revolving figure was not a bodybuilder or one of his newer stars. It was one of the old gang—John Terpak (with Schemansky's body)—who would remain in Hoffman's eyes the perfect athlete, performing a split snatch. Much at York was new, but what prevailed was tradition.

DESCENT FROM GLORY

8

CULTURAL COUNTERCURRENTS

> Money is of absolutely no use to me apart from the power which it brings with it. I, of course, allude to its power for good, when rightfully used.
>
> —Bernarr Macfadden

As Hoffman entered his seventies, York Barbell experienced a clash of two cultures. The first was based on the ego and image of Bob himself. By dint of his remarkable salesmanship and the fortune he had amassed, especially from health foods, he earned from one reader the epithet "man of many labels."[1] Though beset by physical ailments, Hoffman still aspired to recognition as "World's Healthiest Man" and "World's Busiest Man." Already known as "Father of American Weightlifting," he also sought to be "Father of Physical Culture" and once even claimed to have been the "World's Strongest Man," possibly the highest accolade for weightlifters. Through promotion of such images, accompanied by increased philanthropy and involvement in national politics, Hoffman hoped to carve a permanent niche for himself in history. Emerging to challenge the views of Hoffman and his generation was a weightlifting counterculture that reflected changes in American society. The new York gang, whose youth, education, and scientific orientation had inspired so much hope, now demanded a share in the money, power, and glory of the organization—prerogatives heretofore guarded jealously by company elders. Differences between the two groups surfaced over drugs, lifestyle, and respect for authority. The revolt of the flower generation ultimately had a devastating effect on the overt displays of masculinity that so much characterized Muscletown during its golden age.

Emphasis on Youth

The late 1960s witnessed an emphasis in the iron game, as in American society, on youth, liberation, and idealism. At York these qualities were exemplified by a group of ardent spirits who seemed to embody the virtues Hoffman had been advocating for decades. Bill Starr and Tommy Suggs, editors of *Strength & Health*, were the nucleus of a team that rivaled the enthusiasm of the old York gang. Training in Muscletown for the 1967 Pan-Am Games were a host of rising stars who kept "the weights really flying. The York Gym never looked better." Adding to this intensity were a dozen young lifters who attended the second Olympic Development Training Camp at York Junior College. They were coached by Morris Weissbrot, who had recently studied eastern European methods of total conditioning. He contended that his charges "learned more about weightlifting in these two weeks than they could have possibly learned in two years on their own." Californians Bob Hise III and Jack Hill Jr. were group leaders, while Chicagoan Rick Holbrook was named top prospect. At the Duncan YMCA lifters under Gajda and former Hungarian champ Mihaly Huska beat York in the 1967 YMCA championships. Duncan's top performer was middleweight Fred Lowe, in whom Hoffman saw the same kind of physical potential as Schemansky. He had "never seen a more powerfully built lifter. Fred Lowe personifies power by his mere presence." Also impressive was 1967 Teenage Mr. America Mike Dayton of Oakland. "He's an All-American boy," Hoffman proudly stated. His tall, handsome blond appearance caused another observer to call Dayton "the kind of boy I'd trust my daughter with. . . . you can tell by looking at him, he is a real clean-cut type."[2] The November 1967 cover of *Strength & Health* featured Dayton with an insert of the lads from the Olympic Development Camp. Hoffman could hardly hope for finer examples of wholesome youth.

Cultural Countercurrents

Notwithstanding business, family, and training obligations, Suggs and Starr traveled thousands of miles as York ambassadors to meets and exhibitions. At the Winston-Salem Open in 1967 they lifted, conducted a clinic, and met North Carolina AAU chairman Jack King, "one of the 'new breed' of progressive meet promoters." They were impressed by the pool of local talent waiting to be tapped in the Tar Heel State and elsewhere, and by the new "happening" sweeping the country. "From New York to San Francisco and Chicago to New Orleans the new generation 'hippies' are having 'Be-ins,' " wrote Suggs. "This is where it's happening," he said of a "York Lift-In" between heavyweights Gubner, Schemansky, and Ernie Pickett to pick the final member of a team that would attend the Little Olympics in Mexico City. Though it seemed unlikely that Pickett could defeat the two veterans, he had experienced an upsurge in recent months and registered a stunning upset with lifts of 410, 320, and 435. Bednarski, who had had the same kind of dramatic rise a year earlier, was coaching him. Jubilant over his success, Bednarski turned "cart-wheels and the other lifters just stood around wondering how he got so strong so fast." When asked about his gains, Pickett replied that he was "not doing anything different . . . except representing York and training in the York gym once or twice a week." That the new York spirit was merely the leading edge of a broader phenomenon was suggested by a general improvement in American lifting performances. While an 885 total placed third in the mid-heavy division at the 1966 senior nationals, it was only enough for eleventh in 1967.[3]

Further evidence of a resurgence was the fine showing of American lifters at the Winnipeg Pan-Am Games in July and the Little Olympics in September. Especially reassuring were their observations of Communist-bloc athletes, who, at close quarters, did not seem unbeatable. One American, after watching the Poles train, asked, "Where is all that blinding speed I thought I would see? They have speed, flexibility, good form, but nothing really different from our lifters." Suggs agreed: "If there is one thing that impressed me most in Mexico City it was the fact that all the lifters were just normal guys. There weren't any mechanical robots or zombies lifting." While no American placed first against the world's best, Puleo came close to winning, Knipp placed second, Pickett took third, Walter Imahara and Grippaldi came in fourth, and Gerald Moyer was seventh. The American team placed one point away from second, and no one seemed outclassed. With Bednarski

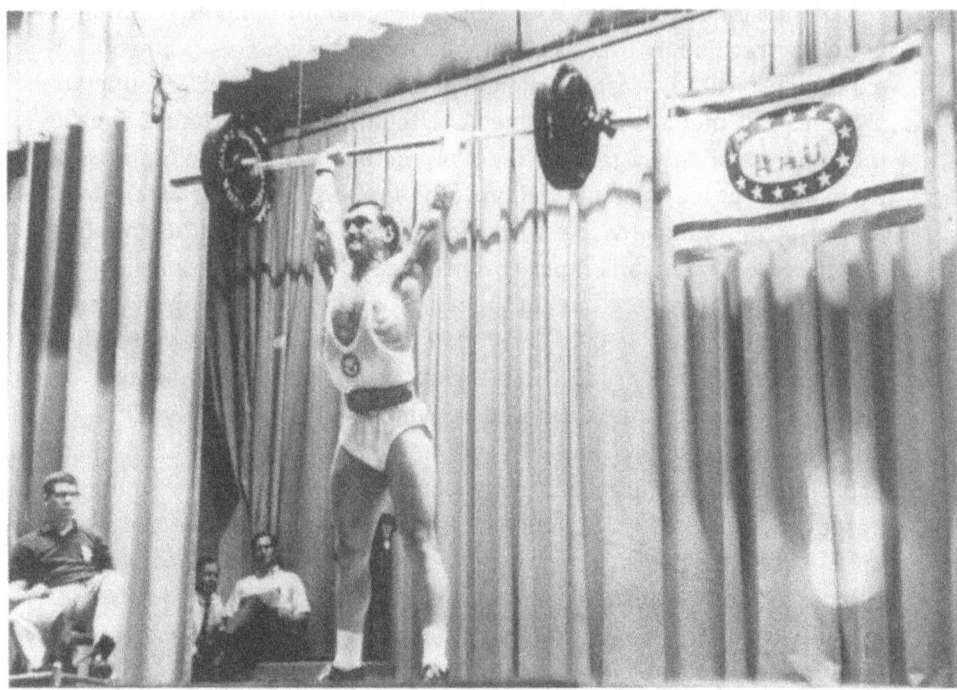

Bill Starr was the most enterprising member of the "new" York gang in the late 1960s. In the early 1970s he experienced an about-face and led an attack on the York establishment. His muscularity is evident in this 310-pound press.

speedily recovering from an elbow injury sustained in Winnipeg, there was optimism all around. Hoffman was "very proud" of his young team and believed it could improve enough to win the Olympics. "The future of American lifting [was] looking very good."[4]

Those athletes attracted to York in the late 1960s seemed to exude the finest features of America's youth-oriented society. Reminiscent of the youthful Terpak and Terlazzo, Starr was idealized in *Strength & Health* as a hardworking employee who taught at the local college in the evenings, was a good father, and still made lifting gains. Suggs, following his promotion to office manager, was portrayed as an astute businessman. But at home he was a gentleman farmer, raising "corn, wheat, evergreen trees, and choice steers." Starr observed that "Tommy's work, family life, and lifting" were "well balanced." After being selected "Lifter of the Year" a second time, Bednarski received a similar eulogy. Like Suggs, he was "an extrovert supreme." As Starr wrote at the time: "He still gets a real thrill out of performing in front of people. We go on many exhibitions together and . . . he gets as keyed up for a cub scout troop or a junior high assembly as he does for the Seniors. He loves to lift in front of groups, both big and small, and he always pleases the crowd. They can sense the enjoyment he is receiving and it catches on. Barski never shortchanged a crowd in his life. He dreads lifting, or for that matter doing anything, alone." Starr recalls that Bednarski came to York as a "clean-cut kid" with a young family and lived in one of Bob's houses in Brookside Park "with doilies on the chairs, etc." It was his enthusiasm that started the York gang training twice a day.[5] Among Starr's editorial innovations was a "Hats Off" section to recognize the sport's hardworking volunteers and a "Speaking Out" column. Starr's views did not always accord with Hoffman's old-fashioned outlook stemming from the 1930s, yet everyone liked the spunk, honesty, and openness of this articulate spokesman of the younger generation.

An additional reason for Hoffman to feel pride was that he had invested a lot of money educating lifters. The list of beneficiaries included such standouts as Frank Capsouras, Barry Whitcomb, Phil Grippaldi, and Russell Knipp. Of those residing in York, Gary Glenney was attending the Harrisburg campus of Penn State, and Bednarski was taking freshman English at York Junior College. Don Reed, a Californian who had worked his way into the organization as editorial assistant, was never an outstanding lifter, but Hoffman assisted with his schooling. Emphasis on education was evident also in the magazine sections "Barbells on Campus" and "Research and the Weight Man" and in the clinics held by Suggs and Starr around the country. In researching his master's thesis in physical education at the University of Maryland, Whitcomb employed the York gang as subjects. A national collegiate weightlifting championship (soon followed by one in powerlifting) was held annually, and Dick Landis of Princeton University was organizing a league in the mid-Atlantic states.[6] Though weightlifting rarely became a varsity sport, higher education and its attendant values had thoroughly permeated the iron game.

Philanthropic Endeavors

Despite Bob's interest in education, the Hoffman Foundation was assuming a more perfunctory role. Following the departure of Ziegler and

Todd, it became mainly a laboratory for chemist Don Nickol to test water and food samples. But most of his work was for outside concerns. After Nickol departed in 1970, the foundation's name served as a heading for outside research articles published in *Strength & Health* and as a tax write-off. Winston Day explains how Dietz also used the foundation to personal advantage in the stock market. Given seven days to pay for a purchase, he would secure it with his own money if the stock went up in that period; if it went down, the foundation would be obliged to invest in it. Small wonder, he reckons, that Dietz lived like a king in one of York's finest houses. What Bob saw in the evolving role of the foundation was an opportunity not to make more money but to give it away and thereby achieve a higher form of renown. Aside from scholarships for his lifters, Hoffman's philanthropic endeavors, accompanied by much fanfare, had been limited to $1,000 bids in the yearly cake auction at the retarded children's dance in York. He also had made periodic contributions to the York YMCA, but in 1968 he escalated his donation, giving a thousand acres for a YMCA camping center. Admittedly, part of Bob's motivation can be traced to his concern for the health and well-being of American youth, but the most satisfying aspect of his generosity was undoubtedly the sign he envisioned over the entrance, recognizing him as "Prominent Educator, Philanthropist, and Friend of Youth."[7]

And renown was not Hoffman's sole ulterior motive. A political motive was evident in his donation of a further 152 acres of farmland to York County Parks just after the election of Richard Nixon. Named the Richard M. Nixon County Park, much was made of the fact that Nixon's parents and brother had lived on a nearby farm after World War II. The transfer took place on January 9, the president-elect's fifty-sixth birthday, in ceremonies at the Yorktowne Hotel with local congressman George Goodling and Pennsylvania's two senators present. It was disappointing that neither Nixon nor Governor Raymond Shafer attended, but it was an important step in catapulting Hoffman into the national limelight. Goodling publicized the event with an announcement in Congress, referring to Bob as "a close friend of Dick Nixon's . . . over a good span of years."[8] Hoffman's gift was also prompted by a realization that, without an heir, the foundation would carry his name, fortune, and work into posterity. Since the 1930s he had found that making a lot of money was one way to achieve fame, but such fame was always tainted by the possible stigma of greed. Now, taking a cue from Andrew Carnegie of his native Pittsburgh, Bob realized that by devoting his fortune to the public welfare, he could gain recognition, tax relief, and a modicum of political influence. If he could not live forever, he could achieve lasting remembrance through the Hoffman Foundation.

What enabled Bob to contemplate grandiose philanthropic schemes was a dramatic upsurge of sales in the late 1960s. Monthly averages, based on extant data, are as follows:

1966—$215,243	1969—$335,068	1972—$616,972
1967—$238,032	1970—$451,813	
1968—$293,078	1971—$540,835	

From 1968 to 1972 sales more than doubled, and from 1966 to 1972 they nearly tripled. In a previous six-year period (1960–66) sales increased only 38 percent. "Business, particularly in the health food field is booming," Terpak confided to a friend in 1971. "Every couple of years we expand our production facilities. We've averaged a 30 percent increase in sales each of the past three years. Looks like we'll be adding about 20,000 more sq. feet of space by the end of 1972 and so it goes." The rise in sales may be ascribed to America's growing awareness of the need for fitness and health. Many of the ideas Hoffman had been espousing for decades, albeit with one eye on the ledger books, were being borne out. Weight training and health foods were gaining public acceptance. Profit margins for the latter were so great that Bob almost never had to make adjustments for inflation! Super Hi-Proteen was his best seller, though (at $5 a can) it was considerably more expensive than his other products—an obvious sign of consumer demand for quality. Bottled water was one of Bob's newest ventures, and it compelled him to add "pure soft bottled water" to his rules for healthful living.[9] Aside from any intrinsic value, a product's worth was based on *his* liking of it and it's enhancement of his self-image.

Bob's Later Books

Hoffman had always used books to promote his ideas and products, and in 1967 he published four of them. *Running for Your Life* was inspired by his recent medical problems. He resorted to running to restore his health, the book serving to memorialize his experiences—real and imagined.

Not only did he extol the virtues of running and his achievements as a runner, but he devoted nearly as much attention to stair climbing, which he estimated to consume as many calories as running ten miles per hour. When he arrived early for an appointment in a multistoried building, he would make "ten round trips, sometimes twenty or more," before the other party arrived. At airports he "did not use the escalator, but carried [his] suitcases up the stairs." Always eager to be a model, he contended that the running he did as a youth led to the development of his deep chest. At age sixty-seven, when he weighed 270 pounds, it "reached the largest size of [his] life, 53 inches." On his sixty-ninth birthday he claimed to have run fifteen miles. He had good reason to doubt whether this feat had ever been done before by a man of his age and size.[10]

Besides self-promotion, the aim of Bob's books was to create a need for his products; they constituted an early version of the "infomercial." Though obsessed with weightlifters, Hoffman was interested in athletes of all sports, especially track and field. Jim Ryun, the young Kansan who dominated the mile in the late 1960s, he highly esteemed. He contended that Ryun used York products and followed the "Hoffman-York System of weight training." Another American success story was Billy Mills's unexpected victory in the ten-thousand-meter race at the 1964 Olympics. In *Strength, Energy, and Endurance*, Hoffman placed his own gloss on Mills's heroics.

> No American had ever won this long race before. Billy Mills was a little known runner, the athletes and coaches of the remainder of the world had never even heard of him. Yet as they rounded the last curve and spread out a bit on the stretch with Ron Clark of Australia, the world record holder, leading, suddenly Billy Mills darted out from the gasping, fighting runners and left them behind as if they were not in the race. . . . Bill Sharp, the famous Triple Jumper, who is now in charge of Physical Training, at the Police Academy in Philadelphia said, "Bob Hoffman's Stuff won that race. Billy Mills and I went to Bob's room at the Biltmore Hotel before we left Los Angeles, on the way to the Olympics, and carried out two armsful of Bob's Food Supplements, almost enough to stock a small health food store, and he used them faithfully."

Likewise in *How to Gain Weight* and *Reducing and Weight Control*, Bob integrated the sale of his health foods into his training advice.

"Hundreds of national championship medals, at least a hundred of gold medals, have resulted primarily through the advice I offered the 'Bob Hoffman boys grown up.'" Even professional athletes were enlisted as York disciples.[11] York products and training advice had, in Hoffman's idealized view, revolutionized American sport.

In both books on weight Hoffman also expounded on his own excellent health. Still using himself as a guinea pig, he claimed to have gained twenty pounds by consuming his Gain Weight Hi-Proteen and was soon "breaking some of [his] lifetime records." Then, in an experiment where he imbibed equal amounts of Energol and Golden Papaya, he allegedly ran "six miles breathing entirely through [his] nose, and at no time was [his] respiration higher than 20 per minute, or [his] pulse rate more than 110." To lose weight, Hoffman suggested fasting. Indeed, he claimed to eat only six meals a week, going Sunday to Tuesday without food, losing nine to fourteen pounds. On his seventieth birthday Bob claimed that his health was so perfect that he qualified for a million-dollar insurance policy. With blood pressure of 125 over 75 and a normal cardiogram, "all of [his] processes [were] in fit order." Bob was capable of believing that he still had the health of his youth and that he could will his heart fibrillations to go away.[12]

In *Drink More Water* (1970) Bob claimed to be an authority on water. His knowledge was established on three grounds. First, he had lived near water all his life and twice came close to drowning as a child. Then he claimed to have paddled a canoe in his youth from the source of both the Delaware and the Susquehanna Rivers to the ocean, and to have paddled from the source of the Allegheny River in Olean, New York, to New Orleans. How much such statements strained reader credulity can only be imagined. Third, Hoffman owned "a sizeable water empire," indeed "more springs and larger springs than any individual in the water business." Bob had to be first in everything, even owning springs! The text also mentioned that he had read countless books on water, but it was personal experience through which he appealed to consumers: "After years of drinking Blue Rock Mountain Spring Water, I feel like 40 million." Since Hoffman ate but one meal per day, he could not drink as much water at meals as others, so he drank it profusely at night. When at home reading magazines or typing letters, he might consume several quarts. Still expecting to live to the year 2000, he was sure that failure to do so would not come from lack of good drinking water.[13] The profit motive notwithstanding, Bob's recognition of the water marketing potential in North America anticipated Perrier by at least a decade.

An interesting feature of Bob's later writings is his frequent attribution of inspiration to Dr. Lorand's *Health and Longevity Through Rational Diet,* which he supposedly received on his tenth birthday, in 1908. It was not published, however, until 1912, and there is little in Hoffman's writings to suggest that he got much from it. On the subject of water, their views are contradictory. On behalf of the soft water he was peddling, Bob stated that "in studying hundreds of books" on water, he had "not found a single kind word concerning the use of hard water . . . or that soft water has anything to do with heart disease." Lorand, however, is explicit on the virtues of hard water: "Not only does hard drinking-water have a most beneficial influence upon the teeth, but in cities where such water is drunk the chest measure and height of the people is greater, as well as their fitness for military service, while where the water is soft the opposite condition prevails." For persons with a heart ailment, such as Hoffman, Lorand considered it inadvisable to consume much water. Contrary to Bob's custom of drinking several quarts in the evening alone, Lorand advised consumption of no more than one and one-half liters a day, lest tissues become "too watery, and the task of the blood-vessels and the heart be rendered too difficult." Lorand also denounced Hoffman's practice of eating just one meal per day. Winston Day confirms that Bob "ate more than I've ever seen anyone eat" at his evening meals. "He ate like a horse, then 20 minutes later he had to poop." Prescribing a quite different regimen, Lorand deplored the custom in his native Austria of eating lightly in the morning and heavily in the evening, especially after seven o'clock.[14]

A Credibility Gap

While there were doubtless many readers who believed in Bob and his products, a credibility gap was opening between himself and many youth in the iron game, including those of the York gang. Later, Bill Starr would assess Hoffman as "a chronic liar—almost pathologically." Within his organization, he became the butt of jokes and was regarded as a hypocrite for not living the wholesome lifestyle he preached. Also resented was his aloofness from the steroid problem while attempting to convey the impression that gains made by York lifters were from nutrition-consciousness and hard work. "Our athletes do not get tired and many can actually train twice a day," Hoffman maintained. The youthful spirits at York were appalled by these simplistic views and became restive, calling for more honesty and openness. Indignation was evident in a response to the decision to print "for the first time" the judges' scores in the 1968 Mr. America contest. Heretofore they had been "guarded like the crown jewels," observed Starr, "leaving many people with the impression that they must hide them because things may just not be on the up and up." A more subtle expression of discontent can be discerned in the "Speaking Out" section of the November 1968 *Strength & Health,* in which Puleo criticized the announcer, always a paternal figure, at the 1968 senior nationals. Puleo chastised the latter for jokes that were "uncalled for" and "degrading." One concerned Bednarski. "Bob holds his arms out in sort of a crucifix when he is concentrating for a lift. The joke was that he was drying his armpits!"[15] In retrospect, this quip seems amusing, but to earnest young men out to change the world in the late 1960s, it was no laughing matter.

Pre-Olympic Euphoria

Before the 1968 Olympics there was little indication that trouble was brewing at York. Business was good, and American lifting was soaring. Intensified by the excitement of an Olympic year, the competitive level in all classes was high, as evidenced by "higher and higher totals." In the lead was Bednarski. Starr noted: "As soon as we report that he has clean and jerked 450, he does 460 the following Saturday." After Bednarski jerked 500 pounds off the rack, Hoffman earmarked him as " 'odds-on' favorite to be the first man in history to clean and jerk 500 pounds." Starr told readers it would be "more newsy to report that 'Fantastic' Freddie Lowe and Bob Bednarski *haven't* broken any records in the last month.... We can almost hear the *Star Spangled Banner* in the background." Additionally March was back, resembling the old March in "appearance and lifting prowess," and Pickett pressed 450 off the rack. Even some of the lesser lights, Whitcomb of College Park, Dave Brower from nearby Hellertown, and bantamweight Roman Mielec from Newark, were moving ahead. Summer trainees included a spate of teachers looking for positions near Muscletown, including Kenny Moore and Frank Saunders from North Carolina, Puleo from Michigan, George Lugrin from Texas, and Pete Roselli from Philadelphia.[16] More than ever, in 1968 all roads in American weightlifting led to York.

A climax to this feverish activity was reached at the senior nationals, held in June at York. A standing-room audience watched the largest-ever crop of national-caliber athletes do their best lifting. Orchestrated by Terlazzo and Smitty, it attracted the most enthusiastic crowd since the 1964 Olympic Trials. Crowed *Strength & Health:* "We have more top notch lifters this year than we have had in ten or fifteen years. Some have just made the jump since last year's Nationals. This was only the second year for Bob Hise to lift in the National Championships. In training a week and a half before the contest he made lifts of 330, 320, and 375 while weighing 190 and cleaned 400. . . . That is international caliber lifting and it all happened in less than two years. Rick Holbrook didn't even lift in the Senior Nationals last year. This year he snatched 310 for a new Meet Record." Other star performers included Russ Knipp, Mike Karchut, and Peter Rawluk (middle); Joe Puleo and Gerald Moyer (light-heavy); Phil Grippaldi, Frank Capsouras, and John Gourgott (mid-heavy); and Joe Dube (heavy). But Bednarski turned in a performance that bordered on the miraculous. He stunned the overflow crowd by pressing 456½ and cleaning and jerking 486½ for two world records at only 247 bodyweight. His final lift could not have been more dramatic. "Just as I took a deep breath before my last attempt," Bednarski recalls, "there was a big flash of lightning, and a thunderclap shook the building. It was as if the gods had been looking down and decided to help me." Hoffman called his clean and jerk "the greatest lift ever made." *Strength & Health* reported that "over 2000 hysterical fans gave the 'Ninth Wonder' a standing ovation for a full five minutes. Records fell like ten pins during the two-day meet."[17]

The euphoria continued into the summer as American lifters combined a cooperative spirit with a competitive attitude. "One actually gets so saturated with terrific lifting," observed Suggs, "that he can't get excited with any lift—even a world record." The York spirit was contagious, migrating not only to hot spots of lifting in Chicago and Los Angeles but to the hinterlands—like Virginia, Indiana, Iowa, Arkansas, and Oklahoma. From December 1967 to midsummer 1968, 124 records were broken by American lifters: American Olympic, 40; American power, 26; American Olympic teenage, 10; junior national meet, 18;

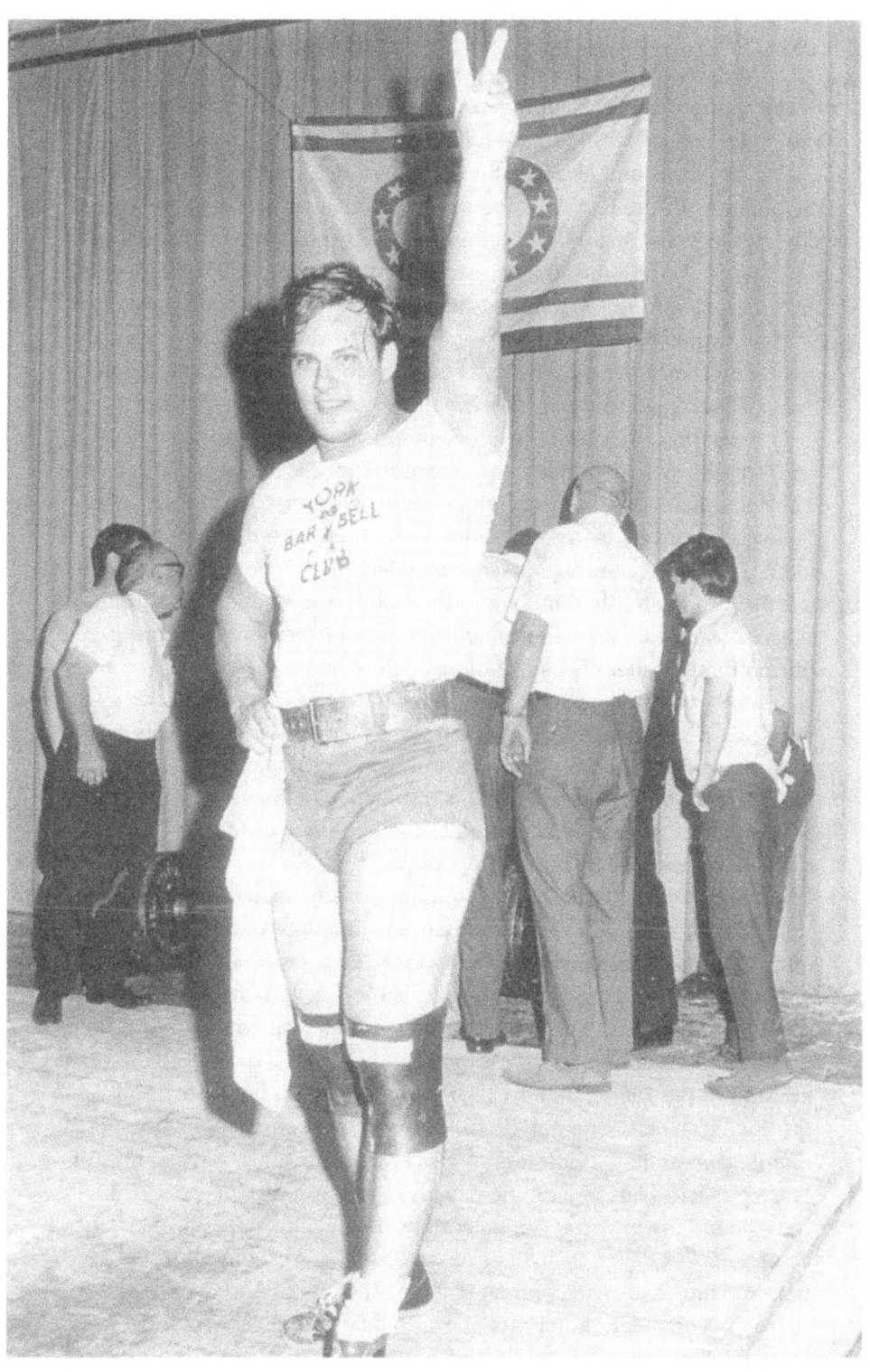

An exuberant Bob Bednarski flashes the victory sign while officials weigh his 486.5-pound world-record clean and jerk in 1968.

senior national meet, 20; junior world, 4; world, 6.[18] Most encouraging, this sudden surge was animated mainly by youth.

Socially the summer of 1968 was euphoric. Camaraderie abounded as members of the new York gang adopted clever nicknames for each other. Starr was "Star Trek," Bednarski "Barski," Glenney "Double G," and Suggs was gaining so much "muscular bodyweight" his pals called him "Super Suggs." When the lifters were not training, working, or studying, they were playing. Some went to the local state park for swimming and boating, while others frequented movies or local auctions. The gang also gathered at Suggs's farm for some "All-American fun," remarked Starr. "Everyone would bring some goodies and Kay and Tommy would provide refreshments and act as social directors. The footballs flew, the soccer balls bounced and so did many of the fellows. Generally everyone begged off squats the day after such an outing." Other gathering places included the bachelor pads of Hise and Holbrook and the family homes of Starr and Bednarski. Countless escapades and incidents enriched the lives of the youthful York gang during this summer of socialization. A crew from *Wide World of Sports* came to shoot footage for a special on the Olympics. Once Starr was introduced on a local television program called *Coach's Corner* as editor of *Sunshine and Health*—the nudist magazine! "Long after each of us has hung up his lifting belt and his trophies have become tarnished he will sit back and remember some of the experiences of the summer of '68. . . . It's going to be hard to top, ever."[19]

Significantly, none of the old York gang were involved, or even mentioned, in these frolics. With their careers, families, and finances intact and business better than ever, they were scarcely aware of the profound changes in the offing. At first the only visible link with the national youth culture, embodied in the civil rights movement, women's liberation, and protest of the Vietnam War, was the slightly longer hair sported by some athletes at the 1968 nationals. Then, as more lifters began to adopt less traditional styles of hair and dress, Hoffman, concerned about the sport's image, commented that lifters should at least be "neat and clean." Terlazzo was more unsympathetic with the change in fashion: "Some lifters have been showing up at contests lately looking like hippies from Haight Street. . . . Let's cut out this nonsense." Soon Suggs and Starr had long hair and mustaches, in contrast to their previous clean-cut appearance. Also, the convivial gatherings at Suggs's farm and elsewhere were no longer just innocent frolics. "Heavy partying and recreational drug use," especially marijuana, became the norm, according to Fred Lowe. In 1968 it was "all kind of a happy thing and having a good time in leisure hours, but the use would become much heavier in the next two years." Starr recalls that "Friday afternoons were sort of a blow out. We might smoke after a meet. It was extremely mild now that we look back on it. We didn't smoke it every day—we had families. We didn't want to do anything to fuck up our lifting." Whether taking recreational drugs was directly related to the steroids York lifters were taking is debatable, but the behavior of the younger gang coincided with that of an increasingly drug-oriented society. Grimek believed Jaqueline Susann's *Valley of the Dolls* typified society's growing dependence on drugs: "People swallow pills for just about anything that ails them, not knowing and caring less about the consequences."[20] Almost any kind of high seemed attainable in the summer of 1968.

The Bubble Bursts

At the Olympics these good feelings ended. A premonition of disaster came in the trials at York in August. Although competition was intense and winning totals were higher than those at the senior nationals in four of six classes, the "ninth wonder," after ascending the heights, plunged to the depths. "Before the contest, if anyone had told me that Bob Bednarski would come in third, I would have thought they were crazy," remarked Hoffman. But he had one of those days when nothing went right. "The man considered by many to be the greatest weightlifter of all time would not be going to the Olympics." Then at Mexico City the American team, whose prospects had seemed so bright, collapsed. Only Floridian Joe Dube won a medal, a bronze, and America placed seventh. "What can I say?" was Terpak's reaction. "We had the strongest team we have ever had in international competition, even stronger than our 1967 team, which came so close to winning the world title last year. But this year we were never in contention." Hoffman agreed that "we had expected to show the world" but ended up "almost the lowest on the totem pole." Obviously American lifters had let him down, and Bob never took defeat lightly. Starr was more reflective. Comparing performances with those at the trials, he found that "not a single lifter matched . . . his total at the Games." He concluded that the trials were too close to the Olympics, the team was relatively inexperienced, and it did not adapt well to living conditions in Mexico. The lifters were "in great physical shape, but it seemed as if they were fatigued mentally." The bitterest irony was that Bednarski, at a Saturday workout in York, became the first man in history to clean and jerk over 500 pounds, weighing only 246. That he had also front-squatted 550 pounds showed that he could do more. Such was the mystique of the "ninth wonder" that it was rumored he had cleaned and jerked 501 backstage at the Olympics![21]

The stunning loss at Mexico City had momentous consequences. Hoffman, despite an outward show of resignation, was deeply troubled: "I maintain a tranquil mind pretty well when only myself is involved. But when the team does not do well, I suffer internally more than anyone will ever know." Gary Glenney confirms that "you had to win." Bob "would not accept second." The only way Bob could reconcile himself to *seventh* place was to conjure up the myth that he had triumphed personally in Mexico City. So, he took credit for accomplishments of foreign lifters, noting that "all the world is following our training systems." Serge Reding, the rotund Belgian heavyweight who eased Dube out of second place, had supposedly purchased a York power rack, which led to "his tremendous power." Hoffman also assumed credit for the victorious Russians. Just after the competition Zhabotinski told him: " 'You are my father, you are my teacher: all that I am I owe to you.' These were strong words, nobly and sincerely spoken. Zhabotinski's interest in weightlifting was awakened through *Strength and Health* magazine." Another accolade in which Hoffman took pride was his designation as "Father of Weightlifting" by the IWF Congress. Additionally, Clarence Johnson was reelected president of the federation; the 242-pound class (where American "pocket" heavyweights would excel) was adopted; and Columbus, Ohio, was chosen for the 1970 world championships. Furthermore, the York barbells that were used in the Olympics "weighed out to the exact gram even when the poundage was in excess of 400." Notwithstanding his lifters' failure, Hoffman was "pleased and a bit proud that I was instrumental in winning all our major points" at the congress. He could therefore rationalize that the Olympics was not a disaster at all but "a worthwhile trip for American weightlifting," and could bask in the glow of self-glorification. The same *Strength & Health* issue that carried the depressing Olympic results was dedicated to Bob's seventieth birthday. It featured a large picture of him

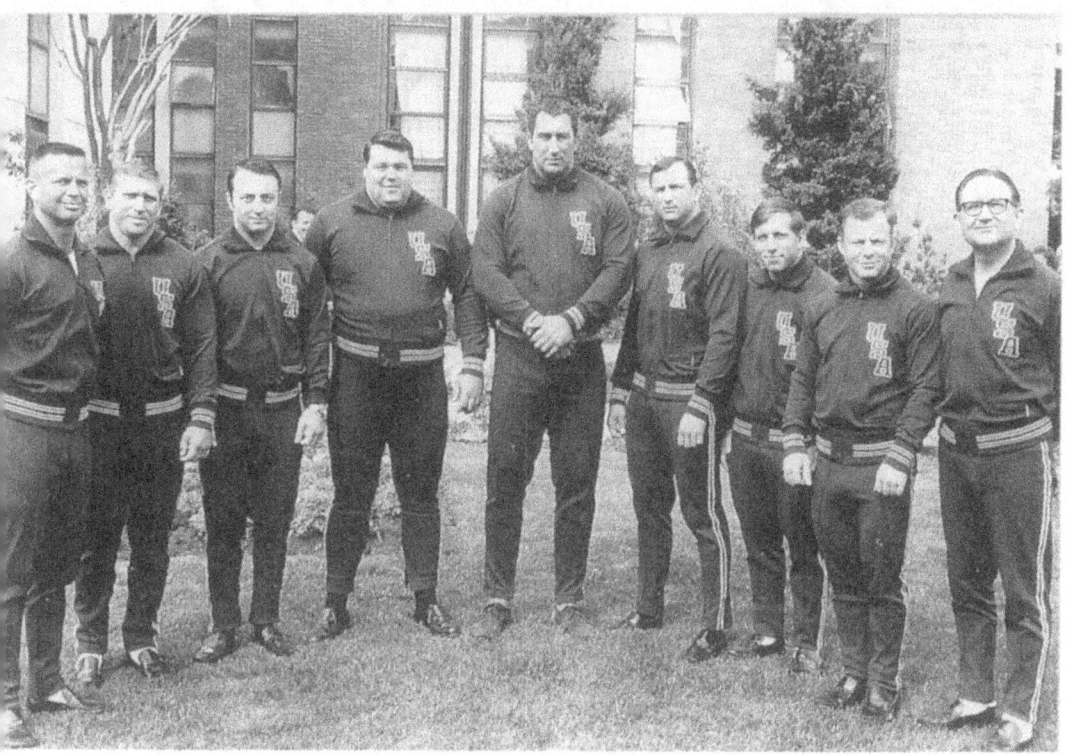

The 1968 Olympic Team: Major George Otott (trainer) of the U.S. Marines, Phil Grippaldi, Joe Puleo, Joe Dube, George Pickett, Bob Bartholomew, Fred Lowe, Russ Knipp, and John Terpak (coach).

on the cover, an autobiographical piece on "The Four Phases of My Life," and birthday messages from lifting notables across the country. Then 225 guests showed up on November 8 for his birthday party at the Yorktowne. In a contest the next day in the York gym, Bednarski made 402, 330, and 462 for a 1,195-pound total. "He had plenty left," Suggs observed, "but why hurry to his absolute limit for the world's his oyster now that there's an international 242-class." The recognition of American greatness that Hoffman was denied at the Olympics was at last realized by Bednarski.[22]

Depression and disillusionment were the most common reactions to the Mexican fiasco, however, and soon various stars in the York firmament began fading. Puleo and Lowe, never more than temporary fixtures, married and returned to their studies at universities in Michigan and Ohio. Russ Knipp joined Athletes in Action, a group of Christian athletes who gave exhibitions and testimonies nationwide. He was later joined by Glenney. Hise returned to California, and Pickett lost a lot of weight trying to become a normal human being again. The biggest loss was Suggs, who sold his farm and returned to Texas. He opened a gym and sold York products, and was soon joined by

Roman Mielec. Don Reed became assistant editor for a while before returning—"disillusioned," according to Starr—to California. He was replaced by George Lugrin, who kept the Texas connection alive. Other newcomers included Charlie Shields, a Shippensburg State College student; Joe Zagurski, Wally's son; and Tommy Kurtz, who joined the art department. His cartoons on the training and travels of the York gang, replete with trendy hairdos and garb, appeared in *Strength & Health* for several years. But the espirit de corps of the summer of 1968 was never duplicated.[23]

An AAU Mr. Universe?

Pleased with his seventieth birthday gala, Hoffman thought he could spark a revival by holding "a really big" strength show at York on his next birthday. The centerpiece would be a Mr. Universe contest. Since the IWF had essentially abandoned its physique shows, and York-sponsored Mr. Americas had not done well at Oscar Heidenstam's NABBA contests, Hoffman decided to launch an AAU Mr. Universe in York. He also envisioned a contest for the world's most muscular man and the world's strongest man. These festivities, as with almost everything else Bob instigated, revolved around himself, but there was an ulterior motive of modernization. In the 1960s Heidenstam and Weider capitalized on the old-fashioned standards Bob had imposed on the AAU. Both emphasized muscles for their own sake, encouraged internationalism, and offered contests with more grandiose titles than Mr. America. Then, in 1965 Dan Lurie reentered the field with his World Body Building Guild, which promoted yet another version of Mr. America (now there were three). Later he instituted a Mr. Olympus title to rival Weider's Mr. Olympia. Hoffman noted that "in the British Mr. Universe contests muscles are the only consideration." In the AAU Mr. America competition, scoring was divided evenly for muscularity, symmetry, and general appearance. The latter included "teeth, hair, skin and face" and such intangibles as morality and ability to project well over the media. The winner must also "be patient enough to sign autographs—in other words he must be the best all-round American we can select." Realization that this concept, modeled on the Miss America ideal of the 1950s, was becoming outdated was dawning on Hoffman.

Soon the AAU eliminated athletic-ability points, and Bob announced that his forthcoming Mr. Universe show would be truly an "international event," with judging based on muscles alone.[24]

When this extravaganza did not materialize, Hoffman became vulnerable to Weider charges that he was "The Bodybuilder's Arch Foe!" After ignoring such accusations for years, Hoffman struck back in 1971 with a three-part rebuttal called "Setting the Record Straight," in which he stated that Weider was a liar and that he himself had "done More for Bodybuilding and Physique Contests than any Man in the World." He tried to substantiate this claim by pointing out that Clarence Ross (1945) "was the only Mr. America until Chris Dickerson [1970], who did not train in the York Barbell Club gym.... No Weider man ever won an AAU Mr. America contest!" However great were Bob's contributions to bodybuilding and unfair Weider's charges, his adversary's "muscle up and make out" approach and emphasis on muscles alone had more popular appeal than Hoffman's philosophy of all-round development. The most serious blow to York was Weider's acquisition of Arnold Schwarzenegger, supposedly after being turned away by Hoffman. In *Muscle Builder,* Arnold called Boyer Coe and other AAU stars "paper tigers" for not entering IFBB contests and accused NABBA champions Bill Pearl and Reg Park of trying to preserve their reputations by avoiding competition.[25] Hoffman could hardly have predicted Schwarzenegger's impact on the pecking order in the world of muscles.

Powerlifting Wrangles

The other front on which Hoffman faced a challenge was in powerlifting, owing mainly to promotional efforts by former hammer thrower George Frenn. Not only was Frenn writing powerlifting articles for Joe, but in 1968 he proposed to the AAU a British-U.S. match in London to be sponsored by Weider. "He has been a very controversial character in A.A.U. track and field," noted Terpak. "It's unfortunate that we in weightlifting have to inherit the guy." But Frenn's actions goaded York to take action. At a 1969 IWF meeting in Warsaw the United States supported a proposal, rejected 3–27, for powerlifting to become an international sport. Also, to parry Frenn's attempts to form his own association, Terpak was setting up a separate AAU powerlifting committee. He assured Peary

Rader that he was "not opposed to powerlifting," but when Weider finally did hold a meet between British and American power men in southern California, York belittled it. Another magazine feud ensued, with Bob denying Joe's accusations that he and the AAU were trying to destroy powerlifting. "This past year there were more AAU powerlifting contests than Olympic lifting contests," was his indignant response. He also claimed that "in the thirties, before Weider even started putting out a few mimeographed sheets," York and others were holding odd-lift contests all over the country. Refusing to admit he had missed an opportunity to be first, Bob trivialized the Weider meet as "a little club contest" and promised to hold "the first World's Powerlifting Championships right here in Muscletown, USA."[26]

Frenn, labeled the "Ralph Nader of power lifters" by *Muscle Builder*, was not intimidated by York's pervasive influence. He scoffed at "the purveyors of jealousy and distrust" and labeled Hoffman an old fogey. Frenn explained how York threw every obstacle possible in the way of the recent international contest. Yet it was a "howling success," with five American and thirteen British records set—a "moral defeat" for Hoffman. York ally Murray Levin was emphatic that Terpak "must respond and rebutt whatever garbage Weider puts out." He thought Weider and Rader were "going to make an all out play to dominate powerlifting. York should keep its lead at all costs." Levin even suggested adding a powerlifting section to *Strength & Health*. "You can't win a pissing match with a skunk," was Terpak's response to York's latest bout with Weider. Furthermore, any libelous attacks would result in court action. "I have been receiving some vicious letters from Ben, only because I have taken [a] 'Rock of Gibralter' stand against IFBB affiliation with the A.A.U."[27]

Unfortunately powerlifting did not always exhibit the all-American image Hoffman had sought to instill with weightlifters and physique men. The 1960s powerlifter was often stereotyped by AAU weightlifting stalwarts as a dull-witted self-indulgent slob who lifted in bare feet, cut-off jeans, and tank top. As Starr observed after the 1970 senior (power) nationals, "[N]o one can get excited over watching a slob even if he squats a million pounds." Also disconcerting was excessive wrap use. Since flexibility and free movement were not required to perform the squat, bench press, and deadlift, powerlifters had adopted extensive knee and elbow bandages, oversized belts, stiff work boots, and body wraps. Some lifters even used bedsheets for added tensile strength. Along with drugs (which became as rampant in powerlifting as in weightlifting) and lax judging standards (particularly in squats), powerlifters often joked about bringing a winch to help them with their lifts. Because of these problems and the newness of the sport, it is not surprising that sixty-eight national powerlifting records were set in 1970.[28] Stricter regulations and officiating ensued under Bob Crist, who became national chairman in 1971, but image problems plagued powerlifting. Hoffman preferred weightlifting to powerlifting, but he could not appear to be giving it less than full support.

York's Public Image

Another problem for Bob was an ongoing feud with the FDA. Originating in 1964 over misleading claims in his books, articles, and advertising, it threatened York's enormous profits on food supplements. By 1968 it was the oldest case on the docket of the Middle District Court of Pennsylvania, but Bob was prepared to fight the government indefinitely. "No compromise" was his initial reaction to a proposed consent decree that called for omission or alteration of fifty-seven statements he had made about his products: "If our attorneys think we should sign crap like this we had better get other attorneys." After a summer of procedural wrangling, the company's attorney, Solomon Friend, provided assurances that if Bob signed, there would be no publicity and the document would merely be filed as a matter of record. Furthermore, if York violated the decree, the government could not sue. No contempt charges would be cited. The judge, he was told, did not want to try the case, the FDA wanted to withdraw from it, and the signed decree was "absolutely worthless." With assurances that were tantamount to victory, Hoffman signed the document just before the case went to trial. But Bob had no intention of changing his promotional material, all of which he believed was true.[29]

Among weightlifting and health-food enthusiasts Hoffman did not lack support. "Without you I am afraid that weightlifting would go to pot," was the opinion of Frank Bates, who headed the Keasby Eagles club in Paterson, New Jersey. Another administrator, Bob Bendel, assured Bob that "thousands of people are living stronger, healthier lives because of you." Gary Echternacht, organizer of the 1969 teenage nationals in Des Moines, was "thrilled" when the "father of World Weightlifting" agreed to serve as announcer. In distant India H. V. Sathyanarayana, secretary of the Mysore Weightlifters' Association, believed Bob deserved acclaim not only as "the 'FATHER OF WEIGHTLIFTING' in America," but as "'GRANDFATHER OF MODERN WEIGHTLIFTING' in the entire Universe." Other tributes centered on Hoffman's products and promotions. Mrs. Frank Duncan of Austin, Texas, was so impressed by his book *Reducing and Weight Control* that she wanted to start using his products, but she did not know whether she "should use all of [his] products or only a few." Don Baxter, a ranch foreman in Lake Luzerne, New York, had gained twenty pounds of muscular bodyweight on Hoffman's protein and vitamins. Now he was interested in selling it to his fellow cowboys. Ed Seeman of White House Station, New Jersey, wanted to order Energol in gallon quantities, not for himself, but for his show horses. In response to magazine appeals for contributions to the Hoffman Foundation, Bob Gans of Joliet, Illinois, "an S & H man for 9 years," sent a $5 check to Bob. He probably did not understand why it was never cashed. From San Quentin prison came a piece of nostalgia. Prisoner Tony Allan reminded Hoffman of the barbell set he had donated to inmates after the York gang had visited the prison in 1939. Now dubbed "The Old Master," the York set, despite heavy use, was "in perfect condition and [had] out worn at least two other sets."[30]

Letters of criticism, however, were also increasing. Warren Miller, a health-food vendor in Severna Park, Maryland, complained in 1970 when less than half his shipment arrived. Also dissatisfied was Ronald Miller of Petersburg, Virginia, who wanted to know "how many Quick Gain Weight bars you have to eat to gain a lb? I've eaten over a box and 1/2 now and only gained 1/2 lb." But J. P. Babinsky of San Antonio was gaining weight by taking reducing tablets. "At the end of 8 days I had gone from 184 lbs to 191 lbs." Part of Babinsky's problem stemmed from lack of quality control at York. Bednarski, who worked in the stock room, explains that Quick Gain Weight and Protein Reducing Tablets all came from the same vat, and Bacon observed regular Hi-Proteen being poured into Super Hi-Proteen containers. "It didn't matter." Customer dissatisfaction was also evident in a letter from Vincent Penta of Highlands, New Jersey, who nearly broke his tooth on a piece of grit in Hoffman's Vigorola: "What kind of standards do you people have any way?" He expected better products from health-food vendors than from the A & P.[31]

Cultural Countercurrents

Most hurtful were assertions that York compared unfavorably to Weider. E. T. of Newark, Ohio, criticized a statement in *Strength & Health* that Chris Dickerson, Ken Waller, and Casey Viator were the "3 best built men in America—ignoring the claims of Bill Pearl, Boyer Coe, Chuck Sipes, Harold Poole, Dave Draper, Larry Scott, Frank Zane, John Decola, and Sergio Oliva," most of whom had Weider connections. Oliva alone, he felt, "could hide all 3 of them behind his left lat. . . . Though Bob Hoffman may have a lot to brag about, it sure gets sickening reading his self glorifying editorials all the time. Let's face it, we've all read it before. . . . Wise Up!" Grimek's remarks in *Muscular Development* about the lack of international physique competition in America invited a similar response. "Just who is he kidding," wrote a South Carolina reader. "International events in the USA take place every year in the IFBB." Charles Evanich of Normal, Illinois, was distressed by Hoffman's political views, including his support of the president's Vietnam policy. Though "one of a thousand diehards that would march into the sea on Bob Hoffman's command," he believed Nixon's policy was "not in the interest of the American people." A writer from Tempe, Arizona, had the opposite view of Bob's position, contending that he was helping "socialists, pinkos, and left-wing liberals trying to destroy our sacred system of free enterprise." Symptomatic of the confused values of this period was a letter from Buffalo with the terse remark "You are sick Bob."[32]

Many more people, however, approached Hoffman with problems. In 1968 a Pittsburgh health-food fanatic, after pouring out her distress for fourteen pages, declared: "Enough of this, I can't calm down. I wish I were dead." A man from Malden, Massachusetts, wrote Bob on a paper towel about the theft of heavy objects from his house—a two-hundred-pound barbell, a hundred-pound cast-iron sink, and three hundred pounds of plumbing equipment. An employee at Hoffman's Blue Rock Mountain Spring Water Company complained that his boss was a "2-face rat." A middle-aged man from Adrian, Michigan, had suffered many ailments until he discovered a treatment to accompany his high-protein diet: "On rising in the morning, I fill the bathtub with water just under 100 F. I remain prone in this for a full half hour. My hips are slightly elevated so the scrotum is out of the water. . . . This treatment is effective in exercising the heart, stimulating the circulation, cleansing the muscle tissue of lactic acid, getting rid of cholesterol, poisons, harmful bacteria, nicotine, alcohol, and other foreign materials."

Jim Williams, a black champion powerlifter, protested the decision to hold the 1971 senior nationals in New Orleans. He did not believe he and his white wife would be able to travel, eat, or find lodging without risking their lives. Finally, old-timer Hank Feldmann of Brooklyn was appalled by the dismal state of lifting. The 1971 world championships in Peru, broadcast on ABC's *Wide World of Sports,* was "a perfect example of a sport gone to *pot!* Alexeev's gut filled the whole screen, and the others didn't look much better." He did not believe anyone could press two hundred pounds more than Stanko and Grimek had done in the 1930s.[33] Hoffman could also reflect on how much the sport had changed since he won the national heavyweight championship in 1927. Vasily Alexeev's winning total exceeded his own (for five lifts!) by 554 pounds.

"Coin of the Realm"

Hoffman's chief claim to fame now was the wealth he was accumulating. But he had no interest in money for its own sake. He believed "riches in the coin of the realm are of little value, you can't take them with you, you can eat so much, drive one car at a time, sleep in one bed at a time and it doesn't require a fortune to do this." As Bachtell notes, "Bob was not interested in money—only the power to make it." When it became widely known that he had no desire to spend it on himself, there was never any lack of good causes importuning him. When the AAU opened its new headquarters in Indianapolis in 1970, Hoffman gave $1,000 to help furnish it. For the closing banquet at the Columbus world championships he donated $750. And in 1971 Bob presented five $1,000 awards for distinguished writing to students at York College. But he turned down a request from East Side Boys' Club of Erie for free equipment and was unwilling to sponsor a young man from Guyana who aspired to come to the United States to study mechanical engineering and become Mr. America.[34] Hoffman never allowed his generosity to exceed the intangible benefits he expected in return. Self-recognition was always paramount.

Gifts to his women most directly flattered his ego. To Rosetta, living in Maryland, he continued to send $200 a month, for which she regarded him "the kindest generous and most finest man in the world." Her request for a diamond, however, was not honored. Alda was more than a wife to Bob. She was a helpmeet who provided him with emotional stability and could even be described as a business partner. That she should fault him for being unfaithful is hardly surprising. But Hoffman never viewed faithfulness the same way. "Unfaithful!" he once exclaimed. "I've been seeing the same four women . . . for over twenty-five years, at least once a week when I'm in town. . . . *The same four women!* If that's not being faithful, I don't know what faithful means." Winston Day introduced Bob to a "Philadelphia girl" named Bunny, who was a "semipro." Hoffman would bring her to York by train for an afternoon at the House on the Hill. Day recalls that he "bragged about his sexual prowess all the time," saying that "he could have three orgasms in a row without ejaculating. Most men go down. He said he continued to stay erect." His superhuman sexuality was yet another means to bolster his ego. When he visited Day's office in a not-so-nice area of Philadelphia, he would "often leave a girl-friend sitting in the car for four or five hours" while he discussed business. By the early 1970s "his libido began slowing down," but Bob remained devoted to his girlfriends.[35]

While Hoffman amply provided for his women, arrangements for those far more able to improve York's standing proved unworkable. Kono, after retiring from lifting, coached weightlifters for the host countries of the Tokyo and Munich Olympics, promoted York products abroad, and sent information regularly to Bob and Johnny. What Kono wanted most, however, was a permanent place in Muscletown: "I want to be productive," he told Terpak, "and my ambition has always been to work for the York Barbell Company if the salary was good." Kono wanted "to see York the way it was 15–20 years ago when you had the strongest team in the world. I'd like to have an active part in the rejuvenation of the York Barbell Club . . . to make it shine in the lifting world like in the past." Exactly why Hoffman never engaged him will never fully be known, but money was a key factor along with some misplaced priorities. "Dietz was really tight with the money and was probably cockroaching it," Kono recalls. "Nobody liked him."[36] Bob never seemed willing to override Mike's judgment on outside proposals, no matter how worthy, and Mike never questioned any of Bob's initiatives, no matter how unreasonable. Kono alone could hardly have turned York around, but its failure to invest in him or embrace national coaching, while much more money was squandered elsewhere, was a lost opportunity for American lifting.

Bednarski's Demise

The key figure on whom all hopes focused was Bednarski. Unfortunately the "ninth wonder" had become dispirited by his defeat at the 1968 trials and let it hinder later performances. According to Bednarski, Hoffman had told him not to train too hard for the trials but to save himself for the Olympics. After all, he stood a good chance of beating Zhabotinski, and there was danger in peaking too soon or too often. "Weightlifters can do their best maybe three, four times a year," he explains. "After the U.S. nationals I asked Terpak how I was going to keep it up by the tryouts, which were themselves six weeks away, and then hold it for the six more weeks until the Olympics. He said, 'Don't worry. Just go to the tryouts and show them you're in shape. That's all you have to do. After your last performance you're not going to stay home.'" Terpak insists that the selection committee acted fairly. Only two heavyweights could be entered. Dube and Pickett had won the trials and would have felt cheated had they been excluded. Yet everyone knew the world's best lifter was left at home, and it was only natural that Bednarski should feel bitter: "I was never the same after that. I didn't have the heart any more." To cope with his depression Bednarski turned to drugs. Since arriving at York he had been taking Dianabol and syndrox (goon juice). From these he graduated to speed (Dexedrine) to get up for lifting and various sedatives to bring him down and induce sleep, a pattern set at the Winnipeg Games to cope with his distress over marital problems. There, due to the sedative, he became shaky and lost coordination, thereby dislocating his elbow.[37]

Complete drug dependency did not occur immediately, not as long as Ziegler was around. Despite Ziegler's role in bringing drugs to York, he remained mostly a restraining influence. But with Ziegler gone and the disappointment of his setback at the trials still fresh, Bednarski's drug intake got out of control. He recalls getting hold of the *Physicians Desk Reference*, a two-thousand-page manual listing every drug available. Initially he just wanted to know more about the side effects of Dianabol, but he "wound up discovering new steroids, like Winstrol and Durabolin, and decided to go ahead." When syndrox was taken off the market, Bednarski and other York lifters,

> armed like medical students with our *PDR*s, did some quick research and found ourselves some other stimulants, like Dexedrine,

Cultural Countercurrents

Benzedrine, Desoxyn, and Biphetamine-20. . . . We would look up a drug, read the description, and say, "This sounds good." Then we'd call the doctor, and he'd give it to us, saying, "Jesus, you know more about this stuff than I do." And when athletes become their own doctors, the lengths they'll go to procure these things are unbelievable. We tried practically every stimulant in the book. After my Olympic-tryouts defeat I became the most adventurous. . . . In the beginning my intention was just to get out of my depression, and later on I just wanted to get high.

Eventually Bednarski became addicted to Soma, a muscle relaxant containing codeine, to counteract his excitable disposition. He nicknamed it Space Fantasy from its effects. "With the kind of pill popping I did, an average guy probably wouldn't have been able to function at all. But when you're a 240-pound lifting machine, you burn out the pills' effects pretty quickly." Bednarski seldom smoked marijuana and was afraid of LSD and other mind-bending drugs, but he and others were developing addictive behaviors.[38] Increasingly their lifestyle embraced the youth revolution of the late sixties.

Schultz's Drug Store

Remarkably all the drugs York lifters abused were obtained from Shultz's neighborhood drug store (around the corner from the gym) and paid for by the company. "Shultz did a hell of a business," Bednarski recalls. York Barbell had "a monthly drug bill of about $1,000." Two factors made possible this arrangement. First, Starr, whom Hoffman trusted, was given carte blanche to get what he wanted there. Second, Bednarski started sending steroids to athletes throughout the country. Soon he and Starr were disseminating drugs to a score of lifters, and "eventually steroids became a tiny item" in their trade. Hoffman tended to ignore problems and relegate supervision to others. Terpak learned something was awry only in 1969, when Dietz brought to his attention a bill for $740 for Bednarski's drugs. Within a half hour Terpak delivered to Roger Shultz a letter stating that no further drugs should be charged to the company without written orders from Mike or John. That Bob or anyone else could have circumvented this order Terpak dismisses as unlikely, since Shultz, a fellow Shriner and boon companion, would have informed him at once. The lifters' procurement of drugs upset Dietz for economic reasons, Starr believes. "For Terpak, it was on moral grounds." Yet the trafficking continued. Aware of the ease with which athletes were getting ergogenic drugs, outsiders began offering acid and even hard drugs for the lifters' amphetamines. According to Yuri Brokhin, "[O]ne weightlifter confessed that LSD charged him with extra 'power' by allowing him . . . to first project an entire lift in his mind."[39] Usually, however, recreational drugs impaired one's lifting. The drug problem intensified when Bob Hise III visited York, with full cultural baggage from the West Coast. Lou DeMarco recalls his demeanor in the spring of 1967—dressed as a California hippie. As the drug culture got into full swing, virtually everyone recognized Hise as a corrupting influence. Though never in residence more than several months at a time, "Bob Hise stayed in York long enough to contaminate it really bad," observes Bednarski.[40]

The Sexual Revolution

Accompanying the cultural revolution and prompted by widespread use of the birth-control pill was a change in sexual mores. Again Bednarski was in the vanguard. He explains that certain drugs, like testosterone, made you horny, and the sedatives he was taking lowered inhibitions. Their joint effect led him to extramarital affairs as early as 1967, when his wife returned to Rhode Island to deliver their second child. Besides, Hoffman, who always had liberal views about sex, gave money to Bednarski and others to "sow your wild oats" after meets. Eventually he became as preoccupied with sex as he was with drugs and lifting. The drugs released him from reality and moral restraints: "My libido was going into sex rather than lifts on the platform." Bednarski was not the only York lifter to experience these changes. At least half the younger gang and even such mature members as Suggs, Degenhardt, and Starr indulged in sexual experimentation—all in keeping with the times. York was "a den of everything that was going on, including wife swapping." A natural outgrowth of this culture, devoid of moral inhibitions and accompanied by heavy steroid use, was a high divorce rate among the young Yorkers.[41]

It is also not surprising, given this cultural upheaval, that American lifting should decline. Following the Mexico City disaster, there was an attempt to regroup for the next world championships. And Bednarski was providing the lead. At first, while still in control of himself, he regularly set world records in the new 242-pound class. "Bednarski would run into the gym and without changing . . . offer up a world-record lift. He went to a garage for a new muffler and traded another unofficial record for the job; he broke a triple record for six girl scouts who accidently wandered into the gym one day." Not only did he become Weightlifter of the Year again, but he set three world records at the 1969 senior nationals in Chicago. His 1,210 total was fifteen pounds higher than that of superheavyweights Ken Patera and Joe Dube. In the previous year he had set twenty world records. To Hoffman, after his win at the 1969 YMCA nationals, Bednarski remained "the world's best weightlifter": "He owns the 242 class. . . . Each time he breaks a World Record he gains worldwide publicity." Hoffman could not mention that he also paid him $100 for every world record made in competition, and Bednarski was sufficiently short on cash to keep the increments small. But the absence of rivals led to loss of incentive. Starr observed that Bednarski "wasn't self-motivated anymore. As the sole owner of the 242 class he became lazy, skipped training, baled out. He'd come to the gym high, when he came to the gym at all, and he'd leave in no time to get even higher."[42]

Bednarski Versus Talts

At the 1969 world championships in Poland, Bednarski got his come-uppance from Soviet champion Jan Talts. No one expected the latter or anyone else to challenge Bob, and after the press and snatch Bednarski was leading by 16.5 pounds. In the clean and jerk, Bednarski's best lift, both lifters made 440 and eventually 468, which should have bestowed victory on the American. But the Soviets registered a protest, upheld by a 3–1 jury-of-appeal vote, that Bednarski had failed to appear within the required two minutes when the bar was originally loaded for 457. His 468 constituted an illegal fourth attempt. Though Talts was crowned champion, American officials eventually proved that attempts had been made to increase their lifter's poundage within the time limit, and Bednarski was later awarded the gold medal. But Hoffman had to admit that Bednarski was "little more than a shadow of what he was last year." Indeed his lackluster performance seemed symptomatic of a deeper malaise that kept American lifters from realizing their potential. Lowe, Karchut, and Patera failed to register totals, while Knipp, Capsouras, and Grippaldi were unable to win. For the failings of Lowe, York's promising middleweight, Hoffman had no explanation: "We had expected some good lifts from Fred, but something was very wrong.... Instead of being his usual self; ie. looking like a monster and fighting like a tiger, Fred had about as much pep as a sick mouse." Only Dube, with a 1,272 total as a superheavy, fulfilled Hoffman's expectations. His gold medal was America's first since Vinci's Olympic victory in 1960 and (with Bednarski's belated award) the last.[43]

The Columbus World Championships

It was hoped that staging the 1970 world championships in Ohio would arouse the dormant ability of American strength athletes. A comparative ranking done after the senior nationals in Los Angeles between American and foreign lifters showed the former in a strong position to reclaim their world stature. York Barbell Club won its thirty-ninth national championship, and a smell of success was in the air. Starr, not normally prone to exaggeration, said Puleo "looked 100% ready," Lowe was "in the best shape of his life," Gary Deal was "primed and ready," Karchut "appeared in tremendous condition," Bednarski was "manhandling near—World Record poundages," Dube was "over-powering the big weights," and Holbrook, Grippaldi, and Patera were stronger than ever. At Columbus, however, Americans did much worse than predicted. The team placed fifth, behind Russia, Poland, Hungary, and Bulgaria, with individual rankings far lower than precontest comparisons. Three Americans—Lowe, Holbrook, and Patera—failed to total. Starr estimated that if Patera alone had finished, the United States would have been third, but that did not happen. Nineteen world records were set, none by Americans, and the five-hundred-pound barrier, which had seemed ripe for Bednarski's picking a year earlier, was broken by Vasily Alexeev with his 501 clean and jerk. The "ninth wonder" fared no better than third. "Bob Bednarski, long our fair-haired boy, had not been fair-haired lately," noted Hoffman. "He had other interests greater than weightlifting." Again Hoffman singled out Lowe, possibly because his lifting, as first American on the platform, seemed an omen for the team: "We had great hopes for him. He fought to win the national championships but has failed miserably in the '68 Olympics, the '69 World Championship and now this year's world meet. Something happens to our lifters in the World Championships."[44] The inability of Lowe, no less than Bednarski, to live up to expectations symbolized for Hoffman, though Father of World Weightlifting, his growing impotence. On another level, these shortcomings reflected a deeper disorientation in American society.

Most noticeable at York were changes in the socialization patterns that had contributed so much to previous triumphs. Long gone were the aspiring immigrant types, and only Bednarski, Holbrook, and Starr actually resided in Muscletown. The rest of the team lived all over the country and were linked only by the travel subsidies, dietary supplements, and equipment they periodically received from Hoffman, and by their sub-rosa drug network. In 1970 Starr noted that "the usual summer Exodus to Mecca has been on a lower keel this year." At Columbus the American team, unlike earlier ones, did not share living quarters. Only Grippaldi, Karchut, and Holbrook stayed in the Spartan dormitories. The others resided at a nearby motel. "Two or three of the team members are hard to live with under any circumstances," commented Starr. "The stress of major competition" made them "unbearable in close quarters." Not only were drugs much in evidence, but Columbus police, on suspicion of harassment, picked up Bednarski one morning at 1 A.M. outside the house of a girl who had earlier entertained a group of lifters. Neither his mind nor his body was in the right place. Humbled by his third place, Bednarski appeared to have "turned over a new leaf for the coming season," noted Starr. "All he needs now is the desire he had in 1966." Despite recent setbacks, Starr clung to the belief that the American team was "getting its sea legs and [would] be a powerful force in Peru in 71."[45]

Never was confidence more misplaced. In Lima the United States fared worse than ever, placing sixth, behind Russia, Poland, Bulgaria, Japan, and Hungary. While only Dube failed to total, five of the other seven lifters did less than at the senior nationals. By this time many weight-game elders were suspecting something endemic to the new generation that kept it from measuring up to past standards. Grimek's implication, in the editorial "These Changing Times," was that younger males lacked masculinity: "[They] wear long hair while many females keep it boyish short.... At one time men's clothing was masculine but now it's becoming more effeminate.... Where will it lead? Many of the 'boys' have now taken to wearing beads and necklaces" and "see-through clothing!" Such tendencies, along with recent urban riots, portended a breakdown in the social fabric. Youth appeared to be "destruction bent." A York follower in 1970 longed for the good old days of real men like Harry Paschall: "After his death, Strength & Health and coincidentally American weightlifting, started to go downhill."[46] To the elders, modern lifters seemed spoiled, self-indulgent, and unmanly.

A Clash of Cultures

Signs of the times included a 1970 picture in *Strength & Health* of York lifter Steve Ziegman doing a 319 jerk with hair completely covering his eyes and a Kurtz cartoon featuring two members of the York gang flaunting long hair and the peace symbol in an office at Muscletown. Another issue carried a picture of Los Angeles middleweight Peter Rawluk with beard and long hair doing a 285 press. The contrast between his athleticism and wild appearance was striking. Hoffman always believed there was a correlation between looking good and lifting well, and he disapproved of the new styles. He was suspicious when Rawluk appealed to him for financial aid to attend Santa Monica City College and to represent York Barbell. "I realize my mistakes of last season as far as lifting for the L.A. YMCA and my appearance," Rawluk told Terpak. "I have since cut my hair and shaven off my beard.... I had many things bothering me last season but all is well now." Hoffman did eventually send a check, but a picture that appeared months later in a rival magazine of Rawluk's hippie-style marriage on Santa Monica beach was hardly reassuring to York fathers. Murray Levin suspected that drugs were behind the failures of American lifters and resented the abuse York had to endure "all these years from members of the team who [were] prima donnas." Levin professed to "have the answer to the problem" and assured Terpak he and "many others" would "back you up."[47]

However much a housecleaning may have been in order, Hoffman chose the less painful course of addressing the ills of society in his magazine. He believed American youth, by their nonconformity and reliance on drugs, were "running away from reality." "The hippies, the yippies, the Students for a Democratic Society, individuals who are trying to tear our country down, are foremost failures. . . . These rebellious youths who are ripping our country apart should be in mental institutions." After the Kent State incident in 1970, Bob's tone became more political, attacking "Senate doves" and blaming the SDS and Black United Students, not the National Guard, for the killings: "I love the United States. . . . When people I meet voice their dissent and speak disparagingly of the U.S., I have one answer: 'I will buy you a one way ticket to any country in the world that you prefer.'" Though others might not agree with his politics, many were dismayed by the drug dependence of weightlifters. "A 'disease' or rather a corruption . . . has crept *slowly* into the sport," warned Barry Whitcomb, a steadfast Christian. He was unable to reconcile the drug culture with ideals he cherished of becoming a star and helping others. Even Starr, though taking drugs himself, could see that steroids were no substitute for hard work: "The Russians are using the same anabolic that brought so much glory to Kono, Vinci, Berger, and Ski in the '50s. They trained hard. Actually, I'm fairly certain that the Europeans, along with the rest of the weightlifting world, do use some form of anabolic, but they do not have anything that we don't have. . . . Strength, weightlifting fans, is still the name of the game."[48] To many the disappointing performance of American lifters (like that of American soldiers in Southeast Asia) indicated an abandonment of the country's hard-work ethic. Gone was the tough moral fiber that had made their predecessors the best in the world. Self-made men were no longer in vogue.

Starr Bright, Starr Gone

Starr occupied a key position at York in the midst of the cultural rift dividing Americans during the Vietnam War. He was key to bridging the generation gap, having earned the respect of old gang and young trainees alike. Through York's influence he occupied several responsible positions in AAU weightlifting. Hoffman thought highly of him, and Terpak and Starr agree that he was being groomed for an important place in the organization. As Terpak started to contemplate retirement, he viewed Starr as his successor. "I was Terpak's right-hand man and did an awful lot of work for him," confirms Starr. He was the "next generation" York had so desperately needed since World War II. Especially after Suggs's departure, Starr was the hub of socialization. He took the lead in staging clinics for lifting clubs, organizing exhibitions at local colleges and high schools, and providing halftime lifting displays at sporting events. On the day of the National Peace Moratorium he accompanied others in the York bus to the District of Columbia Invitational. Lifters gained a sense of the national crisis from traces of tear gas that wafted into their eyes. Five district chairmen attended, and Starr got to see two close friends, Larry Hanneman and Jack King, who were turning Iowa and North Carolina into hotbeds of lifting. "King, breaking out of a 14-year slump, bettered his snatch by 15 pounds. Chances are that Jack will not go into the lifting annals along side of Bednarski and Kono, but no one can match him for story telling. He can do imitations of anyone he has ever seen lift and the ones he does of March, Smitty, Suggs, Pickett, plus others are precious." In Starr's estimation lifting contests were "about 60% athletic and 40% social." Whether recreational drug-taking accompanied these convivial gatherings is open to conjecture, but no one could deny their invigorating effect. Hanneman was planning the first tuition-style training camp in Des Moines for the summer of 1970. King, who had "ignited a fire across the South," had plans for a regional gym. So intense was King's enthusiasm that he was "spending as much time with the sport" as he was "with his livelihood." His inspiration extended to the York gym, where the Art Department hung a sign reading "If King Can We All Can."[49] The following Starr had built up around the country augured well for York and the future of American lifting.

Exactly where he ran afoul of the powers that be is not easy to ascertain. Members of the old gang, especially Dietz, were suspicious of interlopers who might secure a grasp on the company's assets. Terpak, according to Starr, "felt threatened by education and by youthful innovation." Starr may also have undergone some temperamental change from his use of steroids and other drugs. But it is obvious that the disintegration of his marriage was a critical factor, along with the breakdown of many assumptions he had once shared with company elders about business, sport, and morality. Though never a conventional family man, Bob had always emphasized traditional values. It was therefore with dismay that the elders witnessed Starr's infatuation with Gail Tart, the daughter of a prominent York physician. He might have been able to resist the attractions of Ms. Tart had he not also been subjected to the new standards of sexual promiscuity sweeping the country. When he attended the 1970 AAU convention at the Shoreham Hotel in Washington, he watched two of his companions take turns having sex with a young woman they had picked up. They behaved like kids loose in a candy store. Closer to home, Ray Degenhardt took up with a female colleague in the Art Department and, after divorcing his wife, took off with her to California. Soon the name of Starr's wife, Marlene, no longer appeared under the "Tips on Good Eating" column in *Strength & Health*. Yolanda Crist, with whose husband Bob staged major meets in Virginia, recalls how Gail accompanied Starr on lifting trips: "She was a very intelligent girl and had no intention of marrying Bill."[50] Both were exhilarated by the sexual revolution.

This newfound freedom was reflected in Starr's editorial outlook. For several years he merely skirted around sensitive issues by favorable (often humorous) allusions to the youth culture. He became skilled at double entendre. Then, in the February issue of 1971, coinciding with the crisis in his personal life, he printed a letter criticizing Hoffman's hypocrisy for condemning rebellious drug-taking youths while failing to say anything about drug abuse at York: "Yes, 'Mr. Weightlifter sits back and laughs at these kids because he knows better; he has no time for being a hippy.' It is too bad that a 'perfect' society punishes one form of deviance and seems to condone another. If you do not condone it, why not say something against it!" This satire provoked an editorial defense of "anabolics and amphetamines" from Starr.

> Some go so far as to say that it is immoral to use anabolics. It should be considered cheating and any drug user should be banned. Yet, anabolics are being used by just about everyone in the sport. I seriously doubt if there were over two lifters at this year's Senior Nationals who were not using anabolics . . . They have been used by some lifters in this country since 1960, but at that time their use was guarded like a military secret. Those who did know took a tremendous jump in total and moved out ahead of their opponents. . . . I will not mention names as it isn't my purpose to turn this into a witch hunt, but the only immorality in my mind on the entire subject of anabolics is in keeping it secret.

Starr subscribed to the moral precept, then enjoying wide currency, that he had the right to do anything as long as it did not adversely affect others. The only drug-related wrong, he thought, was for some lifters to use them while others did not.

> I believe that discretion and common sense are the answers to the use of both amphetamines and anabolics. I do believe that anabolics are safe when used properly and that they do result in a substantial strength gain. I believe that amphetamines do bring positive results to some lifters and are not harmful when used properly. And I do believe it is the right of the individual to choose whether he wants to use these substances or not. No one should be able to tell me that I can drink 10 cups of coffee, as this is approved of in our society, and not take 10 miligrams of Ritalin, which is not approved of, before I lift weights. I have been told this and know for a fact that the cups of coffee do me more physical damage than the tiny pill. No one should be able to say that I can take Livitol or Vitamin E but not Dianabol as they all alter the body's chemistry—but in different ways. This is my decision and if I think it's worth the risk to take anabolics then that's my personal business.[51]

This candid expression of liberal views, purporting to expose hypocrisy in York and American weightlifting, was long overdue. It amounted to nothing less than a clarion call for revolution.

York elders, having ignored the drug problem and counterculture in the iron game, were slow to react. But Starr's article unleashed a torrent of controversy. "Can you imagine what possible harm you have done?" was the reaction of one reader. "At one time, S&H stood for physical fitness, for overall health, for moral leadership. Why does Mr. Hoffman . . . not stand up for the things he has fought for all these years? . . . Get rid of the old blood at S&H, and the drug advocates and the advocates of the indirect destruction of amateur sports. Resign, yourself, Mr. Starr." Even angrier was a reader who admitted that "the contents of this article have, in a way, gotten the hair on my neck up. . . . Everyone admires a well built body, man or woman. But if I have to take anabolic or amphetamines to obtain a well built body, then no thanks. . . . I think anyone who has to take pills to stay up with or ahead of the guy who works hard for what he has is in my mind a cripple. We all have a crutch of some type, but let it be your wife, mother, father or CHRIST, not DRUGS or NARCOTICS." While some letters agreed with Starr, most probably shared the sentiments of a reader who, while admittedly "old-fashioned," felt that drug use was "a sad way for athletics to go." After a further outburst of honesty in an article entitled "Fall from Olympus," it was time for Starr to leave the York gang. "Star light, Star bright, Starr gone" were the parting words in *Strength & Health*.[52]

Shock Waves in Muscledom

Starr was too outspoken and involved in drugs to suit his elders, but the ostensible reason for his dismissal was a series of fraud charges. Pending a lawsuit, York was beset by problems from others of the younger set. Most distressing was the behavior of 1971 Mr. America Casey Viator. A native of Louisiana, Viator's massiveness set a new physique standard. But he was also the youngest Mr. America ever and seemed to lack the maturity of former winners. Not only did he stop authoring the popular Mr. America series in *Strength & Health*, but he took off for California and reneged on a commitment to appear at a show in Baltimore, though given an advance of $250 by promoter Bill Stevens. "I do not understand what has happened to the responsible person I talked to after Casey won the Mr. America Contest," Stevens wrote to his parents. "All Mr. Americas have obligations to meet."[53] Yet York could do no more than agonize over the behavior of its many wayward sons. Bob Hoffman's "Boys Grown Up" had turned rebellious.

What seems amazing is that Starr was given so much latitude. His departure came so suddenly that *Strength & Health* missed a month's publication. Furthermore, successor George Lugrin continued for several more months Starr's deviation from the traditional *Strength & Health* format, culminating in an iconoclastic piece entitled "The Dream Is Over—I."

> The reaction to Bill Starr's "Anabolic and Amphetamines" was predictable. Those on the "inside" knew. And those on the "outside" didn't want to know. Nonetheless, it shouldn't have been shocking to discover that science and technology had scaled the victors stand. After all, the signs of technological progress are everywhere. We can see it in the air and taste it in our water. Why not in sports? Could it be because the AAU and Olympic Committee, not to mention Wheaties Inc., have perpetuated a myth? Or did the

majority feel the coming of another "Mylai" and just didn't want another American bubble busted?

He especially resented the hypocrisy and lack of leadership displayed by the old York/AAU guard in dealing with this new "age of 'chemo-lifting.' " Lugrin never had an opportunity to publish part two of his "Dream" series. The first cut so deeply into the body of myths that Hoffman had for so long nurtured about himself and York that drastic action was necessary. "When we find that some of our men have changed, and no longer think as we do, we must . . . replace them." The next managing editor was Tom Holbrook, a seemingly unlikely choice given the escapades of his younger brother. But Tom, a journalism graduate from the University of Illinois, was a good lifter and shared York's philosophies of "patriotism and healthful living." As he explained, "[M]y brother's reputation has become tainted because of his cavorting with Hise, and his escapades with drugs. I have never condoned these activities. . . . I suspect that since I have never used alcohol or drugs, my admonitions have seemed somewhat 'square' to him." As Tom began his editorial duties, Rick and his wife, Dede, left York. Starr was stripped of his AAU offices and faced a federal fraud charge that Terpak expected would eventually "put him in prison."[54]

Nevertheless the drug consciousness stirred by Starr and Lugrin remained. "A lot of our top lifters have some pretty weird ideas on how to train," argued Morris Weissbrot. Too many "place all the emphasis on 'little blue pills' and certain other pick-me-ups." *Muscular Development* led York's counterattack, not only by disassociating itself from Starr's opinions but by scaring drug users with tabloid-style articles such as "What Steroids Did to Me!" and allusions to "the risk of going through life sporting a scrotum the size of an acorn, post-squirrel." The most astonishing revelation was how Craig Whitehead, former Mr. America finalist, and his wife had gone berserk on drugs. Sacramento sheriff's deputies reported

> the house was a wreck. The Whiteheads had ripped out the toilet, tore up the walls and fired bullets into the walls, all in an apparent search for imagined bugs of both the live and electronic variety, they said.
>
> Officers said they found numerous lewd books; pornographic magazines and photographs, both commercial and home made;

two films; a switchblade knife; a whip; and a cup with "marijuana" painted across the top.

Scattered about were numerous knives and spears; a large number of syringes and hypodermic needles, both new and used, and a kitchen cabinet filled with drugs. . . . Officers said both Whiteheads appeared to be high on drugs and "related that someone was using high intensity radio waves to control their moods." Both had numerous needle marks on their arms.

Their landlord, Ramey Osborne, said the Whiteheads caused nearly $2,000 in damage to the new duplex.

"Until approximately one year ago," probation officer Gloria Louie said, Whitehead "was considered to be a competent ophthalmologist. He began to use the drug, Retalin, to give him more pep and energy while training and competing in weightlifting contests."[55]

Significantly, Whitehead was one of Bob's "Strength & Health Boys" and a member of the fraternity of doctors in which he took such pride. This incident gave the lie to those who attempted to draw a distinction between lifting drugs and recreational drugs and to Starr's advocacy of controlled use. If a physician with Whitehead's credentials could not control himself, who could?

The *Weightlifting Journal*

In the meantime Starr embarked on a publication called the *Weightlifting Journal*, in which he continued to lambaste York. The first issue stated that it was for "the serious weightlifter"—thus limiting sales. But that was not a paramount concern, since Starr's ulterior motive was to perpetuate the revolution he had started. "The leaders of our sport have hidden too much too long," he insisted. "As the truth comes out it just may carry some sting for those that do not like to look in the face of truth." Unlike *Strength & Health*, Starr vowed to "avoid economic bullshit disguised as factual articles." The next issue called for drastic change.

For nearly forty years the fate of American weightlifting has been in the hands of Bob Hoffman. He likes to call himself the

"Father of American Weightlifting," which is probably a fair reward for his efforts. . . . Perhaps it's time for the American weightlifter to pull his head out of the sand and give a genuine look at the situation. Without Hoffman's domination the sport would be much further ahead than it is at this point. What few people realize is that Hoffman is economically motivated, period. . . . The lifters themselves are going to have to put the skids to this nonsense if the sport is to survive. They still prostitute themselves to York for a dollar and end up being used and abused. . . . It dates back to the days of Grimek, Stanko, and Bachtell. "Yes, but Bob gave them jobs, security." Slave labor. Check and see what these men receive from the most benevolent "Father of American Weightlifting." They could do almost as well on relief. The York power structure is a monster that has to be destroyed for the sport to progress.

Starr later joined forces with George Frenn to argue that powerlifters were treated shabbily and should form their own federation. By this time the youth rebellion had gained momentum. "I'm tired of hearing self-aggrandizing statements that tend to place certain individuals on Olympian heights above all the peons," wrote Everill Taggert. "I never did believe in God, though when younger I was almost swayed into believing we muscle heads had experienced God incarnate, alive and well and living in York." Michael O'Brien of Endwell, New York, argued, "It's not pot smoking or so-called shabby appearance that is ruining American lifting. It's the aged administrators who bungle Senior Nationals, neglect their duties, and protect their positions with seniority."[56] No doubt these youthful spirits believed their predicament was unique, but the "generation gap" was a phenomenon that went far beyond the iron game.

Escape Mechanisms

How much this rebellion affected Hoffman is uncertain, but York elders decided to turn their backs on the escapades of unruly youth. After decades of dedication to American lifting and fitness, Bob could hardly comprehend the cultural countercurrents that were running through York in the early 1970s. He had to distance himself from the reality of his crumbling social order. Like the hippies who embraced drugs, he sought escape, but to a higher obsession. Hoffman became absorbed in his own health and well-being. In 1969, having spent a rare full day at home, he supposedly "ran 18 miles, and still felt fairly fresh." Thus, as he said of himself, "the life I lead is a good one, one that keeps me at my physical peak." But Lou DeMarco relates that once, when he was at the foundation and two strangers drove up, Hoffman spotted them, ran around the corner, appearing winded, and told them he had just done ten miles. Also, "Bob liked cokes and junk food," and he doused his food with ketchup, rationalizing it was good for you because it came from tomatoes! Bob never discussed any of his health problems, but in November 1969 he sought treatment for a shoulder aggravation, probably heart related. In the following spring he had a mild heart attack and was again admitted to the Lahey Clinic. His brother Chuck advised him to "delegate more responsibility to others and slow down."[57] Yet Bob felt compelled to show that by being the world's busiest man, he was also the world's healthiest man.

It is also possible that Bob's mental health was affected by the youth rebellion. DeMarco recalls sharing a room with him at Bob Crist's house in Virginia while they attended the Chesapeake Bay Invitational. Late at night, with the lights out, Hoffman chattered away to DeMarco, and when DeMarco woke up in the morning, Bob was still talking! At a meet several years later in South America, Bob and Yolanda Crist walked down the hall of their hotel one morning to awaken Hoffman. He appeared at the door in his boxer shorts. Anxious to show that he still possessed an ample physique, Bob stuck out his chest and sucked in his gut, but his underwear dropped straight to the floor. "It was then that I saw the real Father of American Weightlifting," joked Yolanda. At the 1971 senior nationals, Bob did not seem well. While judging the lightweights, he fell off the chair and platform. When he crawled back, the audience gave him a rousing ovation. Later, as heavyweight referee, he failed to give the signal for Bednarski's 413 press, and the York lifter, though given another try, bombed out. Compulsiveness was another trait. He not only "drove like a maniac" but "always had to be there first in anything." Once, when boarding an airplane, he even bolted ahead of the elderly, handicapped, and women with babies. Starr could not believe it. And Hoffman was still neglecting to cash checks sent to him. Alda confirms that Bob was careless in his health and hygiene. He rarely took a bath or changed his clothes, thus accounting for an ever present body odor. Also, he never dried his hands after washing them.[58] Always eccentric, he seemed to be getting more neglectful in old age.

Bob's most notable form of escape was softball. While many iron-game followers have been puzzled by his decision to invest a million dollars in this sport, others attribute it to his disenchantment with American lifting. Both views overlook Hoffman's all-around interest in athletics, going back to childhood. Softball might be likened to his early interest in canoeing. Probably he wanted to dominate it as he had weightlifting. The November 1969 issue of *Strength & Health* featured an article on "Softball for Fun and Exercise" in which Hoffman noted that York had thirteen softball fields and would soon host "one of the greatest slow pitch tournaments ever held" in the East. "Weightlifting is my favorite sport. But baseball is a good sport too; particularly softball, which can be played by anyone, regardless of age." Soon Bob announced that he was raising money for a Hoffman Field in York to host the National (World) Softball Championship in 1971. Then he accompanied York mayor Eli Eichelberger to Tucson to bid for the 1972 Women's Slowpitch

Hoffman, disenchanted with his weightlifters in the late 1960s, turned to softball. Shown here with his 1971 team.

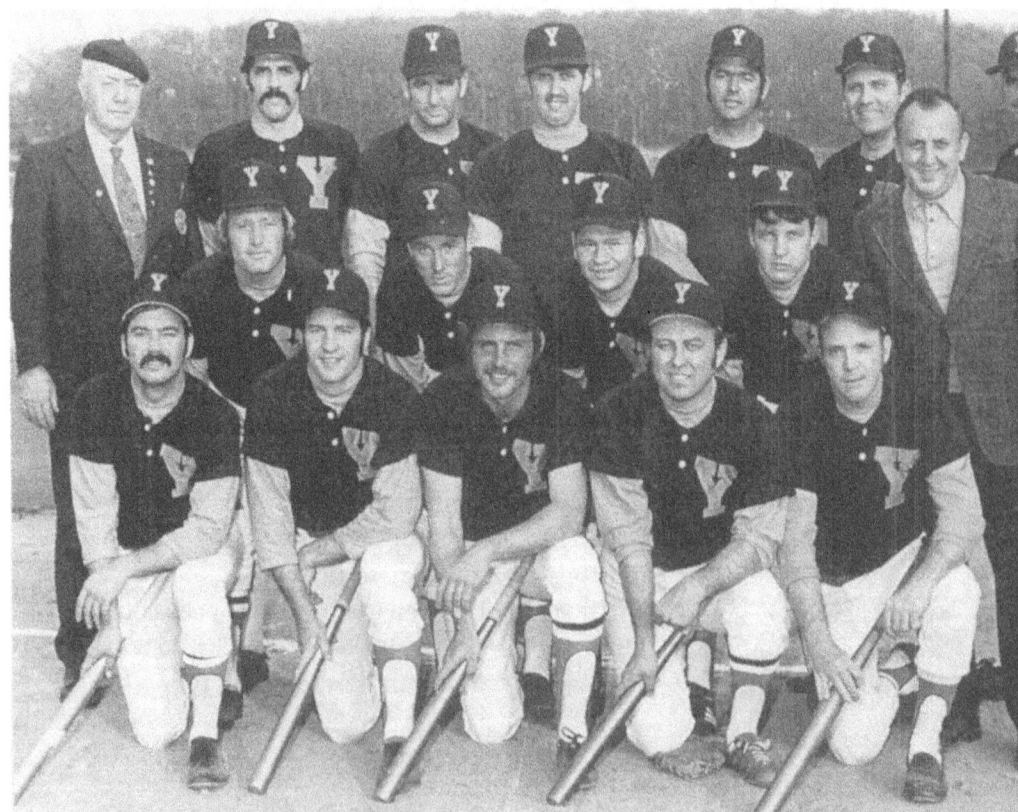

Championship. It was evident that Bob was enthralled by softball and saw the prospect of recovering some of the respect he was losing in weightlifting. In keeping with these broader interests, Hoffman styled himself "Father of Physical Fitness." Henceforth Muscletown would also be known as Physical Fitness City. Accordingly he revamped *Strength & Health* to provide more emphasis on family and general fitness. What appealed to Hoffman in this new approach was wholesomeness.[59] The February 1970 issue featured the all-American-looking family of bodybuilder Carl Smith, and the July issue carried a picture of fitness couple Chris Dickerson (a future Mr. America) and Diane Chapman (a mother of four) with the watchwords "Sports, Fitness, and Beauty." Ironically the "Family Fitness Issue" of July 1971 featured Gail Tart with former Mr. Pittsburgh Robert Lauda and two children named Bebe and Skooter of unexplained origin. It was never easy for Bob to escape those of his enemies who fought guerilla style.

Cultivating the White House

Hoffman's scope was also broadened by his craving for national recognition. In previous decades egomania had driven him to seek contacts in various presidential administrations. Hoping again to exercise influence in high quarters, he encouraged the election of Richard Nixon and showered favors on him. When Nixon could not attend the presentation of the park named in his honor, Hoffman arranged for Bednarski and Dube, gold medalists at the 1969 world championships, to meet the president. They would be "great on the offensive line," quipped Nixon. "Nobody could come through." What Hoffman purported to show the president with these two magnificent specimens was that America's future lay in its youth: "I told him that these boys and girls have doting parents, and these parents make up his great silent majority that is talked about." He also started sending Nixon and members of Congress the "activity report" he prepared monthly for the National Health Federation. Bob boasted that at its annual convention he had met six congressmen and a senator: "I asked the congressmen if they are reading my reports, and without exception they said 'Indeed yes, every word of them.'" He also believed that the president read "every word" and gave them "careful consideration." Hoffman used every opportunity to persuade politicians

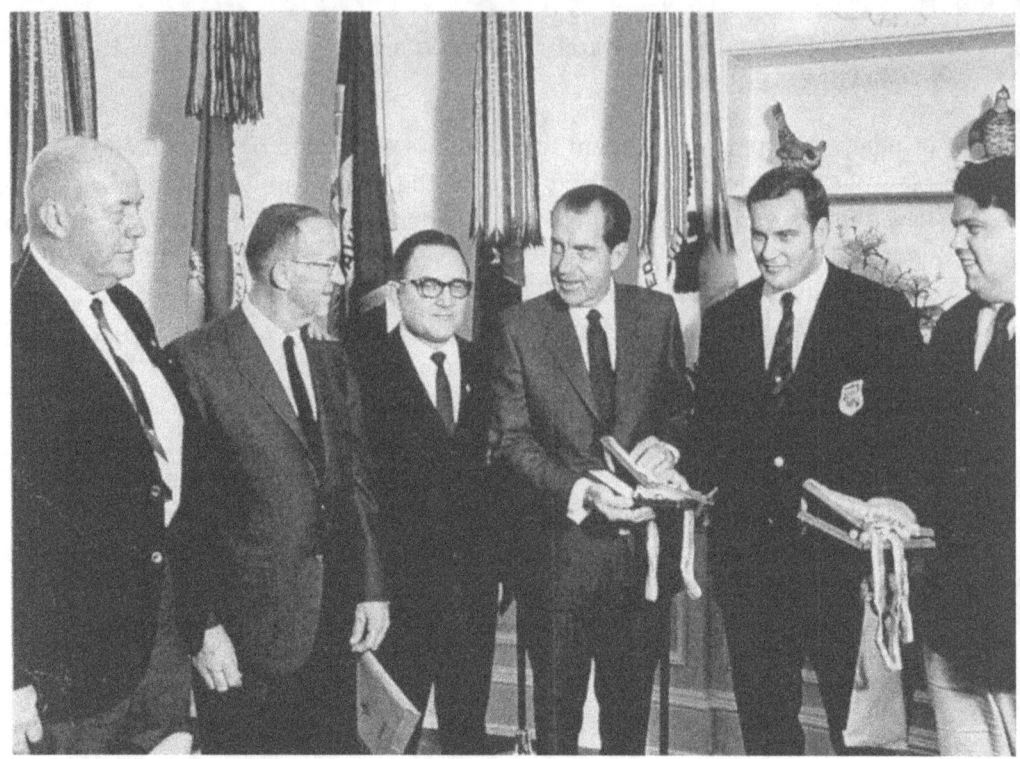

The gold medal victories of Bob Bednarski and Joe Dube at the 1969 world championships in Warsaw were America's last. Accompanied by Hoffman, Congressman George Goodling, and Terpak, the lifters are congratulated by Richard Nixon at the White House.

of the benefits of health foods and to hold forth on the pernicious work of the FDA. Convinced that Nixon was listening to him and following his advice, it is hardly surprising that Bob regarded him as "the most conscientious and intelligent president in modern history."[60]

What Hoffman most coveted was a return to the President's Council for Youth Fitness. He was delighted when Nixon placed him on the Advisory Conference on Physical Fitness in 1970, and reeled off a long letter to the president, making it clear that he took his duties seriously. He outlined an elaborate plan by which his Hoffman-York Plan, the Daily Dozen, and other ideas he had fostered over the years would be implemented by the AAU, the YMCA, and the NHF. To encourage acceptance, Bob emphasized that "getting my favorite President re-elected" was part of his strategy. He felt "sure that millions of Nixon votes will result, to our mutual advantage." He also hoped to "meet with Martha Mitchell, Virginia Knauer, Spiro Agnew during January to talk over this over-all physical fitness plan." To facilitate these plans, Hoffman engaged the services of Gertrude "Trudy" Engel, wife of a Michigan lawyer, who had carved out a career for herself as a Washington lobbyist.

She was full of "big cars and big cigar talk," recalls Winston Day. Trudy knew how to curry the favor of rich people, attract the attention of those with political power, and bring the two together. She could hardly have asked for a more ideal client than Hoffman. Engel gushed with enthusiasm. Far more successful than any previous influence peddler, she exuded a feminine charm that fed Bob's ego and a professionalism that ensured a permanent lock on it. She had him "thinking he was getting close to the President."[61]

Quite aside from Trudy's influence, an unexpected opportunity arose in mid-February, when Hoffman was invited to a meeting of the President's Council by its chairman, James Lovell, the astronaut. The meeting included a reception with the president at the White House. Hoffman arrived as a man with a mission, carrying a pair of fifteen-pound dumbbells, a batch of his own books and courses, and a personal letter proffering advice on nutrition.

> We went in to hear the president speak, finally he appeared and talked extemporaneously for a half hour. It sounded like Bob Hoffman was talking, we have known each other since 1955, when we were invited to the White House when good reports came . . . concerning our visit to Russia. . . . The presidents talk ended and he started to shake hands with all of those present. I had been standing six—eight feet from him, so I was among the first to be greeted by him. I was pleased when he turned to Mrs. Nixon and said, "This is Bob Hoffman, one of our strongest supporters." She said, "Yes I know, in more ways than one." . . . I was a little selfish, as I had so much to say to him, and talked a bit more than my share as we clasped hands. . . . I finally moved on, had some of the "brunch," and looked at the paintings of past presidents. And I happened to notice that the President was still shaking hands but that there were only two or three people in the line. So I walked over to get in the line again. The newspapers made much of the fact that I "got seconds."

Nixon aides undoubtedly knew the type well—the garrulous old man with lots of money wanting to suck up to the president. Yet they could not afford to offend him inasmuch as these kinds of individuals constituted the bedrock of Nixon's political support. Hoffman's professed ambition was to make him (physically) the strongest president in history, and he

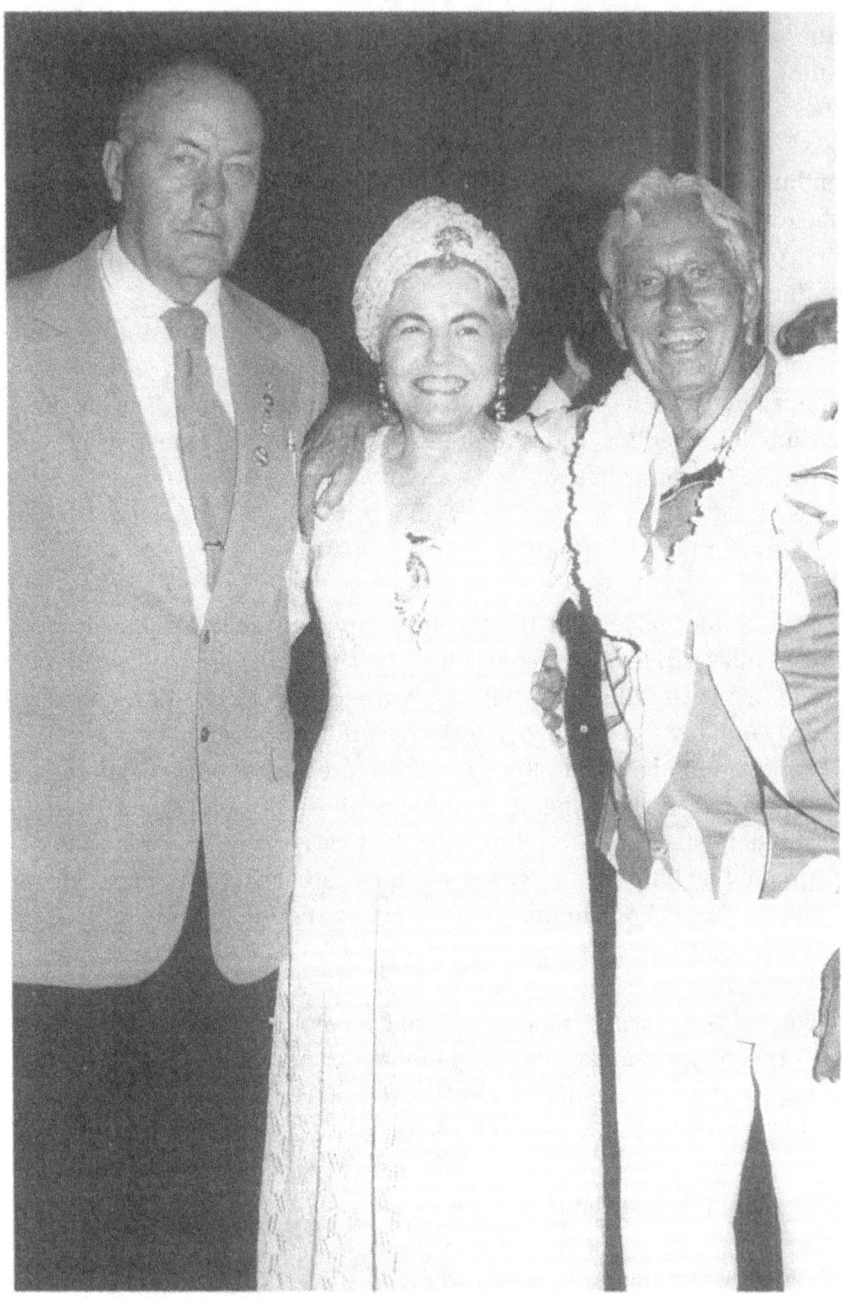

Bob with his lobbyist, Trudy Engel, and California fitness promoter Don Bragg, who encouraged Hoffman to market food supplements after World War II.

proudly published Nixon's thank-you note for the dumbbells in *Muscular Development*.[62]

Celebrity Status

However ridiculous the notion was that Nixon, one of the busiest and most important men in the world, was seriously training with weights and becoming a disciple of Hoffman, the media (abetted by Engel's promotions) had a feeding frenzy on the myths Bob perpetrated at York. No matter how distant Hoffman's stories of his accomplishments were from reality, they became believable when magnified for public consumption by the press. The London *Times* described Hoffman as "Mr. Physical Fitness of the United States," a man who worked sixteen hours and ran three miles every day and "proudly boasts that he is 'the strongest man for my age in the world.' " He boasted that he "got the President indoctrinated on health foods and I'm now working hard on Spiro Agnew." In an interview for the *Washington Post* Bob added some new wrinkles—that he had collected six hundred trophies in weightlifting and a few years earlier had been lifting a 1,600-pound dumbbell eighty times a week. On his seventy-second birthday he had supposedly run ten miles and "repeated the run for four more days." No matter how distorted the assertions, the fact that he was reaching a national audience and that most people believe anything in print brought the kind of recognition he desired. He could thus rise above the dismal state of American lifting to a level commanding respect. What's more, Bob believed he had finally gained access to the corridors of power. "It is evident that the dropping water has finally worn away the stone," he asserted after his White House reception.[63] Little did he know that such commissions, employed by politicians to curry public favor, accomplish little. The president, no less than Hoffman, probably confused rhetoric for reality.

A final way in which Hoffman projected himself was through television. Using his recognition by the president as a credibility base, he wrote to Johnny Carson about appearing with Bednarski and Dube on *The Tonight Show*, claiming that both lifters could break world records on the air. Unable to dwell just on his lifters' attributes, Bob talked mostly about himself. He explained that he had been a weightlifter for sixty years, was the most decorated army man in World War I, and was past president of the AAU, all gross exaggerations. Then, in an outburst of hyperbole, he claimed that many congressmen, senators, governors, the late Robert and Jack Kennedy, the shah of Iran, Gamel Abdel Nasser, and others in high places were "Bob Hoffman boys grown up." However flawed Hoffman's estimation of his self-worth may have been, he got the attention of *Tonight Show* executives, and Dube performed some Olympic lifts for a television audience in the fall of 1970. This coverage was followed by ABC's telecast of portions of the world championships on *Wide World of Sports*. Hoffman himself appeared on the *Mike Douglas Show* and the *Today Show*, and he was featured in *Reader's Digest*. He was also seen by millions on the popular *To Tell the Truth* game show.[64] All of these exposures enabled Hoffman, despite many setbacks, to maintain the illusion that he was still a superman.

Outward appearances of success, however, disguised underlying stresses at York. More than ever, Bob seemed driven to justify himself in the light of history. Having decided to befriend powerlifting, it seemed necessary to trace it back to the Civil War. In 1971 he portrayed himself as both "man of the hour" and "a link with the past" by virtue of his "61 years in the health food business." Hoffman nutritional products, he claimed, were first made in 1930. Such deliberate distortions distracted him from the plight of American lifting. No one was more aware of it than Tommy Kono. There was a time when "York had the magic attraction and the best lifters in the U.S. beat a path to your door. . . . But lately the 'mecca' has been tarnishing . . . and some people are even attacking York." Bob's failure to enlist Kono to his cause indicates, as does his obsession with his patriarchal status, that he was more interested in dwelling on the past than in planning for the future. Bob's conservatism was cast in even bolder relief by the loss of Starr, whose bold, innovative, and farsighted ideas were needed to lift weightlifting out of the doldrums. But Starr's prescription for change included new approaches to drugs, sex, morality, and politics, which created a culture clash at York. Symbolizing the controversy was hair. As Venables reported at the 1971 Mr. America contest, "[T]he fellows with long hair didn't fare so well. Long hair makes the head look larger and detracts from the body." Not surprisingly the youth at York chafed at these attitudes. Under Starr they voiced their resentments and rebelled. "A lifter when he leaves York has little self-esteem left after being abused by the men of authority in Muscletown," wrote Starr after leaving. "Everyone left there changed."[65] Hoffman, of course, had been exuding most of the manly self-esteem at York for years. Now he also exerted a retrograde and divisive influence. Unwilling to allow the new gang any substantive role in his organization and intolerant of the course charted by the youth culture of the 1960s, Hoffman ceased to be a force for innovation or socialization in the iron game. Increasingly he sought escape to a higher ground of general fitness, national politics, and philanthropy, where he could indulge in myths that would obscure reality and transform failure into success.

9

FATHER OF WORLD WEIGHTLIFTING

Form rather than function succeeds in today's world.

—Alan M. Klein, *Little Big Men*

At York in the 1970s there was more emphasis on family fitness, powerlifting, and softball, attempts to recapture bodybuilding, and efforts to combat weightlifting's counterculture. By marketing more health products than ever, Hoffman appeared to have the wherewithal to promote these endeavors and reassert his hegemony in the iron game. But the challenges he faced were formidable. With Weider and the Soviets still far from vanquished, he had to cope with new and more serious issues involving his lifters, his employees, the FDA, and changing American social norms—all of which seemed to threaten the manly culture Bob had created in Muscletown. Much depended on whether the ideology of success he had formulated early in the century could be applied to the harsh realities of the 1970s. It was imperative that he appear in perfect health and not slow down, and that his achievements be elevated to ever higher levels. Hence he eagerly embraced the title of Father of *World* Weightlifting, got a Ph.D. from *World* University, made York the center for *world* championships in powerlifting and softball, and staged a Mr. *World* physique title. But the most grandiose means by which Hoffman hoped to achieve immortality was by exercising influence, with Trudy

Engel's assistance, in the highest echelons of government. Incapable of altering his own outlook, he sought atavistic changes in society through a movement "To Save the United States."

Tests of Strength

A critical test of York's strength took place in October 1971 at the Lake Placid meeting of the national weightlifting committee to elect a chairman to succeed Terpak. Virginian Bob Crist had inspired confidence by his conduct of the Chesapeake Bay Invitational each spring and by his reforms of the AAU physique scoring system. Though sympathetic with York, Crist was recognized as independent, hardworking, and businesslike. At Lake Placid, however, Bob Hise, frustrated by York for many years in attempting to bring his Los Angeles YMCA team to the forefront of American lifting, made a leadership bid. York was determined to block him, especially when it was learned he was acting in league with Weider, Starr, and other disaffected elements. Crist won by a vote of twenty-four to twenty-one, and York prevented discussion of IFBB affiliation, but the Weiders continued their attempts to subvert Hoffman's power base in the AAU. This struggle differed from previous York-Weider bouts. First, it featured Ben rather than Joe. Somewhat more suave than his brother, Ben was a self-made millionaire who shared Hoffman's outlook that money was only a means to greater ends. The IFBB was Ben's "whole life, faith and future. Any man can manufacture things," was his attitude. "Only a few can be international presidents—for life."[1] Second, Terpak was Weider's chief opponent, and the stakes were more international and political than commercial. Finally, the conflict was waged over attempts by Weider to infiltrate the AAU. What encouraged the Weider offensive was acceptance of the IFBB into the General Assembly of International Sports Federations (GAIF), a Swiss-based organization with affiliates in seventy-three nations. This affiliation enhanced the IFBB's standing, especially since the AAU had no international links in physique. Despite repeated rebuffs by Terpak and weightlifting's ruling councils, Ben was able to use GAIF affiliation to gain the ear of AAU president Jack Kelly Jr. Though a longtime friend of Hoffman, Kelly felt obliged to hold a conference between the two sides at his Philadelphia apartment in November 1971.

Terpak, still chairman until the end of the year, was accompanied by Dave Mayor, Pete Miller, and Rudy Sablo, while Weider had Ralph Johnson, Bob Hise, and Jack King in tow. Respective accounts show there was little common ground and that the York side shunned Weider's conciliatory gestures. The IWF did not recognize bodybuilding and had no authority to meddle in the affairs of another GAIF affiliate, but there seemed no reason why the IFBB could not affiliate with the AAU and enter its athletes in the Mr. America contest. Obviously York would never allow such an intrusion. In view of York's deep-seated distrust of Weider, it is hardly surprising that the discussion converged on personalities and ethics. To York's objection that the IFBB (with its life president) was not democratic, Weider stated that he would resign. But he added, "I will be re-elected anyway." Sablo, to discredit the opposition, reviewed IFBB activities since 1946. Weider, "noticeably annoyed, asked that [York] let bygones be bygones, that he was not interested in history but was interested only in helping US bodybuilders."[2] It was evident that the Weiders possessed the necessary energy and determination to dominate bodybuilding in the United States. Hoffman had always exhibited these qualities too. Now, however, time was no longer on York's side.

In Britain an anti-Weider crusade was carried on by Oscar Heidenstam, who regretted that Weider's magazine-distribution system was so superior to York's and that David Webster, a respected iron-game figure, was lending credibility to the Weiders in the history of bodybuilding he was writing. Even more distressing was the conduct of FIH secretary Oscar State, who, though highly regarded in weightlifting circles, was working to gain recognition for Weider. "I imagine that State and the Weider brothers are of the same political and racial fraternity," wrote Heidenstam. As an alternative to Weider, the French had formed an international federation that was supported by NABBA and other bodybuilding associations, but GAIF recognition gave the Weiders an immense advantage. Heidenstam felt that Hoffman should have protested this recognition: "It was a terrible mistake." Therefore the IFBB's formal request for affiliation at the national AAU meeting in Kansas City in 1972 had to be checked. To prevent the Weiders from getting a worldwide "strangle hold on bodybuilding," Terpak lined up a phalanx of persons in key positions. Dave Matlin, former AAU president and weightlifting chairman, informed Ben Weider that he would vigorously oppose affiliation. Crist wrote a similar letter and assured Terpak that the AAU would "be ready for the Weider lovers

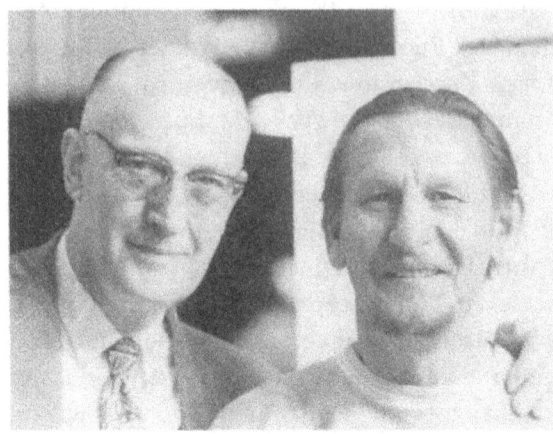

Friendly and unfriendly rivals of York. Peary Rader, editor of *Iron Man* magazine, and Bob Hise, coach of the Los Angeles YMCA team.

and any of their new recruits." As the meeting approached, Hoffman prepared a circular, "We Ask You to Vote No," in which he resorted to scare tactics, pointing out that the Weiders, who for many years had been "publishing pornographic magazines," were only interested in money, and that IFBB affiliation would result in a takeover of AAU operations. When news arrived that the Weider proposal could muster only two votes, Heidenstam welcomed "the good Christmas tidings" as "a blow for 'Mr. Big' himself!" The old guard had presented a solid front. By this time, too, Starr's movement to take the sport back from the tired old men who had so long dominated it was faltering. For survival's sake, he had defected to Weider and moved to California to edit Joe's publications. But he soon realized that working with Weider was hardly better than working with York.[3] Soon his *Weightlifting Journal* lapsed into oblivion.

Drugs and Debauchery

Arguably the greatest setback for the young revolutionaries was their loss of innocence. Starr spoke repeatedly of the intelligence and sense of responsibility of the athletes: "It's time someone realized that there are far more college degrees on the platform than there are on the judges seats." Yet it was obvious that Olympic lifters were behaving more like big children and hooligans. Tales abounded from York about the latest bizarre incident, perversion, irresponsible act (usually drug-related), or the new lifestyles. Nearly all lifters affected long hair or hippie attire, signifying rebellion. Donnie Warner characterized the younger York gang as "family": "We didn't let outsiders know what others in our circle were doing that was bad." The culture at York was totally different from the wholesome values of fitness and family life portrayed in *Strength & Health*. "The public saw X, while Y was the reality," recalls Warner. "We were American heroes, but we had our own little counterculture." Ironically, sustaining this waywardness was Hoffman, whom the lifters, with a mixture of affection and contempt, referred to as "Daddy." Terpak was "Terpsie," and Shultz's Drug Store, à la Joe Weider, was "The Trainer of Champions." "We got to get money from Big Daddy, but you got to watch out for Terpsie," was the word as lifters developed ingenious ways of sidestepping authority to get what they wanted, chiefly drugs and money. "The old gang simply did not want to know about the drug scene." Their attitude was that "if I act like it's not there, it's not there." Bob knew about the steroid abuse and much else, but did not intervene for fear of losing good lifters. Warner likened his attitude to his appetite for hot dogs. Hoffman condemned them to the health-minded public, but confided to lifters, "They're tasty little devils, aren't they!"[4]

Such double standards encouraged permissiveness and acts of moral irresponsibility. Sexual promiscuity, as practiced by Hoffman for decades, or even wife swapping, was considered old-fashioned. Stories circulated about York lifters engaging in sex with eleven-year-old girls, acts of sodomy with teenage boys, and picture parties with baby-sitters. One of the athletes derived a perverted delight from watching his wife have sex with junior high boys, and the ten-year-old son of another proudly demonstrated how to roll a joint. One lifter's apartment was a frequent gathering place for drug and sex orgies. It featured piles of records, a psychedelic light show, and a giant stereo pushed to capacity. There were also piles of trash. "They were the biggest bums I ever met," states Alda, "taking from Bob all they could get." However warped such behavior might appear in retrospect, one must remember it was part of the revolution that descended on the nation in the late 1960s. "Partying became more important than lifting or anything else," Warner relates.[5] Nonconformity, shunned as morally degrading and reprehensible in the 1950s, was considered more admissible, even "hip" or "groovy," in the permissive climate of the Vietnam War era, when all traditional standards seemed to come under protest.

In their crazed state the lifters even turned on their sustainer by vandalizing and robbing Bob's house one night while he was with Alda at the Thomasville Inn. Along with damaging furnishings and doors, they stole jewelry, pocket books, and memorabilia. In 1972 Hoffman's war medals and lifting awards were stolen from the fall-of-fame trophy case. Though he knew the culprits, Bob would not let Alda take them to court. "After all, we need good lifters, don't we?" was his rationale. According to Alda, he let the lifters get away with anything: " 'The only way you can get along with Bob Hoffman is to steal everything you can from him,'" Hooley Schell, a 1930s associate, often said. "And you know, he was right."[6]

The 1973 Nationals

The remarkable aspect of this degenerate saga is that Holbrook, Hise, and others in the drug fraternity seemed to do amazing lifting while burning the candle at both ends. These illusions were shattered at the 1973 senior nationals hosted by Crist at Williamsburg. Cameras from CBS *Sports Spectacular* recorded the sorry spectacle of lifter after lifter bombing out or performing far below potential. Holbrook, who made the highest clean and jerk in his class at the Munich Olympics, arrived in Williamsburg as a heavy favorite, recalls Warner, but he was completely stoned. Profuse sweating from a drug trip reduced his bodyweight to 188. Despite efforts from friends to revive him, Holbrook was in no condition to lift. He made only a 319 snatch and missed all of his clean and jerks. Hoffman refused Holbrook admission to his room the next morning. The latter was so incensed that he kept knocking on Bob's door until police took him away in handcuffs and charged the 1972 Lifter of the Year with disorderly conduct and public drunkenness. To Hoffman "the saddest feature" of the meet was the effect of drugs on Roger Quinn. He attributed Quinn's decline, and three failures with a 270 snatch, to his affiliation with the Los Angeles YMCA team, coached by Bob Hise Sr. Hoffman remembered him as "a clean-cut young man" when he represented York at the start of his career: "Now you should see him." Bednarski, though he won his class, was no less disappointing. Always a sure jerker, on this day he was awkward, and shook while holding his final jerk of 429. It was "not that he was so good," Hoffman explained, "but because the others were not as they should have been." Warner agrees with Starr that lifters, rather than train hard, were relying too heavily on steroids. And by this juncture the steroids were accompanied by a wide variety of recreational drugs, resulting in burnout. At last, "the dissipation caught up with these young supermen."[7]

The devastation was not limited to the lifting platform. Hospitality House, the meet headquarters, was the scene of lawlessness and destruction. Fifteen-year-old Dennis Senay was caught smoking marijuana and passing out pills. After his featherweight victory, Warner was "slipped a mickey" at a party in Bednarski's room on Saturday night and did not wake up until Sunday night. In addition to damage and theft in the rooms of Hill and Holbrook, Timmy Garcia, a follower of Holbrook, "totally destroyed" Warner's room in a rage. Afterward he fell into a deep depression. He was hospitalized for several days in a security unit for fear that he might take his life or someone else's. Terpak recalls that he presented a pathetic sight, lying naked and curled up on the floor crying. Garcia recovered, but the incident sent shock waves through the iron game. "What has happened to us?" asked Tom Holbrook. There was "something drastically wrong."

> Joe Puleo recently told me that when he looked at Ivanchencko and Kolotov at the '70 World Championships, "I could see the handwriting on the wall." He knew we weren't ever going to win again and in his opinion, our lifters have simply given up. . . . The comment of Dick Smith also comes to mind. He said that many of our lifters don't even act like men any more. . . . The sport has been infiltrated by a collection of freaks who are trying to corrupt everyone around them. Like a bunch of demented pharmacists, they can be seen snaking their way around the meets bent on perverting others to the insanity of their world.

"I hate to see so many creeps in Oly lifting," wrote heavyweight Bruce Wilhelm. "The long hair and sweat bands, and all on their own personal psychedelic trip. Ugh." Chicago promoter Fred Schutz attributed weightlifting's woes to a decline in moral fiber at the top. "Haven't any of these big name lifters heard of good sportsmanship or just plain acting like decent human beings?" "Up to this point it was all a big joke," recalls Warner, but the drug culture in lifting was no longer the sport

DESCENT FROM GLORY

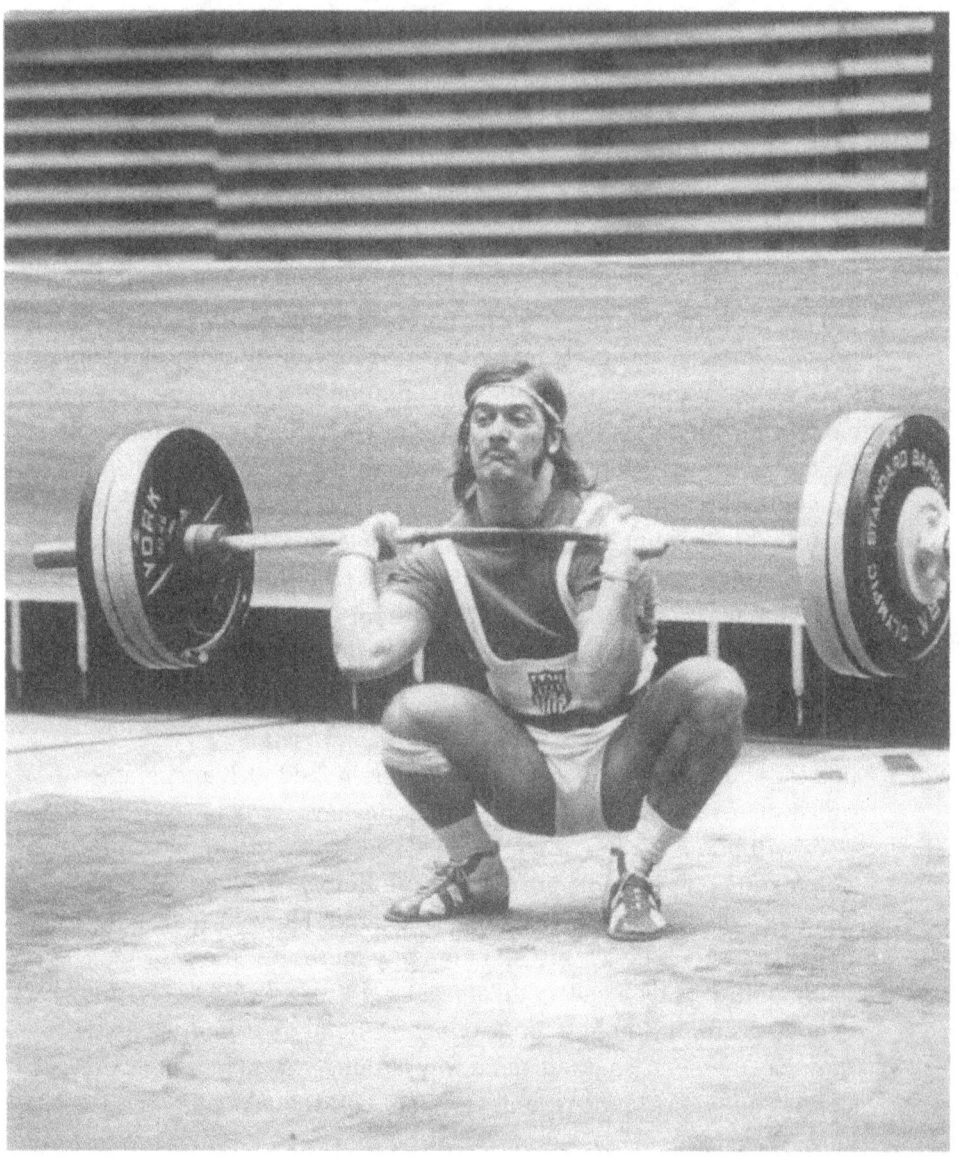

A beleaguered Rick Holbrook struggling with a 418-pound clean at the 1973 Senior Nationals in Williamsburg.

behind the sport. "The Williamsburg Nationals," DeMarco confirms, "was the culmination of it all. By the 1974 nationals in York all the craziness was gone." The wild period that started in 1968 was over.[8]

Reaction Sets In

What followed at York, coinciding with a national mood swing, was reaction. First came AAU suspension of the four York team members who perpetrated malicious mischief in Williamsburg. Bednarski, for his many acts of misconduct, was run out of York. Alda told him, "Never set foot in my yard again or I'll kill you." Holbrook, Garcia, and Senay were also dismissed. To taunts that they would join York's opposition, Hoffman retorted that "the good guys can always beat the bad guys." And there were so many other good lifters eager to lift for him that York Barbell would "win the national team titles at least as long as [he was] around." This was true in the sense that York was still the only team that could provide continuous financial subsidies, but there was less reason for Bob to feel proud. His lifters performed for smaller audiences each year, and the public was becoming disgusted with champions who were drug users. The Williamsburg experience was a revelation to Hoffman on how close to home the drug problem had hit. The "drug addicts" who had their "pot parties up the road a half mile from here and did 14 thousand dollars worth of damage to one of our homes" had "wrecked not only our own team but the team to represent the United States." Hoffman was repulsed by long hair and obsessed with the statistic that 42 percent of the youth in San Mateo County, California, were smoking marijuana. To combat this menace, he was writing a book on drug addiction. And to protect himself against personal assaults, he donated land next to his home for a new headquarters of the Northern York County Regional Police.[9]

It was chiefly Terpak, however, who had to deal with the hard realities of the dilemma. To him, York's problem went back to Starr, and he was determined to bring him to justice. Soon after he learned that Starr had "lined up with Weider" and Frenn had "gotten the boot," Terpak confided to Crist that "Billy the Kid will get kicked out after they play him as a sucker. He'll rap York, Hoffman, myself and others for a few issues as did Frenn—then out . . . unless Uncle Sam gets to him first, which is quite possible. This Starr matter is such a mess that I get indigestion when I think about it. Too bad! (for him). He was a nice guy, once." Not only was Terpak correct in his prediction about Starr, but (to complete the scenario) a 1972 issue of *Strength & Health* featured Frenn on the cover, throwing the hammer, and a complimentary story entitled "George Frenn Really Gets It On." Now Starr was out and Frenn was in! Starr disappeared after his magazine went under, then showed up in 1974 as strength coach for the University of Hawaii football team. He was recognized by Dr. You and Tommy Kono, who sent word of his whereabouts to York. "I hope there is no problem for him," remarked Kono, "for he has been doing a good job over here." But Terpak, determined to bring Starr to justice, instigated extradition proceedings. He told his lawyer, "Pack your bags—mine are ready."[10]

Starr freely admits stealing. It began innocently when he and others started hauling off Hoffman products to meets, with Bob's tacit approval, selling them and pocketing the proceeds. Later the racket expanded as Starr began taking weights from the plant and selling them to friends across the country—Hanneman (Iowa), DeMarco (Ohio), King (North Carolina), Gourgott (Louisiana), and Suggs (Texas), who resold them for profit. At one time, one key opened the whole building, and lots of people were looting. When there was a meet in York with lots of visitors interested in cut rates, lifters ran into each other helping themselves. "It was too easy to pull things off . . . like stealing from a blind man. It was all encouraged by Hoffman," Starr insists, "who knew about the stealing. He knew they weren't paying us enough, and if you figured a way of getting it underneath, then it was alright. If these people had treated us with a little respect, things would have been different." So, he adopted the same code of ethics as Hoffman, who had been "stealing" from his employees and the public his entire career. "We did it because we became like Hoffman," Starr claims. He further rationalizes that "selling the stuff created a demand and improved business." In this sense "the ultimate winners were Hoffman, Dietz, and Terpak." After all, Terpak was earning a 1 percent cut from gross sales.[11] But Terpak never saw it this way, nor was Dietz prepared to condone stealing of money and goods that he might steal himself.

Retribution

Where Starr made his fatal error was in leaving a paper trail. He would receive orders for equipment from his cronies over the phone and record them, after which shipment was made and invoices sent out. Then Bill would come in at night, make an entry for these items under receivables and register the bills as paid. That something was awry came to the attention of office personnel, who noticed that these entries were not in the hand of Nancy, the bookkeeper. When invoices of $57,000, all to Starr's friends, were checked against credits, he was called in and not given a chance to deny anything. For his misdeeds twenty-nine charges of larceny were lodged. At his trial, however, the judge approved a plea bargain whereby Starr paid only $1,725 restitution and $1,628 court costs. Starr in retrospect perceives York Barbell as a microcosm of American culture, in which, as he sees it, "ends always justify the means" in one's climb to the top: "You could do anything." What he perhaps fails to take into account, and the reason for his lasting bitterness toward York, is the conservative backlash that set in after the end of America's Vietnam presence in 1973. Hoffman regretted that Starr's involvement at York ended on "a sour note," but was perhaps more regretful that the involvement had started in the first place. Recalling past editors of *Strength & Health,* Hoffman said, "Three I'm sorry I ever met, are Starr, Suggs and Lugrin"—all once hopeful prospects from the Texas connection.[12]

With Starr in the bag, Terpak went after those allegedly in connivance with him. With Lou DeMarco, who had received goods from York at sixty cents on the dollar, settlement was simple. He paid back $1,900 without protest in 1974. Likewise Hanneman eventually paid the amount he owed York Barbell in monthly payments of $50. Suggs, though full of alibis, paid up "when he realized that his only choice was to pay his bill or go to trial." Gourgott's case was more taxing. To retrieve its $9,214, York engaged a collection agency and lawyers in two states to track "the good doctor" down. His defense was that Hoffman ran "a loose 'family' business," that he was entitled to special consideration for services performed as "an athlete, writer, and agent," that he had remitted $2,000 for some goods, and that in any case he had never been billed. Terpak succinctly denied Gourgott's claims. He told the court that the defendant had been paid fully for articles he had written for York, that as an athlete he had been paid travel expenses only for

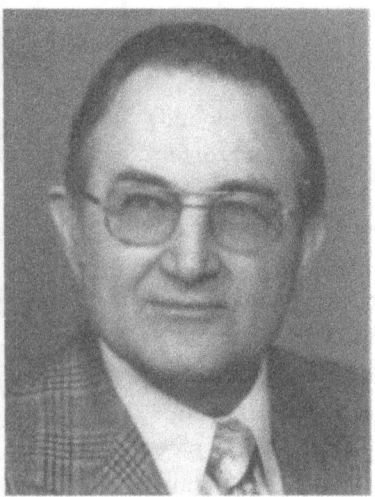

John Terpak, Hoffman's general manager and successor.

contests, and that merchandise was never regarded as payment for any of Gourgott's alleged services to York. Terpak called the defendant's claim that he paid $2,000 "a fabricated lie," and remarked that Gourgott could consider York "a loose 'family' business" only because "his former 'partner in crime'" had been "caught adjusting . . . office records in Dr. Gourgott's favor." Just before trial the parties reached a settlement for $5,500.[13] The judgment against Gourgott proved to Hoffman that the confidence he had placed in education, science, and persons with "M.D." and "Ph.D." behind their names may have been misplaced. Henceforth there would be more emphasis on the company as a business and less on its status as a lifting fraternity.

Jack King proved the most resistant to York's counterassault. Like Gourgott, he stalled and appeared to be hiding assets to avoid making full restitution. King showed little remorse. In response to allegations that he had illegally accepted goods, he claimed that he had never entered any contract for the items enumerated in the invoice and that they were received in return "for certain favors." King argued that York had "requested and encouraged the defendant to promote their line, to open up the South for the company," and had "repeatedly furnished gratuities." He insisted that the litigation against him was simple retribution for his support of Hise at Lake Placid in 1971. Though the judge disallowed a portion of York's claim, King was required to pay $5,000. Worse yet, in the midst of the litigation in 1976 he nearly died from the effects of drugs he had been taking for a decade.[14]

Gary Deal and the AWLA

Terpak denies that he was motivated by vengeance in dealing with these young rebels, stating that York simply wanted to tighten its business practices and send a message to other employees. But Bob's loss from an investment with Gary Deal, a leading heavyweight from Seattle and securities analyst for Walston and Co., seems to have stirred some vindictiveness. In 1970 Bob had sent a check for $10,000 to Deal and was supposedly told, after the 1971 world championships, that the money had grown to $11,000 and had been placed in escrow, since Deal had terminated his association with Walston. Hoffman believed Deal later used the $11,000 to purchase stock for himself and, when it went down to $6,393, had it transferred to Hoffman's account. Dismayed by this chicanery, Hoffman filed suit with his attorney, Dave Matlin, in 1972. Deal denied this interpretation, saying that Hoffman, after discovering that his stock had gone down, "suddenly decided that he had never authorized Mr. Deal to do anything." Furthermore, Deal was considering filing a counterclaim for slander, alleging that Bob referred to him as a "criminal" and "a bunko artist." Deal was, however, prepared to settle the matter by offering Bob the $6,393 that remained in his account. Matlin advised acceptance because a suit would likely take several years to reach judgment, there would be substantial attorney fees, the trial would be in Deal's home city, a counterclaim was likely, and Hoffman could deduct the loss on income tax. On the other hand, if he wanted to teach Deal a lesson, he should go ahead with the case.[15] However much logic suggested the former course, Bob chose the latter.

While their lawyers jockeyed for positions, the opposing parties searched for corroborative evidence. Hoffman recalled telling Deal how "we had been trimmed by many of our associates. He must have got the idea we were easy ... so he decided to take us." In response to Hoffman's suit to recover $11,000 for fraud, Deal filed a cross-claim for $150,000. It was apparent that Deal and his lawyer, Richard Krutch, intended to round up sufficient witnesses to make the claim stick. Although Starr declined to testify, Charlie Shields, whom Matlin called a "'frustrated' weightlifter" and "extremely biased" against York, seemed eager to be involved. After the demise of the *Weightlifting Journal*, Shields took up Starr's cause by forming the American Weightlifting Association (AWLA) to combat AAU/York hegemony. Operating from his Mechanicsburg law office, Shields printed a brochure explaining the current power structure and named a board consisting of Les Cramer, Michael Karchut, Bob Bednarski, and Larry Pacifico. While Karchut perhaps nursed a grievance against Muscletown elders for their stance on drugs, Bednarski, back in York's good graces, denied he had given anyone permission to use his name. Cramer, an Erie promoter, had been thwarted by York in his attempts to gain a leadership role. Pacifico not only denied any knowledge of his name's being used but expressed a desire to lift for York and sue the AWLA for using his name. Where Deal fit into this campaign was evident in a note Shields attached to the brochure he sent him. An appeal had been

> released to all Russian & Polish press, all W/L mags, all major sports mags in U.S. Sports Illus, Newsday, etc.
> We are going to petition IWF to look into your problems as well as Bob's. Keep in touch and make sure Starr realizes we weren't bullshitting. Timing is important—Watergate almost resolved—S3500 passed Senate—will next have fight in House.[16]

Seemingly on all fronts, even national politics, York's enemies were the friends of the AWLA.

Most probably realized that AWLA opposition was largely on paper and that Deal could not orchestrate the many gremlins that were attacking the York monster. Only Shields and Degenhardt, former art director at York, agreed to testify they had overheard Bob slander Deal. Jacob Stefan, a heavyweight who harbored resentments against York, deposed for Deal. After Hoffman flew to Seattle in 1974, the affair was abruptly terminated. Matlin reported to Terpak on Bob's deposition:

> I want to state that I am very proud of the way he handled himself. He was brief, alert and refused to be trapped by any "trick" questions.
> The depositions ended when Bob Hoffman told the attorney for Gary Deal "off" in a very definitive manner, which came as a surprise to everyone, as they had thought that Bob was getting old. He may be old in years, but certainly not mentally or physically.

In all likelihood this "telling off" was the whole point of York's initiative, which had consumed many months of time and much more in lawyers' fees and expenses than the $6,500 Bob received in out-of-court settlement. As always, it was a matter of ego—its aim simply to show others and prove to himself that he was not going to be gulled by, or lose a test of will to, anyone, least of all a young lifter who sided with his enemies. Most remarkable, however, was a letter from Deal to Terpak only four months later requesting two cans of protein and a plane ticket to an upcoming meet, and including a reminder that York was $200 behind on its reimbursement checks for his monthly training.[17] Bob's need to produce a winning team still prevailed over all.

New Low Ebbs

Hopes were high that the 1972 Olympics would bring out the best in American lifters. Tom Holbrook's confident prognosis, after a pre-Olympic training camp in August, was that "our men are in the best shape of their lives" and should do well in Munich. Results again defied expectations. "Quite a few people asked me how many gold medals we won," wrote Hoffman. "I said, those days are gone." He could only rationalize the performance of America's two great middleweights, Knipp and Lowe, by saying, "[I]t is good to get eighth and ninth in competition with 26 of the best men in the world." The United States would have placed fifth had Karchut not been injured and Ken Patera, America's best prospect for gold, not missed all his snatches. Sadly Patera, the first American officially to clean and jerk over five hundred pounds (at the 1972 seniors), retired from lifting after Munich to enter professional wrestling. It must have been painful for Hoffman to concede superiority to the winner, Bulgaria, a nation with the same population as New York City: "What are we to do? We are in the position of a man who is running a race with a man who is well ahead of him and running faster." Although the United States garnered only eighth place, pundit Herb Glossbrenner wanted to believe that lifting was "on the upswing in this country" and that "we should be proud of this year's Olympic squad. . . . Let us have more bouquets and less brickbats."[18]

What no one could understand was why it was impossible to return to the golden days of yesteryear. With almost no remaining lifter/employees at York, Bob produced winning teams at the senior nationals by recruiting lifters all over the country. Yet however much this technique satisfied Bob's ego, it failed to induce the socialization that inspired earlier teams. "People resented York because they could buy lifters," recalls Crist—"a particularly bitter point with Bob Hise." Crist, as much as anyone, saw the need to disperse power, and worked ceaselessly to establish an independent system of financing and coaching. But with little support from the government and the U.S. Olympic Committee, and only a trickle of money from individuals and corporate sponsors, Crist always had to return "hat in hand" to Hoffman to finance overseas trips and national meets. Funding for the youth-development program, resources for the fast-growing physique and powerlifting sectors, and $50,000 yearly for a national coach seemed daunting. The latter position was reduced to a less costly coordinatorship, filled by Carl Miller of New Mexico. To cope with York, Crist exercised tact. Hoffman liked to pick officials for the championships, so Crist gave him a ceremonial post and waved a list in front of him. "As long as you shared things with Bob, he cooperated. If York was opposing me, my method was to set up a committee and outvote them. My strategy was to use York but [not to] let them control [me]."[19] The problem was that weightlifting had always been dependent on the driving force of Bob's ego and money. As other leaders sought to create a new dynamic that was more democratic, they ran the risk of jeopardizing the whole system.

Despite earnest efforts by its promoters, American lifting descended to a new low at the 1973 world championships in Havana. The United States finished thirteenth, behind not only Cuba but Czechoslovakia, Iran, Italy, and Australia. That it happened in the most hated of Communist vassal states made defeat intolerable. Hoffman was so depressed that he abandoned his *Strength & Health* narrative, noting merely the white and red lights given to each lifter. Though four of seven American lifters failed to make a total, Hoffman reserved special criticism for heavyweight Jacob Stefan, who, after missing his snatches, refused to attempt any clean and jerks for a possible medal in the Pan-Am phase of competition. Bob noted how Stefan, "with his waist-long hair, had gone back to his pool," where "his co-conspirators could see what they had done to American weightlifting. NO OTHER AMERICAN TEAM EVER MADE SUCH A MISERABLE FAILURE, U.S. WEIGHTLIFTING IS AT IT'S LOWEST EBB." The lifters responded by sending an "Athletes Report" to Jack Kelly. They complained that in addition to seven athletes and six officials, twelve other "tourists," all well-meaning local promoters, accompanied the group. "Their lack of knowledge and awareness" irritated the athletes.

Father of World Weightlifting

Besides, Hoffman and Terpak had "no regard for the lifters' personal aspirations for the world competition" and coached simply to beat Cuba. Trainer Karl Faeth and physician Frank Corbett were allegedly insensitive, and Terpak supposedly misguided athletes in selecting weights. Most galling were Hoffman's remarks to a *Sports Illustrated* reporter "that the lifters were a bunch of louses; you could see that by their hair." He believed there was "a conspiracy" among them to "do badly in order to embarrass the U.S. weightlifting hierarchy in front of the Communists." Harshly rebutting the lifters, Terpak insisted they were "not in top form," and ascribed the many bomb-outs to unrealistic aspirations. Privately, the more passionate Levin stated what Terpak could not say in public: "When several of our lifters refuse to carry the American flag, then in my old fashioned opinion they should be thrown off the team." In the same spirit, Crist submitted guidelines to the International Selection Committee to ensure that any athlete would be a team player, loyal to his country, and obedient to his elders.[20]

With only four lifters attending the 1974 world championships in Manila and five at Moscow in 1975 (accompanied by twice as many officials and tourists), no one expected much. Indeed no American placed higher than fifth at either meet. Being "treated like a king" (as Father of World Weightlifting) distracted Hoffman from events on the platform in Manila. But he could not ignore the humiliation of his team's eleventh place finish in the birthplace of Communism. Most humbling was the separation of the lightweight and mid-heavy classes into A and B groups because of so many lifters. All three Americans in those classes were relegated to the inferior B group, a virtual admission that they could not hope to win medals. "Never before in our weightlifting history had we sunk so low," Hoffman admitted. "Remember that I am the Father of American Weightlifting but I'm not too proud a father at present." The incident perhaps most indicative of this malaise occurred at a meeting of the national committee in Culver City, California, in June 1975. For years resentment had been growing among Bob Hise Sr. and others over York's control. On his home turf and with frustrations coming to a head, Hise hit Terpak in the face and broke his glasses. According to Crist, "Hise got up across the table and asked, 'Why have you always persecuted me and my son?'" Terpak was going to have him arrested, but later he told Pete George that the incident was "best forgotten": "In addition to having a 'short fuse' the guy needs psychiatric help." The issue was resolved at the national AAU meeting in November, and an apology was extracted from Hise.[21] Nevertheless it illustrated the hostility rising against York and its years of domination.

Softball Diversions

It is hardly surprising that Hoffman sought consolation in softball. Clair Bollinger, who worked for the York Parks and Recreation Department, was its chief promoter before 1969. Then he met Bob, who wanted to know the cost of bringing a national championship to York. For $5,700 he won a bid for the men's "A" championships of the American Softball Association (ASA). Eventually he won bids for all five competition categories and modernized the city's softball facilities. The Hoffman Memorial Stadium comprised seven fields. Bollinger estimates that up to 1973 Bob devoted $25,000 yearly to the sport and over $100,000 in later years. He not only sponsored as many as seventeen teams at one time, but sent them on extensive trips. Twice he sent a women's team to Hawaii and once even brought one from there to York. "Bob was very liberal," states Bollinger, "but got nothing except plaques and praise." Softball was the one area where there was never any problem getting money from Dietz, probably because he was a softball fan and because support for it came from the foundation, whereas money for the lifters came from York Barbell. Softball brought out some of Bob's best qualities: those of a real sports enthusiast with big plans and dreams and a genuine desire to help young people.[22] He aspired to make York the "Softball Capital of the World." But Bob's philanthropy was always tied to self-promotion. So he adopted the moniker "Mr. Softball," and in 1975 he was inducted into the Pennsylvania Softball Hall of Fame. He provided housing for it in the barbell plant and financed the publication of *Softball News*. In addition to the pleasure he took in having his name flashed around, Bob delighted in traveling to distant cities and outbidding other promoters. Bollinger recalls a bidding duel between Hoffman and Richard Howard of the Charlotte Speedway at San Jose in 1972. They eventually compromised, swapped championships, and exchanged signed dollar bills. In contrast to weightlifting, which lacked spectator appeal and whose athletes behaved unpatriotically, softball, Hoffman believed, was totally wholesome: "It is a game that is good for all who play it, and for those who watch it and for the United States of America."[23]

Father of World Weightlifting

Powerlifting Triumphs

Still, Bob could not escape the iron game, perhaps never fully comprehending the grip it had on him. One night in 1973 one of the girls on his team "hit a beautiful home run." As Hoffman reports, "[I was] astonished at what I felt when I patted her upper back. 'Where did you get all of those muscles?' I asked. 'Why, I train with weights,' was the reply." The grip of weightlifting was evident also in a 1975 caption to a picture of him, dressed in a softball blazer and cap, standing in front of a statue of himself outside York Barbell: "Bodybuilding, Olympic and powerlifting remain tops with him." That he turned his attentions increasingly to powerlifting was owing in no small part to his disillusionment with Olympic lifting, ruined by drugs and showing little sign of recovery. As Crist explains, "Bob wanted to go out with a winner." To preempt Weider, Crist appointed a national powerlifting chairman and a body of regional chairmen, and he enlisted Hoffman's support for an international organization. Bob now became more interested in powerlifting and staged the first world powerlifting championships at York in 1971, replete with a Mr. World contest. It was he who "bankrolled the IPF and really got powerlifting moving" in the 1970s.[24]

Hoffman must have known that powerlifters were just as heavily into steroids as Olympic lifters. Yet these Americans were winning international contests by wide margins. Another factor that kindled Bob's interest was the reinvolvement of Todd, who reported on championships for *Muscular Development*. Unlike some others at York, Bob had always liked Terry. According to Jan Dellinger, who joined the company in 1976, "Bob had a size complex. He loved Texas and Terry Todd." Todd's articles were inspirational and defended powerlifters. In reporting the 1972 world meet in Harrisburg, he took the emcee to task for belittling the lighter lifters. As one was approaching the bar for his final deadlift, Morris Weissbrot informed the audience that "Alexeev or Patera or some other behemoth could lift 50 pounds more than that all the way over his head." Todd was "deeply offended" by this comment, but one must wonder how mid-heavy champ Jerry Jones must have felt about some Texas-style humor unleashed at his expense: "To come bluntly to the point, the boy has a set of glutes on him that the Quarterhorse breeders at the King Ranch in Texas would give half a section of land for if they could breed stock with hindquarters to match his." Clearly Todd was as impressed with the awesome size and muscularity of lifters as with the great weights they lifted. The 1972 championship was memorable too for the creation of the International Powerlifting Federation (IPF), with Crist as president and Hoffman, who had underwritten almost all national and international power competitions thus far, as treasurer. While others took Bob's generosity for granted, Terry appreciated his drive: "I think it would be fair to consider him a force of nature, in the same category as wind, fire and tidal waves."[25]

That Todd's impressions had an impact was indicated by reader reactions. One stated that his "colorful descriptions and impressions matched mine, as a spectator, exactly." Further assurance that powerlifting was gaining stature was evident in Crist's report of the 1973 nationals at Scranton: judging was "consistent, firm and fair throughout the two day affair." At the 1973 world meet at York the irrepressible Todd (for whom powerlifting was as much art as sport) again held forth, this time on the antics of "the one and only Joseph S. Spack of New York, New York."

> *Mister* Spack is well named, as he seems to friend and foe alike to be truly other worldly. At a bodyweight of 164½, Spack is only moderately strong in the squat and bench press, but in the deadlift he really shines. And, for excitement and grins, I'd place him at or near the top of *any* list, pound for pound. In all his lifts, he has an elaborate, *highly* vocal method of psyching himself up for the big weights. He strides across the platform, glaring at the bar, giving himself a running stream of instructions. And the audience loves him, as do most of the lifters, and love him they should as he is a creature of wonder and delight. Often, after a lift, he'll point *immediately* at the scoring board and shout "Three Whites, please!" And he usually gets them.

At the opposite extreme was light-heavy Bob McKee of Birmingham, who was "extremely quiet" and "unemotional." His "bespectacled, bookish appearance and his lack of showy muscles makes him less of a 'personality,'" but "when the chalk dust has settled to the floor and the totals are posted, old Bob is up there on the winner's pedestal." Then there was Ohioan Vince Anello, "the human derrick, Anello the forklift, Anello the all-powerful, the strongest deadlifter, pound for pound, in the world. Forget his other lifts, for the crowd came to see him yank huge poundages from the clutches of gravity."[26] For Todd, no less than for Hoffman, lifting was more than lifting. It was part of the larger saga of life, a supreme test of human will.

Thus Hoffman, though "father" of Olympic lifting, was drawn to powerlifters. His interest was stirred also by the coincidence of the 1973 world power meet with his seventy-fifth birthday. Bob was honored with a special party at the Yorktowne, where the York gang, old-timers, and current friends showered him with gifts. The Texas connection, revived by Todd's articles, was reinforced by powerlifter Clay Patterson, who presented Bob with a ten-gallon hat. Hoffman wore it proudly as he danced a fast polka around the hall with Alda to show his agility, youthfulness, and fine physical condition. The Mr. World contest, won by Englishman Roy Duval, was given an entire evening, and the powerlifting meet was won decisively by the United States over Britain, 74–56. All of this activity and adulation left Hoffman with a sweet taste for the sport: "The Olympic lifters have been so ungrateful for what we have done to help them, even the men for whom we have done the most. We have sent them through college, helped them get a start in life, bought them houses and so forth, and now they are our greatest complainants. What I am getting at is that the powermen are a different breed. . . . If the Olympic lifters don't want to support the York Barbell Club in competition, we can turn full force to powerlifting!" Winning was everything for Bob, even after seventy-five years, and if he could not win in one game, he would switch to another. Todd encouraged his defection, pointing out how Olympic lifting had "really hit a Death Valley low," and how much "more appreciated and productive" his support would be in powerlifting. "The Powerlifters are ready, Bob, so let's go."[27]

An attractive feature of powerlifting was its team spirit. Patterson, who accompanied an American team on its trip to England in 1974, reported that it was "a real team. From day one to day twelve when we bid adieu, we were fourteen people working as one." Much the same kind of feeling prevailed when the English team lifted at the 1975 world championships in York. But the best example of the spirit of powerlifters, in contrast to the Olympic lifters, was their ability to endure adversity at the second annual Pan-Am meet in Venezuela. George Lugrin reported:

> If you have never taken your squat warm-ups off an elevated bench press apparatus . . . if you have never lifted in the middle of a sandy, open-aired horse pavilion . . . if you have never in your life

lifted in the dark, with the platform lit only by an arc of car headlights . . . if you have never attempted to psyche yourself while artillery fire could be heard in the surrounding mountains . . . if you have never had to sidestep horse dung, or if you haven't had to be careful about where you waited, exhausted and dehydrated, in your three-minute recovery period, then you, hombre, have never really lifted under adverse contest conditions.

What helped the lifters tolerate such hardships and made them proud to represent their country was that they won virtually everything. Americans held thirty-one of the forty world powerlifting records, including a sweep of the five heaviest classes. Little wonder that Bob was reminded, on returning from a power meet in Puerto Rico, of his remark thirty-five years earlier: " 'I like weightlifting and weightlifters.' After this trip I like them even more."[28]

Until 1975 all world power meets and Mr. World contests were held at York in conjunction with Hoffman's birthday. Though it moved to Birmingham, England, in 1975, Bob continued his support, calling it a "thrilling, exciting, satisfying and happy experience." Todd reminded powerlifters that the trip cost Hoffman over $15,000: "None of us who are serious about the game should ever forget that a lot of canisters of Hi-Proteen, bottles of energol, and barbell sets have to be sold in order to raise that kind of money." Terry made every effort to put a silvery gloss on events in Birmingham to assure Bob that York money had been well invested. Although the United States won eight out of ten classes (with no "bomb-outs"), there were fourteen countries represented on the victor's platform, seven more than in the latest Olympic world championship. The true spirit of powerlifting was embodied in one of the most remarkable lifts ever performed, by ten-time British light-heavy champ Ron Collins. At forty-one he was well past a lifter's prime, but Collins had secured victory over challenger Dennis Wright of Oklahoma with his first deadlift of 623. Though slightly injured and cramping badly, Collins was eager to please the home crowd with a world-record total. So he hobbled back and made a tough 672 second attempt, cramping so badly he could barely walk off stage. "As he limped off, . . . most people felt that the injury, the cramping, the new world record and the world title record would mean that he would forego his last attempt," but Collins then requested 700 pounds. Todd's description of what followed is a classic of lifting lore.

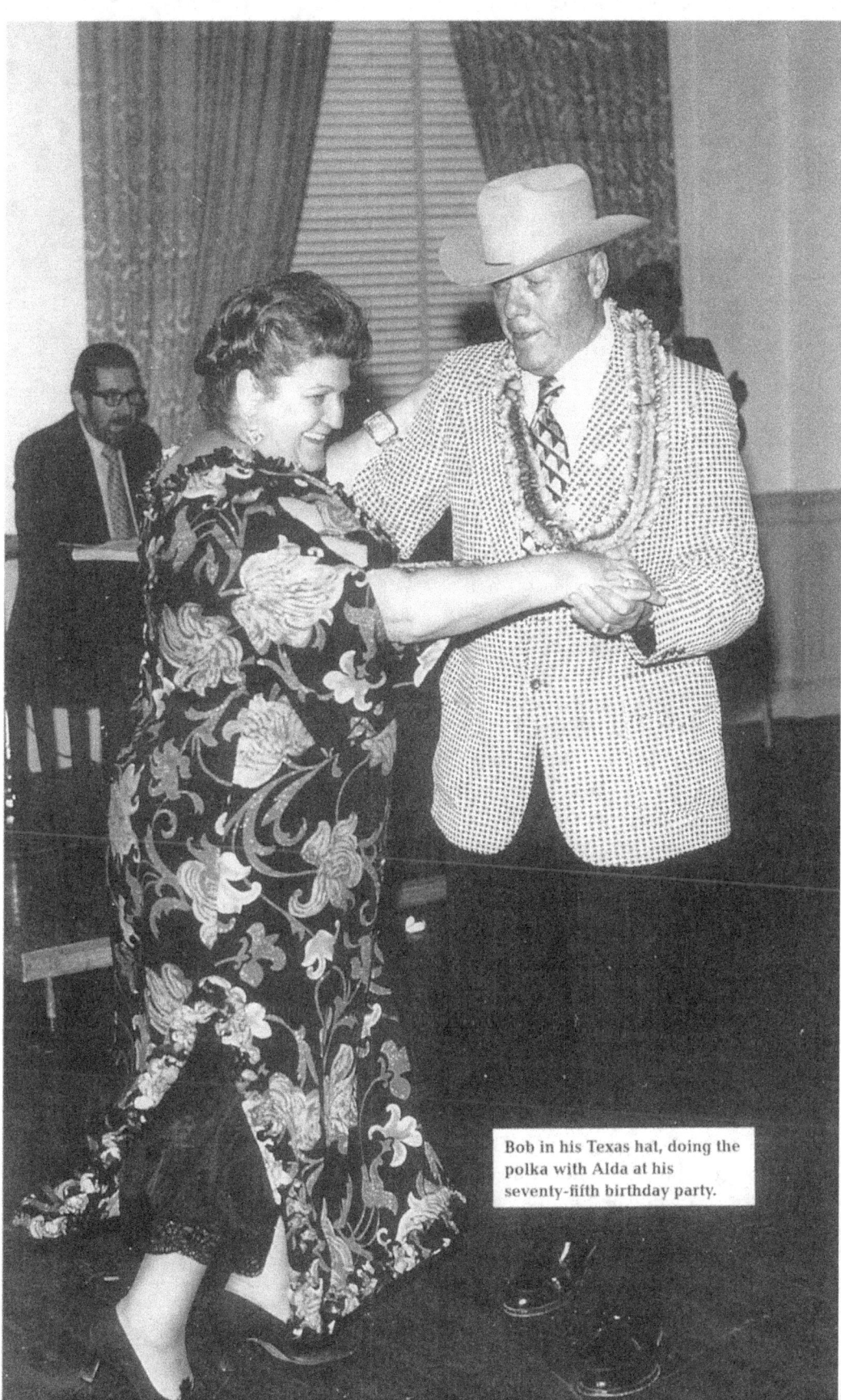

Bob in his Texas hat, doing the polka with Alda at his seventy-fifth birthday party.

He steps painfully onto the platform for the 700. I think he's got a shot at it. The crowd is shouting, helping to psyche him for the effort. He limps to the bar, pains showing on his face, but he is careful not to rush the lift. As he bends to grip the bar, he has only 10 seconds left on the clock. He sets, looks, pulls, and simply *masters* the weight; and as the weight goes up, so does the crowd, brought up by the awesome courage and tenacity of the man. And I, for the first time in my life, feel tears come unbidden to my eyes as I join in paying tribute to this man who has as much right as any man ever has to be called history's greatest powerlifter. The ability to make such a lift with only the pressure of pride driving away the pain moved me as I have never before been moved by a lift.

Todd could look back as one who had done so much to initiate powerlifting a decade earlier, and say with satisfaction, "Our sport has come of age."[29]

Whether holding the world meet in England detracted from Hoffman's influence seems doubtful, especially since it returned to York the following year. What's more, Weider and his allies soon ceased their powerlifting initiatives. In physique, where Weider had a firm foothold, it was different. British organizers, in deference to Heidenstam's concern that the Mr. World contest would conflict with his annual Mr. Universe show, did not stage the contest. Allowing it to lapse a year enabled Weider to make further gains and hamper York efforts to attract top competitors in 1976. Tom Wrange, secretary of Finnish Bodybuilding and Powerlifting, expressed astonishment to Crist that "some kind of a Mr. World contest" was going to be held at the 1976 world power meet. He believed the "IPF should keep only to powerlifting in the same way as IFBB has decided to keep only to bodybuilding." After all, the IFBB was the only bodybuilding federation recognized by GAIF. "All European bodybuilding people I know think it would be high time for AAU to join the IFBB so that all American bodybuilders can take part in the official World Championships. Perhaps you do not realize in AAU how big organization IFBB really is." York held its Mr. World contest, but on the same weekend Weider staged a Mr. Universe show in Montreal, attracting higher quality and more international entries. That 1976 AAU Mr. America Kalman Szkalak defected to Weider and became the 1977 IFBB Mr. Universe was yet another sign of the times.[30]

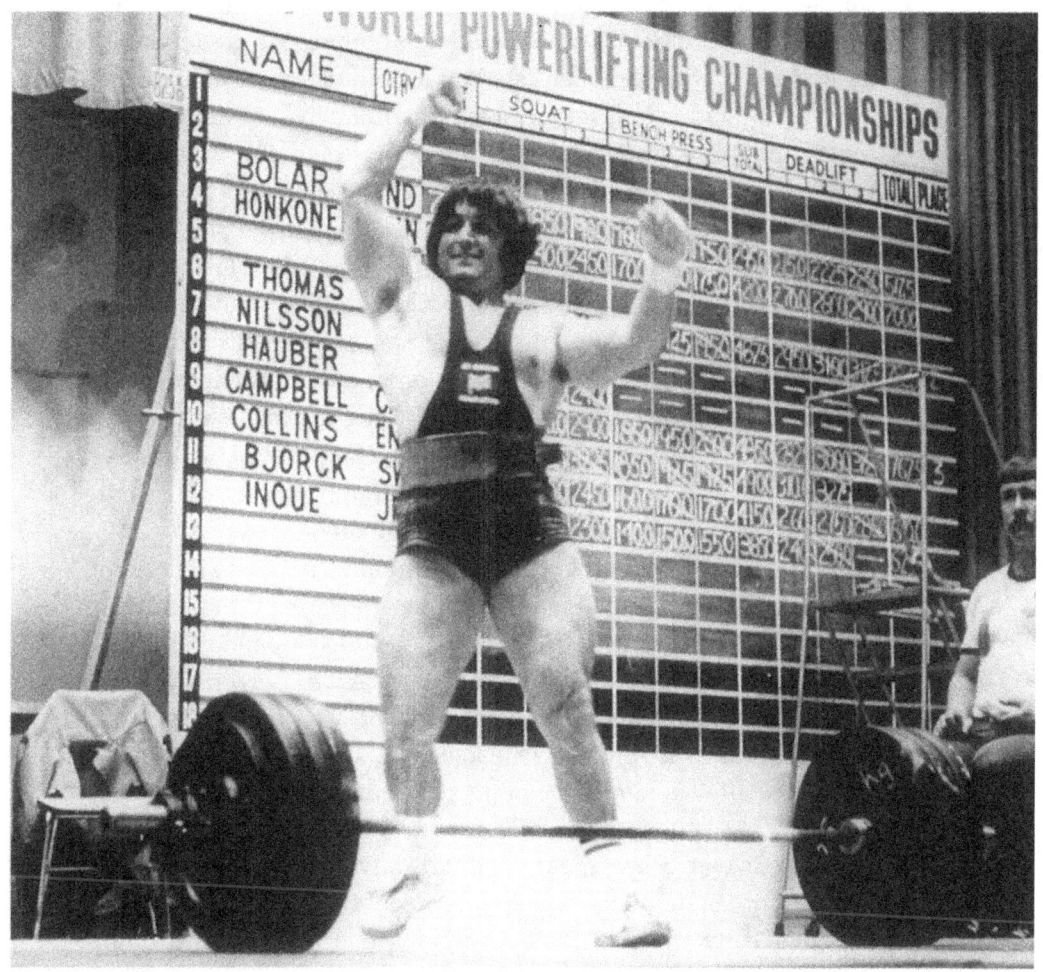

Briton Ron Collins celebrates after completing a 722-pound deadlift for a world record total at the 1976 world championships at York.

Self-Made Accolades

To stay abreast of the times and attain more credibility, Hoffman acquired a Ph.D. Through Trudy Engel, he was "awarded" a cultural doctorate in Therapeutic Philosophy by World University in Tucson, Arizona. Bob never visited it, but for his "generosity" he was recognized by John Zitko, its president, as a "Founder for life." Though knowing nothing about the institution, Hoffman flaunted its credentials. By counting the number of offices listed on its letterhead, he assumed that the university had campuses in twenty-five nations. World University officials probably knew little more about Hoffman, yet Zitko lauded his "contribution to the cause of physical fitness and sports" as "beyond calculation." Nor did Bob understand, though he started using the initials behind his name, the concept of a Ph.D. He thought he had acquired three or four degrees, proudly telling readers, "I have University degrees in Physical Fitness, Sports and Nutrition. . . . My most important degree is Doctor of Therapeutic Philosophy or Ph.D." Hoffman concluded that it was "the first time a triple PhD has ever been awarded." Terpak had to keep telling him that his degree was pronounced "p-h-d," not "phee-h-d." Remarkably, Bob used his degree to dispute other writers and to establish credibility for his products. Employing the phrase "With the Rights and Privileges thereto Pertaining" on his diploma, he refuted claims by other nutritionists that only forty essential nutrients were needed for a good diet. Reminding readers that he, too, was a Ph.D., he argued that there were seventy-five such nutrients, and that this requirement could best be met by taking his Vitamin and Mineral Tablets. He also used his degree to strike back at critics who scoffed at him for having "no scientific background": "But it is believed that my books have been copied by more experts than any other books except Shakespeare and the Holy Bible."[31]

Such absurd statements can only be understood by accepting Hoffman for what he was—a promoter extraordinaire. That even Bob realized he was no scholar and held no degrees was evident later in testimony under oath. But his contributions to fitness and his struggles with supposedly better-informed opinion in medicine and government cannot be so easily dismissed. Unlike many doctors, he regarded the heart as a muscle needing exercise and helped expose the fallacy of the "athlete's heart." He encouraged ambulation after surgery and childbirth long before it became acceptable. He insisted, contrary to coaches' beliefs, that weight training improves athletic ability in any sport, and he did as much as anyone to expose the muscle-bound myth. He popularized isometrics and was a major figure in winning acceptance of high-protein and natural-food products. A pioneer in weight training for women, he was also innovative in sponsoring women's softball teams and encouraging women to powerlift. Alda, who allegedly deadlifted 325 pounds on her first visit to the gym, was his first female powerlifter. His, however, was the best example of an active life. He boasted that he belonged to the "Go-Go club" and covered more mileage than Secretary of State Henry Kissinger. In 1974 only the burial of his brother Chuck made him late for the Philadelphia Open. On turning seventy-five Bob professed to feel no different than he had at age fifty, twenty-five, or even fifteen. He was "super-strong, super-healthy and super-enduring . . . working 17 to 18 hours-a-day, sleeping 4 to 5 hours-a-night, and feeling young in everything but experience." Always needing to set some new record or pass a milestone, at 255 bodyweight he claimed to have run ten miles while wearing a fifteen-pound belt and carrying two twenty-pound dumbbells. "Who else in this world can run 10 miles weighing over 300 pounds?"[32]

Bob's Final Books

No matter how egocentric and commercially motivated, Bob's ideas on exercise, diet, and weight training had a broad impact. Even President Nixon subscribed to the myth that Hoffman, on his seventy-fifth birthday, was at "the height of his powers." Books continued to be a major publicity medium. *The Best Natural Food* extolled the virtues of three ingredients found in Hoffman products—honey, peanuts, and soybeans. Much was made of America's addiction to junk food and the fact that York products were "made of the best of everything." He insisted that York was "more interested in you and . . . your family's health than in making more dollars." Still, without a price change since 1950, York was making a handsome profit. *Energol Germ Oil Concentrate* focused on a single product, with nutritional information drawn from the Department of Agriculture yearbook. More conscious, with his Ph.D., of the need to provide correct information, he regarded the yearbook as "entirely authentic and scientific," so much so, he insisted, that none of its data had ever been questioned! *Why Men Die Younger* was autobiographical almost to the extent of being a memoir. He ascribed to stress the fact that men die younger than women: "The man because he is a man, so often has to prove his masculinity. By getting in a fight, by changing a tire, running for a train, shovelling snow, doing so many things he is not in physical condition to do." To live longer, men needed to exercise more, eat nutritious foods, and avoid life-shortening habits. But the best way of ensuring longevity was to emulate the life Hoffman led. When he had to "meet someone" at his "mansion on Hoffman Hill," he arrived early so he could "climb the stairs." While waiting, he might "walk up and down the stairs fifty times, which is the equivalent of climbing the Washington monument and walking down again." Since the House on the Hill was where he entertained his girlfriends, one can only imagine the sweaty condition, in addition to his usual effusive body odor, with which he must have greeted them! So perfect was his health, he explained, that he ran six miles breathing only through his nose. A doctor who in 1972 conducted tests on him at the Ochsner Clinic in New Orleans said, "I don't know why you are here, you are the healthiest man we have ever examined."[33]

In *How to Keep Your Husband Alive Longer* Hoffman related more examples of his superhuman health, and provided pictures of himself in various life stages. Never content to be second best in anything, even sleep, Hoffman argued that he required less sleep because he slept "faster than most people." Equally idiosyncratic was his view that "sexual intercourse without ejaculation" leads to greater satisfaction and longer life. He also discussed the merits of a couple's sleeping in separate beds. "My wife is not so far away. . . . It's a walk to the next room but I believe in exercise and we can call that physical fitness." He further advised men to remember "your 'love' likes affection even when you are not in bed. Don't forget to kiss her good-bye, and kiss her hello when you come home. Wives, be interested in your husbands work, his business, ask him what kind of a day he has had. . . . Men, don't forget flowers, little gifts, candy if weight is not a problem. A Hoffman food bar, will smooth away a lot of troubles." Increasingly he referred to Alda as his wife, and in many ways they experienced the joys of married love. "We have never had a cross word," he noted. "The life she has made for me is the principal reason why I am a leading contender for the title, World's Healthiest Man."[34] But if Hoffman's patronizing, though sincere, comments are any indication, the real secret to "keeping your husband longer" was to take care of him, as Alda did for Bob.

Confronting Mortality

But Bob did not take care of himself. Notwithstanding his long-distance running claims and a 1973 statement in the *New York Post* that he still lifted weights two hours a day, he was too heavy and in poor physical condition. Closer to the mark was an admission in 1972 that for years he had been averaging a half hour each of weight training and running *per week*. In any case, distance running was precluded by a condition called hammertoes where his second and third toes rubbed the insides of his shoes. It was operated on about 1980, Alda recalls, "but Bob would never admit there was anything wrong with him." He "hid everything inside." At most he would do a fast walk in the basement, during which "he would get awfully red"—hardly the image of the world's healthiest man. Ernie Petersen recalls that the last time he saw Bob break chains with his chest, at a demonstration in Oklahoma, Hoffman slumped over and looked like he was dying. Though he made it on a second try, the gang later hid his chains and belt. As for Bob's report of perfect health from the Ochsner Clinic, a letter from Dr. Oscar Bienvenu reveals a different story: "As you know, we probably accomplished nothing on your brief visit," but "we have multiple means of testing for heart conditions, and we are in a position to give advice about exercise, after certain tests are done." Imagine a doctor advising the father of physical culture on exercise! Bob hid from the truth about his condition, but he could not overlook others among his friends who were dying off. On Memorial Day weekend of 1975 Larry Barnholth and Gord Venables passed away. The following weekend Win Franklin, a health-club operator from Plainfield, New Jersey, noted for his distance running, died of a heart attack. Like Bob, he had practiced denial. Several weeks later the grim reaper claimed Peter Karpovich, the Springfield College educator whose conversion to weight training attracted notice in the 1950s. In June, physique photographer Gregor Arax died in Paris, and Serge Reding, the Belgian superheavy who was the second man to break the five-hundred-pound barrier in the clean and jerk and first to snatch over four hundred, died at the world championships in Manila. These losses, Bob said, only strengthened his resolve to work harder, but in April 1976 his own death was reported in the *Washington Post* by a physician who insisted that protein supplements were valueless, except to Hoffman's pocketbook, and that York lifters had made their gains from anabolic steroids, not Hi-Proteen.[35] Bob was so incensed that he sued the newspaper.

Combating the FDA

Indeed the government seemed to be in league with doctors to debunk those products which contributed most to the wealth and power of York. Though Hoffman had signed a supposedly meaningless consent decree in 1968, the FDA reinstituted twenty-four contempt charges in 1972 on grounds that York had made no labeling changes. In 1974 it seized a cache of Hoffman products not covered by the decree, alleging further violations. Bob's lawyers told him that costs and fees could run as high as $25,000 before trial and $100,000 afterward, but he was determined to win at any cost. As a major health-food producer, Hoffman believed that he was being singled out by the government: "They work about like the Unions. . . . They attack one company at a time." Instead of restricting beneficial products like vitamins, the government should be limiting consumption of tobacco, alcohol, coffee, processed foods, licit drugs like aspirin and sleeping pills, and illicit drugs like marijuana and cocaine. "The FDA, the AMA, the Processed food people and the Devil, have formed an unholy alliance to put our country down." Americans should fight for "nutritional freedom." Freedom of choice was a right deeply ingrained in America's heritage, and he invoked the expression "Give me liberty or give me death" in a pamphlet entitled *If Patrick Henry Were Alive Today*. Hoffman produced a million copies of this screed, likening it to Lincoln's Gettysburg Address. In combating FDA tyranny, Bob cast himself in the same role as the founding fathers.[36] No longer able to test his strength on the lifting platform, and with his erstwhile feuds with Weider and the Soviet Union in abeyance, his struggle with the FDA seemed yet another way to prove his manhood.

He joined other health-food-industry leaders to support a bill introduced by Congressman Craig Hosmer that would curb the powers of the FDA and another by Senator Warren Magnuson to abolish it. Critical to Hoffman's initiatives was the lobbying of Trudy Engel, whom he called "the best known and the most popular female in Washington, outside of the First Lady." As a York employee, Trudy lived near the Watergate Hotel, knew many politicians well, and attended health-related hearings. She also accompanied Bob to health-food conventions, where they usually stayed in adjacent hotel rooms. Hoffman sent her jewelry and frequently danced with her. Opinion is divided on whether their relationship was sexual, but Bob did state at one point that she had the body of a sixteen-year-old. Dave Matlin's first encounter with Trudy occurred in 1972, when he took her and Bob to dinner in Los Angeles. "Trudy is a very charming, fascinating and lovely lady," he reported to Terpak, "and between the two of us, Bob did not have much of an opportunity to talk." She was known as the "candy and cookie lady" in the offices of the high and mighty in Washington. In 1973 Bob boasted that she had made three trips to the White House in four days: "She is almost a member of the family." Dellinger recalls Trudy and Max Huberman, president of the National Nutritional Foods Association, once acting like big children as they vied for Bob's attention: "Trudy was a real motormouth. She could talk incessantly about nothing." Equally obvious to Dellinger was Hoffman's need to "be seen when they went anywhere."[37]

Nowhere were these qualities more evident than at the health festival Trudy orchestrated in October 1973 at the Kennedy Center Atrium, where two hundred guests danced, dined, and celebrated Bob's seventy-fifth birthday. Leading the singing and toasting was Senator Richard Schweiker, a sponsor of legislation to curb FDA powers. Clinton Miller, legislative advocate for the National Health Federation (NHF), awarded Hoffman a Humanitarian of the Year trophy, and York Barbell presented him with a silver plate embellished with a likeness of his favorite person—himself! Trudy also assembled promotional floats for Bob at the Cherry Blossom Festival in 1973 and 1974. The former, on "Health, Exercise, and Nutrition," featured Mr. Americas Chris Dickerson (1970) and Steve Michalik (1972) along with Christy Mizell, the parade princess. Washington Redskins running back Larry Brown and Mayor Walter Washington appeared on the latter. On both occasions Trudy demonstrated abdominal exercises. So confident was Hoffman in Trudy that he attributed some of his own miraculous qualities to her, merely on the basis of shared values: "Trudy Engel has not had a headache in her entire life, even more remarkable for a woman. . . . She tells me that she has never been sick. She has been a Bob Hoffman girl, following the Bob Hoffman system of living for the last 40 years."[38] However unfavorably Trudy's effrontery may have been viewed by others at York, she was a kindred spirit to Bob and undoubtedly opened many doors.

Complementing Trudy's insider influence were pressure groups inspired by Bob's crusade against the FDA. After his birthday gala, food manufacturers, retailers, and consumers demonstrated outside FDA offices against labeling and formula requirements for vitamins. "It wasn't the usual group of protesters with knapsacks, blue jeans and long hair," reported the *Washington Star News*. "Most were middle-aged." Their placards read "FDA Pushes Drugs," "FDA-AMA Stink," "FDA Worse Than Watergate," "FDA Against Health." In addition to Schweiker, Senator William Proxmire and Congressman Paul Rogers provided support in securing passage of the "Heart-Lung, Blood Research, Vitamin Bill" in 1976. Hoffman's generosity was significant in this success. Not only did he underwrite the work of Trudy, but he repeatedly helped the NHF with its legal expenses. *"No single individual in America has contributed more over a longer period of time than you have,"* noted Clinton Miller. Soon, however, Bob was confronted with a more serious challenge from the Federal Trade Commission. It concluded that protein supplements were not only "a total waste of money" but in some cases a "serious health hazard." The FTC proposed rules requiring manufacturers to state on labels and promotional material that "protein supplements are unnecessary for most Americans," to warn of health hazards, and to list protein content. Bob could not comprehend why products so conducive to health could be so misunderstood by bureaucrats and physicians: "Few doctors want people to do well since well people do not help their business and the processed food people want no interference with their merry life of selling foods filled with chemicals and robbed of natural food ingredients." Equally misguided was the press. "I have before me a package of chicken stroganoff, which bears a famous brand name and contains 45 additives which are not foods. Yet, this chemical-laden 'food' bears the Good Housekeeping seal." To dodge the government's Big Brother tactics, Hoffman started calling his products "natural foods."[39] Though a drain on his time and fortune, Bob seemed energized by these encounters with a vastly superior enemy.

The Nixon Connection

It was in the executive branch, however, that Hoffman sought supreme fulfillment. He did everything possible to gain Nixon's attention, admit-

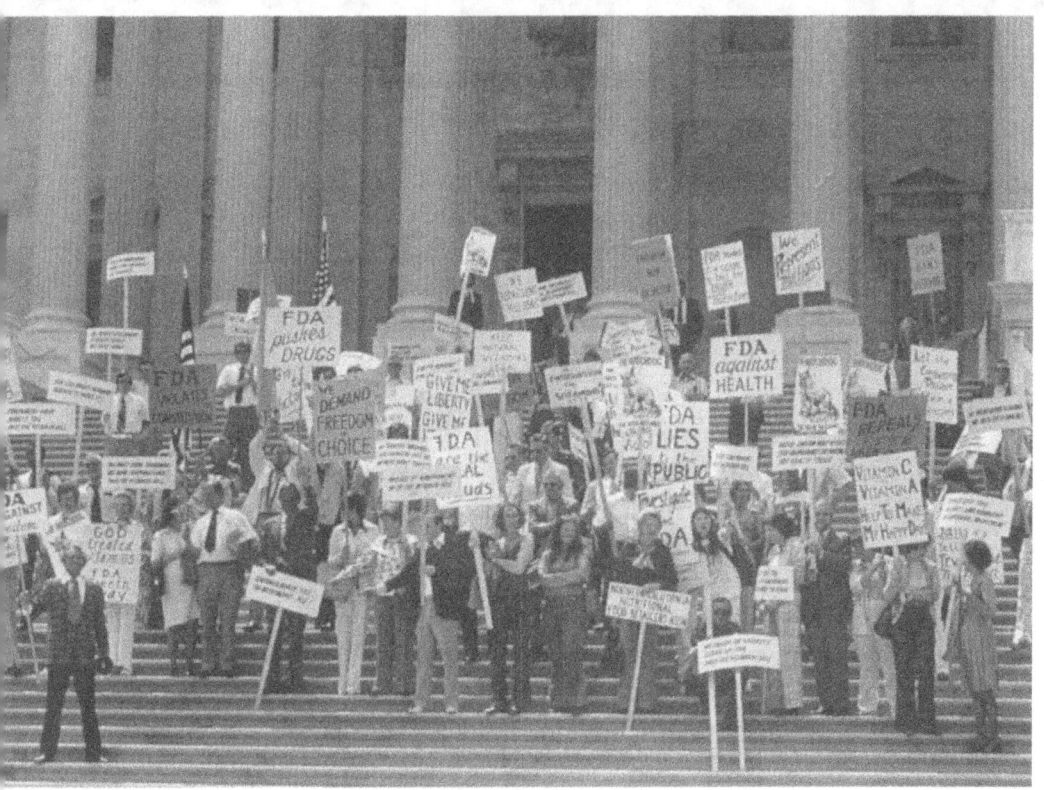

A Hoffman-inspired protest against the FDA, 1973.

ting that he had donated the Nixon Park to gain presidential influence in combating FDA regulations: "I had to get and keep the President's attention and now he says, 'Bob Hoffman is a great guy.' . . . This can mean so much to our industry in the next five years." In addition to acquiring a Ph.D., Hoffman sought notoriety by membership in the National Press Club and an entry in the National Social Directory. As the 1972 election approached, Bob intensified his efforts to gain an inside track at the White House. He planned to invite Pat Nixon to York to throw out the first ball at the world softball championship for women in September. He envisioned a spectacle with thousands present, including the president, and "a hundred or so cameramen and newsmen there to commemorate the day." When Mrs. Nixon declined the invitation, Hoffman still sent a silver-plated bat and ball to the White House with Trudy, "her very personal friend." Bob also campaigned vigorously for Nixon. He was appointed to the president's campaign committee and was invited to the Republican Convention in Miami. Unable to attend because of the Olympics, he sent Trudy as proxy. She showed up with "her nine suitcases" and even took in the Apollo 17 launch that Hoffman had been invited to attend at Cape Kennedy. Bob's campaign assignment was to talk to young people in the YMCA, Boy Scouts, and softball. He estimated that he reached fifty million, including parents: "I am actually in touch [with] and known by half the people in the United States." Claiming to have made over three hundred speeches, he bragged that he "talked more in behalf of the president than the president did himself." In the glow of victory, Bob and Alda attended a Prayer for Peace Ceremony at the White House. He attached great significance to being seated in the front row, between Mamie and Julie Eisenhower, and to Trudy's position beside the president: "I was next to the people who live in the White House. It was a terrific experience, not one of those things that just happen, but arranged, for we stand very well with the 'powers that be.' "[40]

Afterward Hoffman was first in the receiving line. "Four more wonderful years coming up" was his greeting to Nixon. " 'We can do some wonderful things during those years.' He patted me on the shoulder and said, 'Bob, you are doing good work.' That was worth more to me than any of my many decorations." The president then introduced him to John Cardinal Krol as "one of the great athletes of his time." Encouraged by these accolades, Bob and Trudy devised bolder schemes of gaining influence with Nixon. Rationalizing that his decision to institute mass bombings helped shorten the Vietnam War, they tried to secure for him the Nobel prize. When Secretary of State Kissinger won it for the opposite reason of helping instigate peace talks, they took credit for that nomination. Less successful were attempts to place Bob on the contingent accompanying Nixon on his precedent-setting trip to mainland China, but he was not dismayed: "Even being on the list of those who may be a part of the China trip, makes me known." So extensive was knowledge of Bob's ties with the White House that the *Cleveland Plain Dealer* printed a cartoon of "Strength and Health Magazine" showing a caricature of Nixon flexing his muscles on the cover.[41]

Bob seemed convinced that he was gaining access to real power. He still hoped the president would fly up from Camp David to visit Nixon Park: "[W]e could talk as we formerly did, man-to-man. . . . Many times the President took our advice as we wrote him letters and sent long telegrams. We had a lot to do with making present history." Aside from the psychic satisfaction Bob received from these assertions, he received little else. Nixon soon became mired in the Watergate crisis, and Hoffman's nutritional concerns were ignored. Predictably Bob came to Nixon's defense, stating publicly that the investigation was "pretty

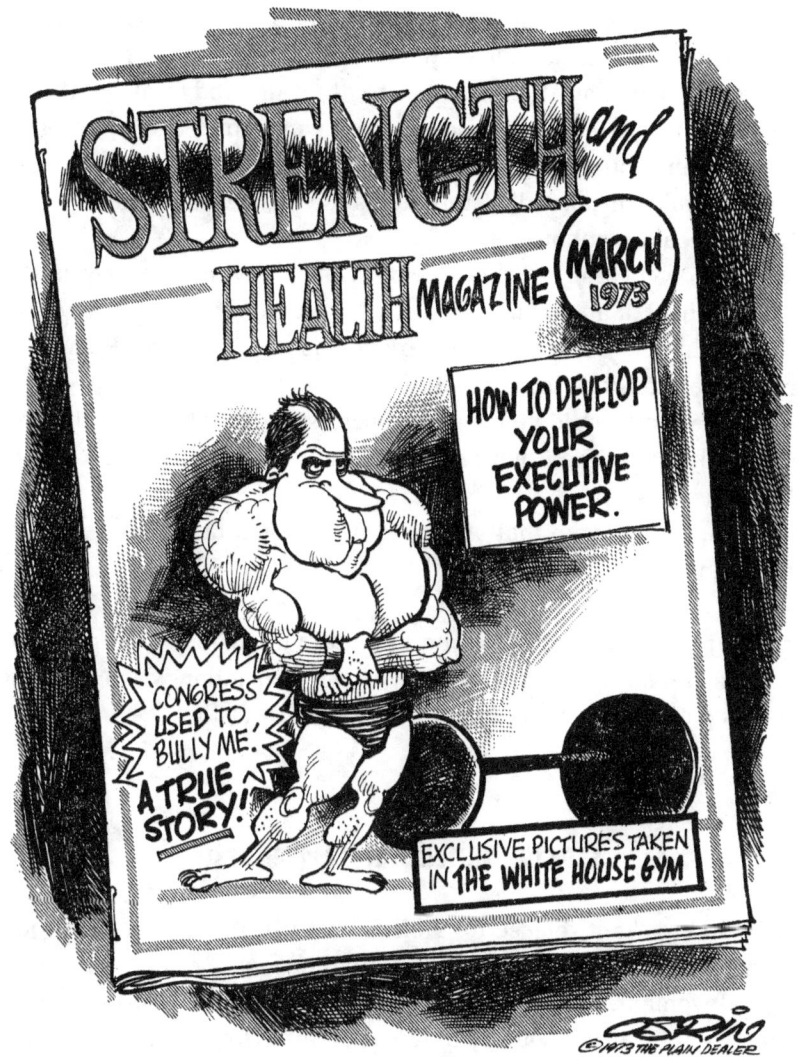

A satire on York's influence behind the Nixon presidency, March 1973.

silly" and that "thinking people [were] overwhelmingly in support of the administration." He was "convinced that the president knew nothing of the Watergate breakins. 'I don't always know what is going on in my own corporations. I have to rely on other people and if they don't tell me, I don't know what they're doing. But I don't call it a 'coverup.' " It would be difficult to imagine a greater setback to Hoffman's hopes than the next year's events, culminating in Nixon's resignation. An Oakland reader no doubt shared the sentiments of other York followers:

I'm in a state of shock. Last year in Strength & Health you wrote an article about Richard Nixon titled MY FAVORITE PRESIDENT. As one of the thousands of American weightlifters and bodybuilders that look to you for leadership and advice, I was impressed [by] what you said and could truly look upon MR. NIXON as a great and honest man. I totally dismissed Watergate as the mistake of some of Mr. Nixon's zealous subordinates.

And now?! He's resigned and everyone is saying that he was a thief, a cheat, a mad man, a liar, etc. My friends even say that you should change the name of the park you gave to York from Richard Nixon Park to Bob Hoffman Park.

Please, Bob, could you set the record straight. There are thousands like me in the American Iron Game who look for your intelligent leadership.

P.S.—Is it really true that you have never even taken an experimental puff of a weed?[42]

Unwilling to admit he was wrong about anything, Bob never tried to set the record straight. Burned badly in his association with Nixon, he proceeded cautiously with the new Ford administration.

Save the United States Movement

The most important release for Hoffman's frustrations over Watergate was the creation, again with Trudy's guidance, of the Save the United States Movement. Reasoning that neither he nor Nixon was misguided, he believed it was the country that was on the wrong course. Foremost of his concerns were health issues and his battles with the FDA and FTC: "We must change our mode of living, for it is apparent that we are not living in the proper way." For an agenda he took his five essentials of good health and added seven: abstinence from tobacco, stimulants, and alcohol; consumption of natural foods; adherence to good-health rules; and avoidance of drugs and sexual indiscretions. These were the twelve commandments of the Save the United States Movement. The last two items, however, went beyond health to address Hoffman's deeper concern, based on experiences with the younger York gang, that America was losing its moral strength. America's greatest threat was no longer the Soviet Union but an internal enemy, manifest in the drug culture, the antiwar movement, and the conspiracy that toppled Nixon from power. He compiled one hundred reasons for the Save the United States Movement and enlisted support of the major health-food federations as well as the AAU and the ASA. In 1975 Bob confided to Don Porter, ASA executive director: "The first thing in my life this year must be softball. I see an opportunity to do more To Save the United States through softball than in any other way."[43] He expected much from its thirty million players and two million teams.

At the 1976 Cherry Blossom Parade, in accord with its bicentennial theme, the York entry was the "Declaration of Health." It featured Bob at a desk signing the declaration, with Terpak behind him as a witness and Trudy, dressed in red, white, and blue, in front of a Statue of Liberty. At the rear was Olympic lifter Mark Cameron performing dumbbell exercises, flanked by two attractive ladies. By such means, along with radio, television, and press interviews, Hoffman publicized his message. He envisioned a grassroots movement in which followers ("Bob Hoffman 100 Percenters") would form neighborhood committees and receive Bob's monthly activity reports. It resembled the Strength and Health League he had formed with Jowett in the 1930s. But there was little indication of what his followers were supposed to do, except be healthy and good and be impressed by Hoffman's dynamic lifestyle. The Save the United States Movement seems to have been Bob's last attempt at immortality, but the American public, especially after Vietnam and Watergate, was too savvy to take seriously a movement whose real motives seemed to be blatant self-promotion and sale of Hoffman products.[44]

Business Initiatives

Financial reports show considerable growth in the early 1970s. Monthly sales-average data show that volume more than doubled in seven years.

1969—$335,068	1972—$616,972	1975—$671,293
1970—$451,813	1973—$578,173	1976—$749,338
1971—$540,835	1974—$592,015	

The most important observation to be derived from these figures is that sales, coincident with the Arab oil embargo and economic recession, slumped in 1973 and took three years to return to the 1972 level. Bob pointed out that paper was scarce and expensive and that scrap iron had recently gone from $35 to $97 a ton. Lacking abundant and cheap iron, York resorted to producing vinyl barbells and purchased two foundries, but still fell behind: "It is almost impossible to get small things such as set screws, washers, other small parts. Everything we need is in short supply." What's more, profits were down, owing in part to a rise in costs and a lag in price adjustments. But Bob, who always dealt with adversity by moving forward, even in the midst of national economic dislocation, made plans for expansion. At the 102,000-square-foot plant along Interstate 83 there was activity "such as there [had] never been before and so much more [was] to come": "Our new additions give us another 100,000 square feet of useful floor space, to EXPAND!!!" Envisioning further growth, he bought nine acres adjacent to the plant. By the mid-1970s York's business was evenly divided between the barbell and fitness line and products that were consumed or applied to the body.[45]

Next to availability and cost of materials, Hoffman's biggest problem was marketing. Obviously he could not sell his "excellent products if the stores [did] not stock them": "And it gripes me no end when the distributors do not have an item." Bob was dismayed that many of the seven hundred health-food stores throughout the country stocked no more than five or six of his 140 products. He wanted more "100% Bob Hoffman—York stores." Richard Pruger, a western Pennsylvania lifter of note who held a master's degree in business administration, suggested a plan for a chain that would carry Hoffman products exclusively. He projected that one hundred stores (at an investment of $2.5 million) could earn as much as $2 million per year. Pruger was hired as York's marketing manager and was allowed to oversee the operation of five Hoffman Health House stores in Pittsburgh. He tried to be loyal by working hard, training regularly, and even submitting quarterly "activity reports" in the Hoffman manner. Unfortunately the reaction to his "MBA techniques and fresh ideas" was almost wholly negative, especially from Dietz, who was "very disapproving." At an early board meeting, Pruger saw that Dietz manipulated Bob and that he was "feeding Bob fallacious figures." Afterward Mike told Ernie Petersen, "This guy Pruger and I are gonna lock assholes." Soon Pruger discovered that "Mecca wasn't what [he had] envisioned it to be." He believed that Dietz was doing all in his power to ensure failure of the Health House experiment. After three years of meager profits and closures, Pruger returned to Pittsburgh to provide closer supervision over the operation. Profits were maintained into 1976, but there were always problems, including stealing and inefficiency by employees, difficulties in acquiring supplies from York, and cutthroat competition.[46] It is little wonder Bob proceeded no further with Pruger's idea of a chain of York company stores.

York Enterprises

Another proposal urged on Hoffman from many quarters, including Terpak, Levin, Day, and Matlin, was that York should become a public corporation. That it did not may be attributed to Bob's preference for power over money and his not wanting to answer to stockholders. Most observers agree that Dietz was also strongly against the proposition and talked him out of it. Most suspect that Dietz (and Hoffman) would never have survived public scrutiny of the financial records. Day estimates that "for every $5 Bob made, Dietz got two or three of it." Bob always said, according to Alda, "I know Mike is stealing, I just don't know how much." It was also widely known that Mike and his sons had established an alternative manufacturing operation called York Enterprises, which took its supplies from York Barbell and was in direct competition with it. As Ernie Petersen puts it, "York Enterprises was living as a parasite off York Barbell. Mike was simply stealing from York." Bob and Johnny first learned of this conflict of interest from Bruce Randall, a former Mr. Universe, at a health show in the early 1970s: the Dietzes were assembling benches at a machine shop in Emigsville and enticing York customers. On returning from the show, Terpak confronted Mike with this information in Bob's presence. But the latter simply sat in Mike's office during the heated exchange, staring out the window. This noninterference, concludes Dellinger, "was a semiblessing" allowing Mike to continue his wayward course.[47]

Unfortunately the problem only worsened. In 1975 Warren Miller, a Maryland distributor of York products, confided to Bob that "Dietz and his two sons" were "operating their own little barbell and equipment factory" and had "offered to sell [him] equipment": "Bill Starr and the other petty thieves that have come and gone at York Barbell, are nothing

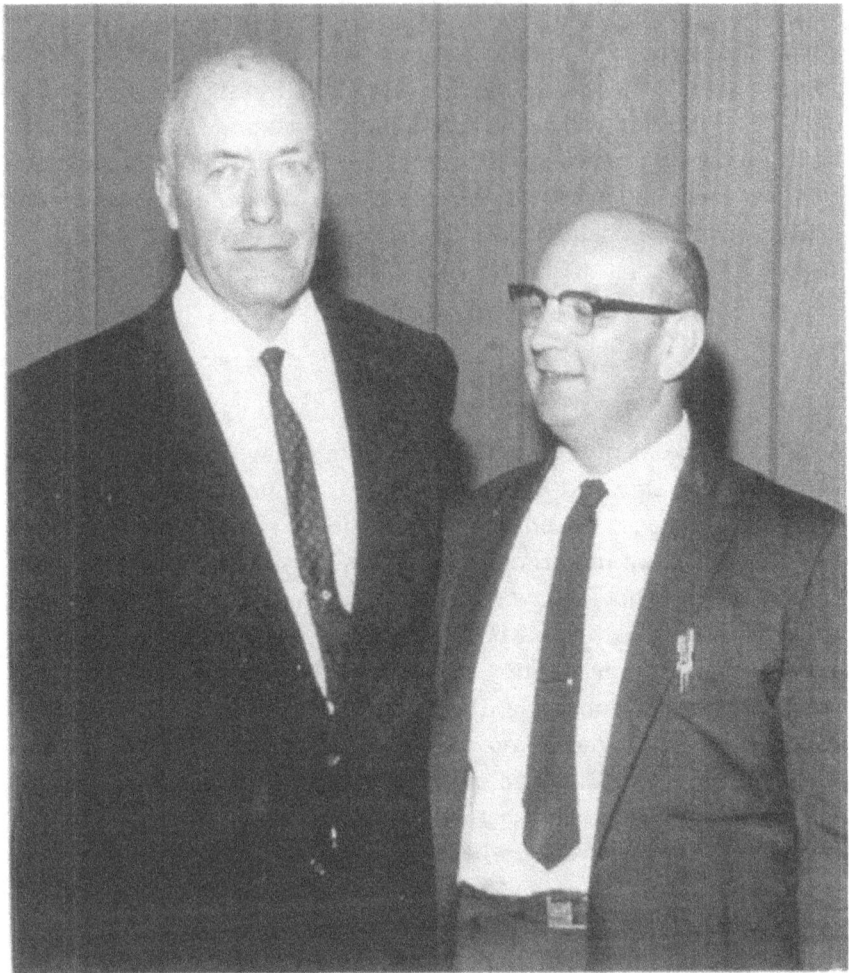

Bob with Mike Dietz, his company's treasurer and successor.

compared to the insidious evil that is now lurking behind the scenes. . . . I would simply fire the whole corrupt trio of the Dietzes." But Bob did nothing. His attitude is typified by the following exchange between Bob and Alda, as reported by Grimek: Driving through the countryside, on their way to an AAU meeting in Philadelphia, Bob pointed out some dairy animals. "They look like our cows," Bob commented to Alda. "What do you mean," she replied, "we don't have cows. Mike has cows." To which Bob casually stated, "Oh, Mike's cows, our cows, what's the difference?" A similar disregard for distinctions between personal and company assets was evident to Bednarski when he occasionally met Dietz at the Spring Garden Hotel bar after work. When Mike got drunk, he would get talkative and friendly, especially with women. Bednarski, who sometimes lined him up with prostitutes, recalls how Mike would pull rolls of twenty-dollar bills out of his pocket and hold them out, saying with a sly grin, "This hand holds the barbell company's money, and this hand holds mine. Occasionally they get just a little mixed up."[48] Evidence of conflict of interest was overwhelming, but Bob's management of the company was so loose, and that loose management had been going on so long, and Mike had such total control of records, that Hoffman's employees either grimly accepted the arrangement or went elsewhere.

Consumer Demands

Corruption, along with low wages, undoubtedly took its toll on morale, efficiency, and ultimately quality of York products. Customer complaints, a few resulting in lawsuits, usually related to food items. As a result of a consumer's discovery of a mouse carcass in a can of Weight Gain, the Pennsylvania Department of Agriculture investigated the York plant. Finding much evidence of insect and rodent activity, it ordered immediate compliance with the state's General Food Law. But a reinspection of the facility a month later uncovered still more instances of sanitary neglect. Other consumer complaints focused on Hoffman's technique of advertising products through himself. An anonymous annotated copy of his "Father of World Weightlifting" editorial addressed him as "Father of Con*seat* and good old American Bull shit": "He must have felt bad this month. He only refers to himself 103 times." A woman reader from New Jersey wrote, "[I am] *appalled* that a man of your background and accomplishments should be given to *common bragging!* . . . Every book and article tells about the great 'I am' (a name given to you by the local club). This out and out bragging has lost you many readers."[49] No longer could Hoffman rely on boldness alone to win acceptance.

Would-be followers began to scrutinize what he was saying and compare it with other versions of the truth. Hoffman's article "The Dope Scene" in *Muscular Development* drew an angry response from a reader in Olympia, Washington, who disputed his linking marijuana to crime:

"Where are your brains? . . . So what if killers use marijuana? Most of them (at least in the U.S.A.) use toilet paper, but I doubt if that incites them to murder." Dismissing what Hoffman wrote as "hearsay," he echoed the moral line Starr had taken: "Don't try to pass your personal value judgements onto others. Their bodies are their's to do with as they please. . . . So cut your simple minded preaching: Not everyone wants to be a bald headed old 'weight-pusher' with a mean glare." Nowhere did Bob feel the waning public acceptance of his traditionalist views more than in the changing fortunes of his magazines. With Holbrook as editor, *Strength & Health* became more diversified. Articles on such themes as swimming, tumbling, Athletes in Action, kickboxing, ice fishing, and even Disney World showed that the magazine was no longer the lifter's journal it had been under Starr. Unfortunately sales continued to fall. These bad tidings coincided with a series of letters from Tom Fleming of Pittsburgh, who described himself as "a York 100 Percenter since the middle forties." With all the brazen wit of Harry Paschall and fifteen years experience in advertising art, writing, and production, Fleming told Hoffman what was wrong with York's marketing approach. Using words such as "corny," "old-fashioned," "lousy," and "unprofessional" to describe *Strength & Health,* he believed Degenhardt had "the imagination of [a] 5-year old" and that his "knowledge of even basic magazine layout [was] zero." Eventually changes were made in the magazine, but hardly in the modernizing mode recommended by Fleming. In 1974 Bob decided that his magazines, to cut costs, would appear bimonthly—one of the few times in his life he backed away from a problem.[50]

Magazine cutbacks provided a rationale for staff changes. Holbrook, in a "forced economy move," was dismissed in March 1974. Two months later Degenhardt resigned and, with his new bride Sandi, went off "to build an art service." Soon, however, he was working for Joe Weider at his new quarters in Woodland Hills, California. Upon hearing of Degenhardt's departure, Fleming offered his services. Aware that no amount of truth could free Bob from the myths that imprisoned him, he appealed to Terpak to save York: "You are working for a company that is not keeping pace with today." To the departed Holbrook he insisted, "The whole problem at the Hoffman empire is Hoffman! He has got to be put to pasture, in order for the company to grow. Apparently everyone at York is afraid of him. Because he was successful in the twenties, he still thinks the techniques used then, will work today. They don't and they wont!" Even with Hoffman an anachronism, the magazines tried to stay current. Dennis Karpinski expanded treatment of women's concerns in *Strength & Health*. A 1974 article entitled "The Gals Take Over" was inspired by Billie Jean King's victory over Bobbie Riggs on the tennis court. "Now womankind is challenging mankind in every field."[51] Soon a "For Women Only" section appeared. In October 1974 it featured Vera Christensen's "To the Ladies" column and articles on weight training for women athletes. *Muscular Development*, on the other hand, enhanced its masculine appeal with a department called "The Arm Benders," dedicated to wristwrestling. Both magazines offered more coverage of softball for men and women. Those who had followed Hoffman for decades were pained by the magazines' problems and York's failure to maintain its traditional orientation.

Eternal Hopes

Not all news was bad for Hoffman. "American weightlifting got a much needed shot in the arm," wrote one *Strength & Health* reader of the ABC *Wide World of Sports* coverage of the 1971 world championships in Peru. Though weightlifting was usually accompanied by another sport, such as water polo or car racing, ABC and CBS responded to viewer interest by covering major meets in the early 1970s. It appeared the sport was finally getting the attention it deserved and that this limelight might stimulate a lifting revival. In 1973 one of the networks produced a movie called *The 500 Pound Jerk*, inspired by Alexeev's record lift in Columbus. It evoked much viewer interest. "Three white lights for Alex Karras and his movie" was one reaction. It "gave the American public a close look at the sport, something the Olympic coverage failed to do." But the fascination of television audiences with weightlifting was short-lived, its decline hastened perhaps by the spectacle of a "dying sport" at the 1973 senior nationals and the unspectacular international performances of Americans. "We need stars!" Holbrook ruefully remarked.[52] But potential weightlifting stars were being lured into sports with greater money-making opportunities. Soon the networks defected to wristwrestling and powerlifting.

Failure hardly came from want of trying. Chairman Crist and such dedicated volunteers as Morris Weissbrot, Rudy Sablo, Frank Bates,

Dave Mayor, Marty Cypher, and Bob Hise seemed to be doing everything possible to resurrect American lifting. To this end, the national committee organized clinics and training camps around the country. Chief motivator was Carl Miller, a New Mexico physical educator and protégé of Frank Spellman. "Already results are being felt," he proudly announced in 1973. "Lifters on one side of the country are finding out what lifters on the other side of the country are doing." Most important, a "vast technical knowledge" was "reaching young lifters." Over the next several years hundreds of clinics instructed American lifters on the latest training methods, especially the double knee-bend pull, from eastern Europe. No one expected immediate results, but there was reason to believe this latest group would make its mark at the 1976 Olympics in Montreal. American lifting did experience an upswing. At the 1975 senior nationals Mark Cameron of Rhode Island set a national record with 451 pounds in the clean and jerk at only 220 bodyweight. He became an immediate celebrity. Hoffman was elated, predicting that he would "be a world class lifter" and win "glory for himself and the United States." Best of all, he enabled York Barbell to win its forty-fifth national championship. For his achievements Cameron garnered 94.5 percent of the votes for "Lifter of the Year." Pruger estimated Cameron would have "an excellent chance of becoming the first American since Joe Dube to win a gold medal" in an international meet. But just how far he was from this feat soon became clear. At the 1975 world championships he surpassed his record, but Bulgaria's Valentin Christov won the class with a 523 world record, 67 pounds more than Cameron's best. A genuine coup for American lifting, however, was the second-place finish of Lee James from Albany, Georgia, in the mid-heavy class at the Montreal Olympics. In the snatch "Lee made sensational success with 363 3/4 for a new Olympic and American record," reported Hoffman. "The crowd went wild! Some long-time friends from Great Britain were sitting around me and they yelled, 'The United States is on its way back!'" Grippaldi, Cameron, and Bruce Wilhelm also nearly snagged medals, and the United States finished eighth. But coach Tommy Kono saw less reason for optimism. Every effort had been made to provide ideal living and training conditions, including precompetition camps at York and Plattsburgh, New York, "to establish team spirit." Team officials stressed this point, reported Kono, but "personality clashes among several team members made this virtually impossible."[53]

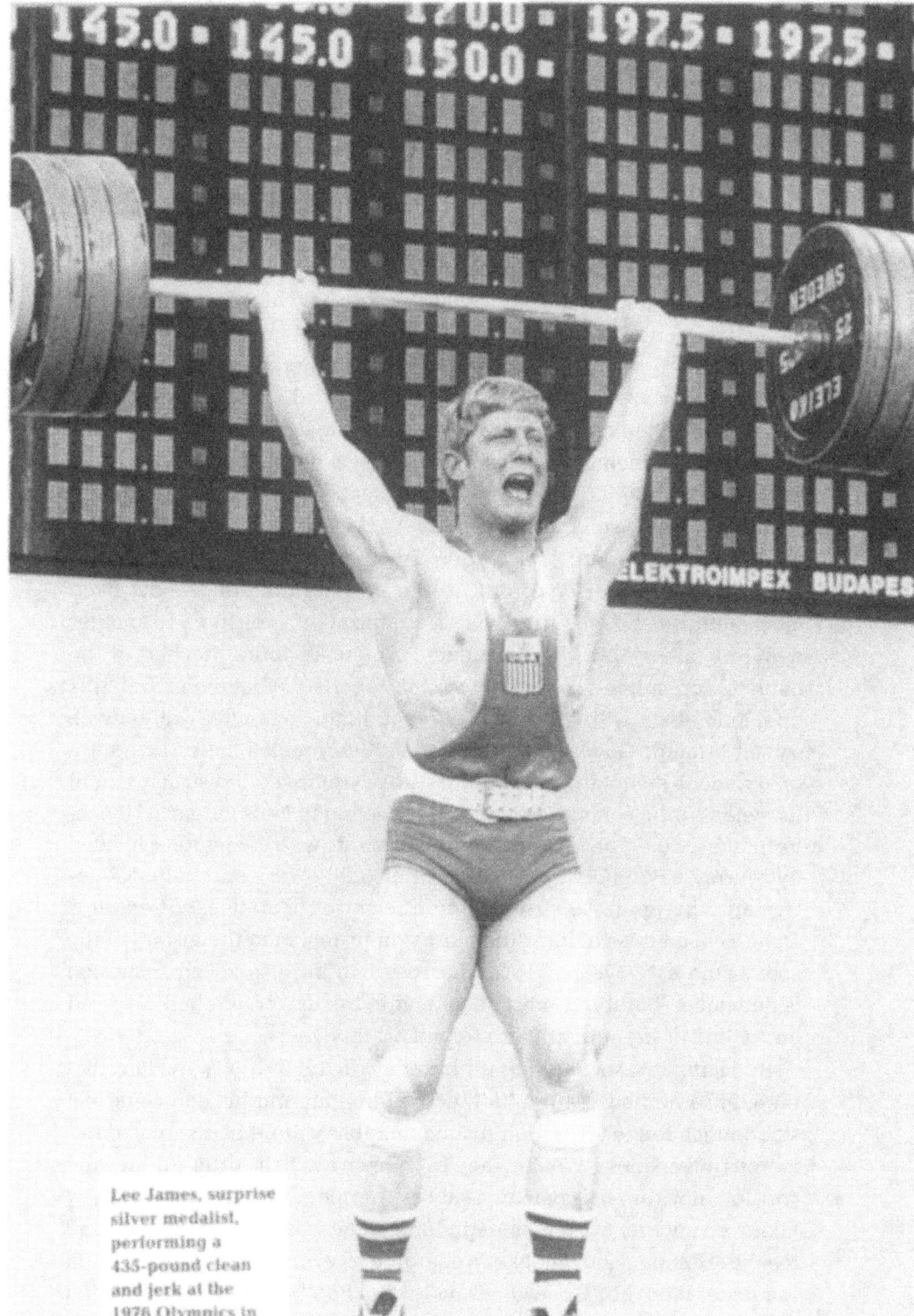

Lee James, surprise silver medalist, performing a 435-pound clean and jerk at the 1976 Olympics in Montreal.

AAU Restructuring

By now many of the internal divisions that plagued American weightlifting were systemic. Crist, trying to be fair, always recognized the equal status of weightlifting, powerlifting, and bodybuilding, but he also insisted that a strong organization was possible only by maintaining unity under the national committee. "To coin an old phrase—'United we stand, divided we fall,'" concurred powerlifting secretary Milt McKinney. But countervailing forces were at work. A constant irritant was Charlie Shields's American Weightlifting Association, which attracted York's enemies. To destroy Hoffman's power base in the AAU, the AWLA supported Senate Bill 3500, sponsored by John Tunney of California, which sought to break the AAU into smaller, self-governing organizations by sport. Anticipating passage, Shields drew up a charter and planned to bid for control of the new weightlifting body. Even more enthusiastic was the Weider organization, sensing yet another way to subvert York. Ben attributed America's lifting decline to the national committee's control of too many sports. "What the I.F.B.B. was unable to effect with the A.A.U. Weightlifting Committee will now be solved through Government legislation," he predicted. To stave off a government-mandated breakup, the AAU approved a restructuring of its weightlifting committee at its 1975 meeting in New Orleans. Henceforth there would be three independent sports with committees headed by Murray Levin (Olympic), Clay Patterson (Power), and Ralph Countryman (Physique). Crist would be director of operations. *Strength & Health* called this change "the most significant . . . in the history of the sport in the last 30 years."[54] Whether restructuring also sowed dissension is debatable, but it did presage an end to the unity York had enforced on American strength athletes for almost fifty years.

By Hoffman's seventy-eighth birthday, in 1976, it was evident that the edifice he had spent a lifetime building around his ego could not stand much longer. Through his indomitable will he had survived numerous adversities—Weider, the FDA, Nixon's fall, the drug culture, and corruption within his company—always surmounting one challenge by taking on another of greater magnitude. But it was obvious to friend and foe that Hoffman could not keep charging forever. A New Jersey pundit fondly recalled the "Good Old Days" when Bob "could count on stoking his lifters with mounds of high-protein pills, pat them on the rear, and send them onto Olympic platforms with every confidence in their ability to beat the rest of the world." Now "his 'era' [was] obviously over." Less sympathetic was the director of the AWLA, who viewed Hoffman's longevity as

> hardly a healthy situation.... "A father will never die so long as he has sons, he will live on," is a statement often made by a well-known W.L. figure who claims to be the father of W.L.
>
> I must ask—does a real father give his sons the learning and capabilities to ... make their own way in an often cruel and harsh world, or does he make them so dependent on him for his own ego-gratification that they are doomed to die with him because of their total dependency on him and their inability to fend for themselves.

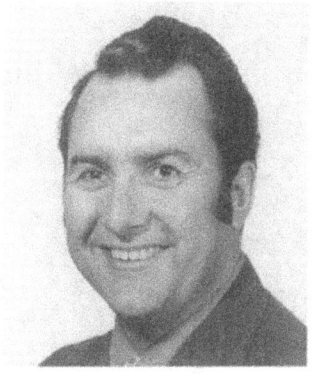

Virginian Bob Crist, national chairman in the early 1970s, who initiated critical changes that helped redefine York's role in the iron game.

Embedded in these agonized expressions was a wisdom that surely surpassed the comprehension of the Father of World Weightlifting. Clearly, the harder he tried to control the system he created, the more it slipped from his grasp. It was not so much that Hoffman failed to lead as that others refused to accept his leadership. He simply could not help himself. Almost as if he thought himself immortal, he gave no thought to passing the reins. Being "it," after all, was the only approach he had ever known. Bob was "the great American success story," but the story became meaningless as he went beyond a patriarchal construct sometime in the 1970s to become an anachronism.[55]

10
BOB HOFFMAN'S DEPARTURE

> As each generation turns to make its exit from the stage it hears a disagreeable sound. People in the audience are talking, not listening; they are indifferent to what their elders are saying on stage, worse they are uttering heresies. That is the inescapable penalty of growing old.
>
> —Noel Annan, *Our Age*

The Founder's Decline

For nearly a half century Bob Hoffman and York Barbell had dominated the iron game. In his last decade of life, however, the founder experienced the ultimate tragedy of witnessing his own decline. With the growing obsolescence of his promotional techniques and diminution of his leadership capacity in the 1970s, he had to relinquish power over his company, and his place in the fitness world. Despite an outward show of vitality, a prolonged period of stagnation set in. As Terpak observed, "We lost our mouthpiece."[1] With the loss of the spiritual force that had placed York first in strength and health, other forms of decline soon followed. The Weiders, who had been vying for a "place in the sun" for decades, wrested control over bodybuilding. Powerlifting abandoned its York roots, and Bob never lived long enough to bring his grandiose ambitions for softball to fruition. Only in Olympic lifting did York retain preeminence, but as participation and performances of American athletes diminished, it became a meaningless distinction. As Bob approached his eightieth birthday, he lost his drive—mental, physical, and sexual—and ultimately his purpose in life. No longer able to uphold the body of manly myths he had created around himself since the early years of the century, Hoffman was at last faced with the reality of his own mortality.

Despite frequent proclamations to the contrary, Bob suffered from many ailments as he entered his twilight years. His worsening heart condition contributed to a general debility of body, mind, and spirit. Not surprisingly, it was most evident during travel. Terpak recalls a time in Florida when he and Bob were running late for their return flight and had a long trek to the departure gate. Always a fast walker, Bob "couldn't keep up, but he would never admit anything was wrong." On another occasion, in St. Louis, Dellinger observed he was suffering angina pains, and as they walked about the city, he tarried frequently to catch his breath. That he stopped to stare at vacant shop windows betrayed his condition. In 1978 Hoffman underwent open-heart surgery, but York publications made no mention of it. To allay suspicions about his health, Hoffman walked around the day after his operation, assuring everyone that he was the "world's healthiest man." To the public it was necessary to portray himself, even at eighty-one, as the most perfect human specimen that ever lived. Such fictions nurtured in youth were impossible to sustain with age. No longer could Bob willfully deny the laws of nature. And as the gulf between public ideal and personal reality widened, Hoffman's mental health deteriorated. On returning from the 1975 world championships in Moscow, he accused the stewardess of stealing his luggage. Then he disappeared at La Guardia airport and was found with a black woman, insisting he owed her $38. Phil Redman recalls that when he became York's advertising manager in 1974, Bob was in "pretty good shape," but "by 1976 he was having problems." Hoffman called Phil the "advertising guy," then could not recognize him at all. "He remembered the weightlifters better." Most appealing to Hoffman's manly instincts were the 135 parachute jumps Ernie Petersen made during the Vietnam War. Soon Bob was introducing him to outsiders as having done 300, then over 1,000, and eventually sinking battleships. As John Terpak Jr. once put it, "[T]here were no battleships in Vietnam except ours." In the late 1970s a consensus developed that the organization would be better off if the Father of American Weightlifting was relegated to the closet.[2] But this ostracism from the York gang worsened his plight.

Bob's abdication of responsibility did help the company in its relations with the government. His lieutenants showed no interest in continuing to fight the FDA. With patience and forbearance Redman, Terpak, and their legal counterparts worked conscientiously to meet FDA/FTC requirements and to negotiate their way out of impasses. The result was a partial consent decree in 1978 on Hi-Proteen Powder and Energol and York's willingness to adhere to all new regulations. "Once Bob ceased to play an active role in the business, there were no more problems with the FDA," observed Terpak. There remained, however, a backlog of cases that required ongoing attention. Bob's flagrant violation of regulations made York the target for endless sanctions and suits. Legal expenses for May 1979 alone exceeded $3,000. Such was the strength of the founder's will that no opponent was too formidable for him. As Alda repeatedly stated, "It was either Bob Hoffman's way or no way."[3] It took his successors a decade to extricate themselves from the clutches of the federal bureaucracy.

York Barbell's Decline

The business weakened during Hoffman's decline, though not immediately. Sales and net profits for York Barbell climbed steadily until Bob reached eighty, then stagnated until his death. Interestingly the margin between sales and profits (in parentheses) widened significantly after 1978.

1974—$6,887,004 (333,054)   1980—$12,165,046 (305,754)
1975—$7,004,996 (352,632)   1981—$12,333,705 (214,762)
1976—$8,393,494 (335,032)   1982—$11,950,465 (155,814)
1977—$9,736,616 (488,319)   1983—$11,558,647 (392,793)
1978—$11,995,489 (837,970)   1984—$11,869,854 (48,363)
1979—$10,947,811 (351,000)   1985—$9,999,925 (153,138)

Other entities owned by Hoffman—York Precision, Swiss Automatic, Hoffman Laboratories, and Ridge Corporation (properties)—also exhibited a decline in the 1980s. Figures on subsidiary operations are

A still robust Hoffman in the 1970s outside the York Barbell plant, beside a statue of himself and beneath the revolving weightlifter sign that was visible from Interstate 83.

unavailable, but 1977 board minutes indicate that the directors (Hoffman, Terpak, and Dietz) were encouraged by the corporation's overall profits and sought further development. Mike wanted more floor space to make barbells, and Bob talked about acquiring a Miami subsidiary to manufacture a device similar to the Universal Machine. "Business was really good in the '70s, especially on protein," observes Claudia Keister, Terpak's secretary. "Big distributors would haul three tractor truckloads away per week. Nineteen seventy-eight—seventy-nine was absolutely our best year."[4]

Concurrent with the loss of Bob's leadership, marketing problems set in. At first it did not matter, but competition became intense in the early 1980s. Redman observes that the health-food industry grew dramatically, from several hundred million to about four billion dollars total sales in a decade: "A lot of companies went mainstream in the way they were marketing products—Celestial Seasonings, Twin Labs, and Weider. LA Gear has grown incredibly. York got lost in the shuffle." Board minutes from 1978 to 1984 record steadily declining sales and profits, first in the lucrative health-food sector, then in old-line barbell products. The company also tended to rest on its laurels. Redman contends that there had "always been almost an arrogance here about being York." An indifference to what was going on outside seemed prevalent. Computerizing late was an example of such indifference. And there were no inventory controls, enabling employees to steal. "Only receivables and payables were handled by computers. Mike Dietz never understood any of this."[5] Entrepreneurial spirit was by no means absent, but York was no longer a leader in health and fitness.

Michener Associates

To compensate for the loss of Hoffman's promotional zeal, York officials engaged an advertising firm, Michener Associates, to bolster the company's public image primarily by stressing the venerable York tradition and Bob. A 1979 AAU award recognizing him as "one of the oldest active amateur athletes in the U.S." was publicized in eight regional newspapers and fourteen radio stations and five television stations. Similar arrangements were made for media coverage, including *Sports Illustrated* and ABC Sports, when York Barbell Club won its forty-ninth national championship in Totowa, New Jersey. The most important tribute to Hoffman's lifework was the new corporate headquarters constructed at the barbell and food plant off I-83. The thirty-four-thousand-square-foot Y-shaped structure included a museum along with a weightlifting and softball hall of fame. For $250,000 the York firm of Marketechs, assisted by iron-game enthusiast Vic Boff, hoped to revive the organization's sagging image by projecting the color of competition and Bob's personality. The facility, including a snack bar and store selling York products, was opened in the summer of 1981. By 1983 company officials seemed pleased that attendance, especially by families, exceeded that of the previous year.[6]

Michener then used this strategy, promoting tradition, to develop a "New Look" in York products. To jump-start sales, three new items—a high-protein-fiber candy bar called Carola and two soft drinks—were introduced in 1979. This was followed by a "face-lift" of six other products. An editorial, "In Search of New Horizons," called it "the first major change in appearance since our health food line was conceived." Market surveys, unheard of when Hoffman was in charge, were part of overall modernization plans, but Michener had difficulty securing cooperation from some stores. Steve Fiedler of the Health Food Center in Dallas criticized York for poor writing and "'junky labels.' He felt the company was 'not with it,' not competitive. His biggest complaint was with Hoffman's use of sugar. . . . He was about to go along with the survey then reconsidered because he didn't want to be associated with Hoffman." Other concerns, however, were more cooperative, and the 1980 report showed a high percentage of consumers in Chicago, Dallas, Philadelphia, and San Francisco preferred Hoffman products. From this "'hard' knowledge" a marketing plan was formulated. Michener recommended that York target major trade magazines and supplement this thrust with attractive support literature and special promotions such as product sampling, couponing, and demonstrators. Public-relations suggestions included a "Hoffman Healthline" newsletter, a "Distributor of the Year" award, and high school essay contests on nutrition and exercise. Total cost for the modernization program would be $521,000.[7] Though some recommendations were adopted, company elders resisted radical innovation. Tried and proven methods prevailed.

After the opening of the hall of fame in 1981, management tended to rely on in-house marketing techniques. They were hindered, however, by the decades-old personality conflict between Terpak and Dietz, who were now running the company, and by the latter's fiscal conservatism. Notwithstanding these constraints, Johnny pursued various low-risk initiatives to improve distribution of York products. He engaged KAF Associates, a manufacturing representative service, to increase business in New England. But a wrangle developed over commission percentages, leading KAF executive Kenneth Fischer to warn that "when people stay where they are, they really go backwards because competition moves ahead." Fiscal restraint and distrust of outsiders was also evident in Dietz's reaction to Terpak's attempt in 1984 to establish accounts with major retailers. "What is this about Sears and Penney's? In my opinion doing business with these Accounts is no step forward. They are too big—they can make or break a Company over night." As an alternative to dealing with powerful high-volume outlets, and in order to reckon with cheap castings from Asia, Mike suggested they establish a low-quality Milo barbell and retail it through discount houses. He also believed York was handling "too many poor risk accounts, slow paying and uncollectable," and that the $2,000 fee paid to Dun and Bradstreet was "being wasted." Also distressing to Mike was the "pitiful" sales of Hi-Proteen.[8] However well intentioned Dietz's proposals for retrenchment—fewer commission accounts, reductions in the labor force, resort to discount houses, and magazine cutbacks—may have been, they were a far cry from Bob's fearless initiatives.

Legal Liabilities

In the 1980s York was beleaguered by consumer complaints and lawsuits. The most serious of the latter, *Tinsman v. York Bar Bell*, involved accident with serious injury. Paul Tinsman dropped a 220-pound York barbell on his neck while he was bench-pressing alone at the YMCA in Macomb, Michigan, in 1978. With the blood supply cut off from his brain, he became mentally incompetent and a quadriplegic. The plaintiff sued for negligence, claiming the YMCA had no supervision and that York provided no instructions or warning with its equipment. Testifying for him were Bill Reynolds and John Henderson. The former, though editor of Weider's *Muscle and Fitness*, was supportive of York, saying that it was "a question of maintenance," not manufacture. He even stated that York sold "the best barbell available and that Weider [was] still attempting to match its quality." On the other hand, Henderson, a Michigan State University professor, stunned the defense by estimating that $16,907,182 would be an appropriate amount of compensation. With Hoffman incapacitated and Dietz recovering from triple-bypass surgery, Terpak was the only York employee providing deposition. He was not aware of research or government reports on the dangers of bench-pressing, but he pointed out what is known to every experienced weight trainee, that "it is common sense to provide for one's own safety." Eventually, after years of negotiation, York settled the suit for $175,000.[9] Not surprisingly, in light of mounting insurance premiums, York decided that it could save money by insuring itself. During the 1980s suits were so numerous that they became a corporate hazard, resulting in lower earnings and higher prices.

The Pruger Case

Not all judgments, however, were adverse or featured York as a defendant. In the late 1970s a controversy developed with Richard Pruger, who, feeling stifled by Dietz and unable to advance his cause at York, created his own (Pitt Barbell) company, founded his own health-food store, and started selling products from other firms in the Hoffman Health Houses. In May 1978, Terpak ordered that locks be changed at the three stores, impounded all goods and records, and fired Pruger. In Allegheny County Court the latter filed a complaint that York had failed to supply adequately the stores he managed. So he ordered, with "full knowledge and consent" of the company, goods of other firms for a monthly fee of $50 per store and was allowed to sell them for his own profit. Furthermore, he alleged that York owed him $19,000 for goods and equipment it had seized. York issued a counterclaim requesting the return of wrongfully appropriated assets, arguing that Pruger had placed "in Defendants' three stores, *for his own personal gain,* a line of goods and equipment in direct competition with York's goods and equipment. . . . These goods were discounted below the prevailing price of York's goods in an effort to undercut York sales. Moreover, Health House employees were extended generous commissions on the sale of Pruger's line." The plaintiff's inability to produce court-mandated records undoubtedly weakened Pruger's position and led to a court order for Pruger to pay York $14,290. The remarkable feature of this expensive, lengthy, and tortuous litigation is that it did not lessen Pruger's devotion to York. As with Gary Deal, he soon was back in touch with Terpak, wanting to know, now that "past problems" were settled, if Terpak was "interested in restoring normal business relations." Noting that some customers preferred York equipment "over any other brand," he sent regards to "Bob, Grimek, Ernie, and all the other folks."[10] The York bond, though antiquated and strained, retained some of its old magic.

Bodybuilding Matures

The area where York was always most vulnerable was bodybuilding. In just this area, in the mid-1970s, the company inadvertently stumbled into a case that tested its strength against the Weiders. It concerned Grimek's statement in the April 1971 issue of *Muscular Development* that Mike Katz, IFBB Mr. America for 1970, had "never won the Mr. America title." Katz viewed Grimek's statement as libelous, and his attorney demanded that York "retract this statement in as public a manner as that in which it was made." Grimek merely replied that Katz had "never won an AAU Mr. America title, which is the only official title we recognize." That he did not publicize this clarification, or publish a retraction, led Katz, claiming injury to his reputation, to sue for punitive damages in Connecticut Superior Court. In the 1977 trial York's case was vitiated by its inability to show the AAU's exclusive right to the Mr. America title and service mark. The plaintiff, on the other hand, insisted "the pot of gold at the end of the rainbow, after winning the Mr. America Contest," was denied him because of Grimek's comment and lack of recognition of his title in *Muscular Development*, then, "without question, the bible of the sport." This treatment prevented him from turning professional, and "posing exhibitions, seminars, training camps, and endorsements were allegedly denied him." The most damaging evidence against York, however, was a 1977 letter showing possible malice. Pruger, then a York employee, had to withdraw an invitation (in the $500-to-$1000 range) he had extended to Katz to pose for a show he was staging in Pittsburgh. In the letter, Pruger wrote, "I had a letter of agreement all typed up when I spoke with my boss concerning the meet.

It seems that you and York have some sort of legal disagreement, all of which is tied in to the authenticity of the I.F.B.B." Terpak attempted to downplay the bad feelings between Hoffman and Weider, but the plaintiff's attorney, with Pruger's letter, was able to show that Katz was "a victim of Hoffman's competitive interest." As a result, the court returned a verdict of $75,000 in damages. York protested on grounds that its testimony had been "unduly circumscribed," while the judge had permitted the plaintiff "undue latitude in presenting his." The final settlement, after two more years of legal sparring, brought a reduction of the award to $17,500.[11] In an immediate sense, it constituted a York victory, but the settlement amounted to tacit recognition of the power and moral weight of the Weiders.

This question was being tested simultaneously in other sectors of bodybuilding where Weider stock was growing dramatically. What had enabled Hoffman to remain paramount in bodybuilding and power-lifting was the loyalty of the weightlifting clique that controlled the AAU power structure. With the decline of Olympic lifting, however, the ground started to shift. The National Sports Act of 1976 divided the three sports into autonomous bodies, leaving the AAU as a service unit. This reorganization provided an opportunity for the Weiders to bid for AAU affiliation and possible takeover. The earliest discussions of this possibility took place in Chicago in February 1976 between physique members of the old weightlifting committee and IFBB officials. Then Notice No. 76–182 from the main AAU office in Indianapolis removed the ban that prohibited crossovers of athletes between the two jurisdictions. "With that obstacle gone, there seemed to be no technical reason barring affiliation," and bodybuilders had a heyday. Independent control by the AAU Physique Committee had an auspicious beginning with the 1977 Mr. America contest in Santa Monica. In the parade preceding the event there was a blend of all elements. Led by Bert Goodrich, the first Mr. America (1939), it featured a cavalcade of musclemen on elephants and a hundred units, including seven marching bands. Over a hundred thousand spectators witnessed the two-hour extravaganza. In the evening Ken Sprague, Physique Committee secretary and owner of Gold's Gym, staged one of the most successful physique contests ever for 3,200 muscle fans in the hotbed of bodybuilding. Special touches included a twenty-piece orchestra, an original Mr. America overture, a handbalancing act, and guest posing by Robby Robinson and Bill Grant. The new Mr. America, Dave Johns, was escorted on stage and presented a

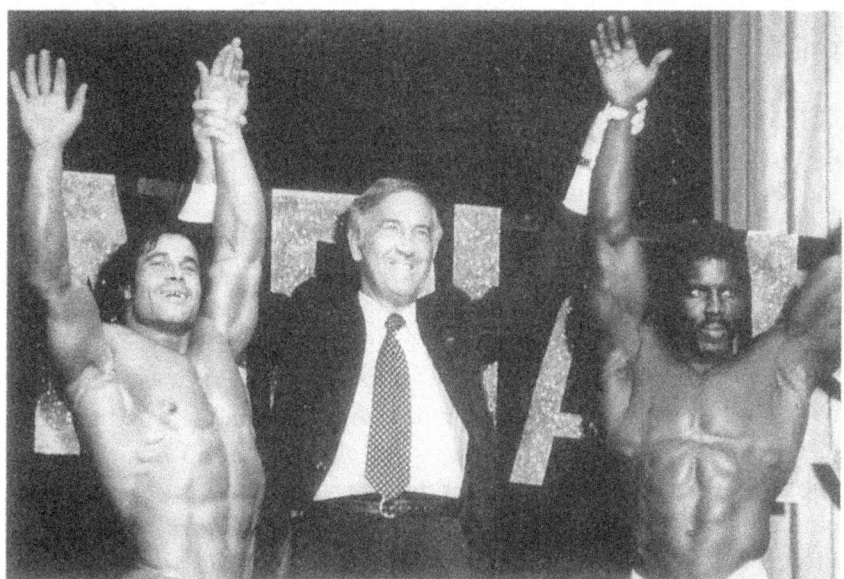

IFBB president Ben Weider with two of his physique stars in the 1970s—Franco Columbo and Robby Robinson.

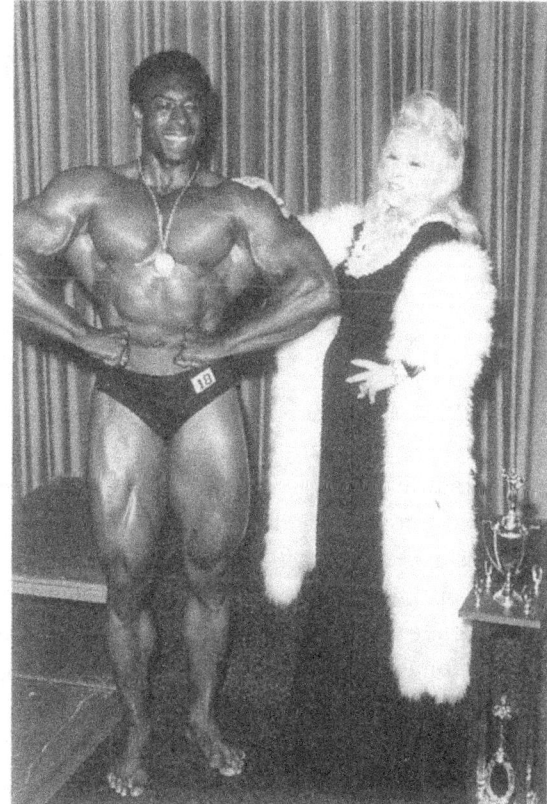

The legendary Mae West with 1977 Mr. America Dave Johns—"Oh, what perfect parts."

six-foot trophy by silver-screen star Mae West, who sighed, "Oh, what perfect parts."[12]

A unique aspect of this spectacle was participation by all factions of the physique community, including Lurie, the Weiders, and Terpak and Grimek from York. On the following day Ben Weider made a bid for AAU affiliation. Peary Rader reported that he was "a very effective and convincing speaker and he faced some . . . difficult questions. . . . The basic difference seems to be that Mr. Weider feels he has a completely democratic organization while some in the audience felt that it was not democratic and said so in pointed terms. Quite a few hot words were exchanged during the course of the five and a half hours of deliberations." Weider stressed that his only motive was the good of the sport. This was hardly the view of former IFBB associates Ed Jubinville, Lud Shusterich, Serge Nubret, and Dan Lurie, who castigated his organization. Jubinville subscribed to the York line that the Weiders were merely striving for "credibility." Although the Physique Committee voted 16–13 in favor of affiliation, it fell short of the required two-thirds majority. Still, for chairman Clarence Bass, an Albuquerque attorney who was instrumental in wresting physique from weightlifters and powerlifters, it was a liberating experience. "Just think of it," he told Ralph Countryman, "casting a vote in favor of Weider right there in front of Terpak, Grimek, God and everybody." It was obvious to Rader "that changes [were] going to take place."[13]

The Weider Takeover

At the 1978 Mr. America contest in Cincinnati the vote in favor of affiliation was overwhelming. Credit for this disruption of York influence was attributed to Sprague, who, according to *Muscle Training Illustrated*, "crashed upon the bodybuilding scene like a comet, a veritable meteorite slashing and burning through the physique world atmosphere. Aside from being known for his merchandising of a small 'pumping iron' palace called 'Gold's Gym' of Santa Monica, California, into a giant, internationally-known fitness household word, Sprague in a period of roughly two years consolidated a political punch that slipped the AAU 'Old Guard' a severe crack which changed the face of bodybuilding in America for all time." Dellinger called the vote an "ambush of the

Bob Hoffman's Departure

old AAU crowd." Though IFBB affiliation lay in limbo for another two years, awaiting final sanction, athletes immediately benefited from the freedom to compete in both AAU and IFBB contests. Bass noted that ever since the Physique Committee had become a separate entity, the Mr. America contests had "been vastly improved." Indeed physiques soon attained a new level of perfection. Grimek was overawed by the muscular massiveness of 1981 Mr. America Tim Belknap, who weighed 191 pounds at 5' 5": "He not only has size but his muscularity is sharp and his proportions blend symmetrically to show flowing lines. . . . He is the only one who approximates the drawings we use by Gilbert."[14] Soon the incredible legs of IFBB champion Tom Platz would leave fans wondering if this stage of development could ever be superseded.

The breakdown of barriers was particularly noticeable at the 1979 Mr. America contest in Atlanta, described by *Iron Man* as "the most spectacular, quality-wise, of any over its prestigious thirty-one year history." It was evident that "the faction benefitting most by the affiliation [was] the amateur bodybuilders." *Muscular Development* concurred, even conceding that while York was known as "muscletown," Atlanta "seemed to be the 'new muscle capital' over the September 8th weekend." The competition was held in style at the historic Fox Theatre, and the headquarters in the Atlanta Hilton gave committee meetings an ambience of class. Random selection of judges guarded against regional bias, while contestants could voice any gripes about judging in a special room. Soon an AAU Physique Committee for Women was formed. Lisa Lyon, its chairwoman, organized its first national contest, in Atlantic City, along with a couples competition, another precedent.[15] Freedom from York's patronage seemed to open endless possibilities of innovation and growth.

Such hopes, however, proved short-lived. Appearances suggested that the Weiders intended to make the AAU their exclusive domain. Despite a pronouncement from Jim Fox, AAU liaison to the Physique Committee, that there was as yet "no affiliation between the IFBB and the AAU," Ben Weider threatened to suspend 1978 Mr. America Tony Pearson from the IFBB *and* the AAU if he performed at a 1979 contest sponsored by Lurie in North Carolina. Weider then claimed that *Muscle and Fitness* was the official magazine of the AAU Physique Committee. That Weider was arrogating power was evident to Sprague, who believed the Physique Committee was becoming a "parrot" of the IFBB.

The closer I became involved with the AAU-IFBB affiliation, I see that Weider—if the AAU is not kept very, very strong—will take advantage of his power position. . . . Traditionally it's been observed, that if you don't train in certain gyms, or align yourself with certain magazines, you will not do well in major contests. The fear was among bodybuilders, and first revolved around York publications, and now it's the Weider publications. . . . Ben is not using the IFBB political position for the honesty of bodybuilding. He's using it to enhance the Weider position commercially.

But Sprague was unable to stop the drift he had instigated from York to Weider. At the 1979 AAU Convention in Las Vegas it was decided that the Physique Committee would be affiliated with the IFBB. Both Hoffman and Joe Weider were there. "The world changed and moved on that November day in Las Vegas, where two Caesars met at 'Caesar's Palace,'" quipped *Muscle Training Illustrated*. "Not a word passed between them. Bob Hoffman, 'The Father' of American weightlifting watches his stepchild grow up and away from him. . . . Joe Weider looks on as a concerned rich uncle." It was also noted how Sprague's machinations had led to a California-slanted committee. On most measures the East Coast representatives (formerly led by York) were outvoted by the westerners. Further changes hastened the drift of amateur physique to the Weiders. In 1980 the AAU Physique Committee (NPC) was fully incorporated, and in 1981 "USA" was substituted for AAU. The extent to which the IFBB now controlled this supposedly independent organization was illustrated by a melding of the former's rules into the latter and the use of the Mr. America contest as a qualifying event for the IFBB Mr. Universe. It was no surprise that Gary Leonard, 1980 Mr. America, received his trophy from Ben Weider.[16]

The AAU Physique Committee

Predictably, York reacted negatively to this course of events. First, it supported Jubinville, Tom Minichiello, and Harold Gibson, who had formed an American Federation of Amateur Bodybuilders (AFAB) to counter the IFBB's newfound strength. They appealed for an end to the feuding and factions that plagued American bodybuilding. "It appeared that all this might be over with the AAU-IFBB affiliation. Instead, the situation has grown worse." Dismantling power blocs and instituting democratic procedures were the group's goals. More successful were countermeasures instigated by the AAU. Its physique representatives, meeting in Indianapolis in 1981, objected to the NPC's suspension of athletes who competed in non-NPC contests, and ruled that the award of any Mr. America title to the NPC be contingent on discontinuing this practice. Further to lure bodybuilders back to the AAU, they denied NPC the right to issue AAU membership cards and urged athletes to register in local AAU associations rather than with the NPC. Not satisfied with the NPC response and convinced that it was merely a front for Weider, Bob Crist organized an AAU Mr. America Committee of twelve. At the 1981 AAU Convention in St. Louis it took a "strong stand" by adopting a new set of rules, agreeing to license the Mr. America trademark out yearly, and making possession of this title contingent on acquisition of an AAU card. Furthermore, steps would be taken to establish links with NABBA, WABBA, and other international organizations outside the IFBB. To establish a legal right to conduct physique competitions, the AAU successfully sued the NPC in federal court in 1982 for violating federal antitrust laws by coercing athletes and attempting to drive the AAU out of business. In 1983 the U.S. Olympic Committee secured a court injunction prohibiting Weider or the IFBB from using the term Olympic in its advertising.[17]

Having established its legitimacy, the AAU Physique Committee held its first Mr. America contest in 1982 at Worcester, Massachusetts. The winner, Rufus Howard, was then flown to London for the NABBA Mr. Universe competition. His second-place finish did not help the AAU cause and led to NPC-IFBB criticism. In *Muscle and Fitness* Jim Manion denigrated the AAU, suggesting that it attracted mostly mediocre contestants and that NPC competitors were far superior: "If the competition between the NPC and the AAU were based on the ability of each organization to present significant and exciting contests, the NPC would win hands down." Joe Weider, in *Flex*, called for elimination of the title "Mr. America," suggesting the competition was merely a "pinup contest" that detracted from bodybuilding's recent progress. Yet in just two years the AAU Mr. America Committee, on the strength of its entitlement to the Mr. America trademark, boasted that it had enlisted ten thousand athletes, officials, and coaches and was "firmly organized in all states and territories." Further to keep pace with the times and growth of women's bodyduilding, it changed its name to the "AAU America Committee."[18]

Next the York/AAU faction decided to develop some international ties to satisfy bodybuilders' aspirations for a competition level above Mr. America. Here the IFBB had an edge inasmuch as the client NPC had inherited the AAU mantle after the 1976 breakup. Furthermore, winning an AAU event in the United States did not qualify an athlete to enter IFBB international events, such as Mr. Universe or Mr. Olympia, which had grown enormously in prestige, media coverage, and remuneration. The AAU sought international stature by reviving its historical links with Oscar Heidenstam's NABBA. Unfortunately NABBA, though it attracted contestants from many countries to its Mr. Universe contest, was just a national organization. So NABBA and the AAU Physique Committee joined Serge Nubret's World Amateur Bodybuilder's Association (WABBA), based in Paris, which could truly attest to international representation and rival the IFBB. Though Heidenstam was made president of WABBA, he resented Nubret's control over it. A break in their alliance occurred at the WABBA's 1983 world championships in Switzerland. It was a "scandal," Heidenstam alleged, how the competition "was dominated by Serge Nubret and his wife." Using "the worst 'tricks' of Weider," Nubret had manipulated a victory for himself in the professional class. Likewise the meeting of national delegates was a "farce," spent mostly haggling over money.[19] These internecine quarrels led to Heidenstam's resignation and a breakup of the united front against the IFBB. By the time of Hoffman's death in 1985, the world of bodybuilding seemed a hopeless muddle. Physique for its own sake had never been Bob's highest priority, and with the National Sports Act and decline of his health, York no longer exercised much authority in this field. The Weiders, whose corporate assets grew as those of York declined, had always devoted their energies almost exclusively to bodybuilding. It is hardly surprising that they were finally able to break the inner citadel of York power in the AAU and attain international hegemony.

Powerlifting Matures

Powerlifting underwent a similar metamorphosis from its disciplined York upbringing to a state of conflicting jurisdictions. Like bodybuilding,

Bob Hoffman's Departure

it was a sport in which the United States led the world and other interests would vie for the power and prestige held by York. The English especially used powerlifting to regain their standing in the iron game and in 1976, for the first time, beat the United States (95–92) on Hoffman's home turf. The following year IPF president Vic Mercer staged the first European power championships, in Birmingham. Though York was losing its grasp, American powerlifters reasserted their superiority at the 1977 world meet in Perth by winning more gold medals than the rest of the world combined. Furthermore, America, with such stars as Lamar Gant, Ricky Crain, Vince Anello, Larry Pacifico, John Kuc, and Don Reinhoudt, held thirty of forty world records. Anello, "Mr. Erectors," held the deadlift record in three classes, and Reinhoudt held all superheavy marks. The reason for this harvest of records was that powerlifting, unlike Olympic lifting, was attracting youth. The 1978 National Collegiates at Louisiana Tech attracted 180 lifters from seventy-eight schools in twenty states. Many American, teenage, and meet records were broken, and nine officials passed national referee tests. Todd was impressed by the 178 lifters who competed at the teenage championships at Evansville University that year. Powerlifting was "a true turnon for teenagers in the U.S."[20]

American lifters figured prominently in a 1978 power extravaganza in Hawaii, where six world records were set before four thousand spectators. There were thirty-three such attempts, including Jo Jo White's dramatic assault on the thousand-pound squat barrier. The audience was also treated to guest appearances by Bruce Wilhelm, who won the televised World's Strongest Man competition, and Arnold Schwarzenegger, who raised bodybuilding to a new level of popularity in the 1970s. When Arnold appeared, "flashcubes popped like firecrackers and many a female heart throbbed." That powerlifting was not just glitz but a respectable sport was evident at the 1978 world championships in Finland. The United States not only defeated strong teams from England and Finland, winning seven of ten classes, but accounted for five of the meet's nine world records. The IPF selected two Americans, Larry Pacifico and Bob Hoffman, and Briton Ron Collins as the first members of its hall of fame. Todd recalls seeing an Indian group in Turku approach Bob, who was bedecked with medals. Some knelt and chanted, " 'Bob Hoffman, Bob Hoffman' like a mantra." Small wonder that Bob's "thoughts on powerlifting" were pleasant.

Overall, I'd have to say that powerlifting is in a wonderful position.... It's been approximately ten years now since I heard the *Star Spangled Banner* played and the Stars and Stripes raised in honor of a world championship being won by a U.S. Olympic lifter, yet in the World Powerlifting Championships in Finland I was treated to no less than seven playings of our national anthem and seven raisings of the U.S. flag.... I like to see our men prevail over the rest of the world as they now do and I intend to redouble my efforts for both the men and the women in powerlifting so that we maintain our supremacy for many, many years. After all, the *Star Spangled Banner* is my favorite song.

Afterward the Finnish federation hosted a banquet, and the ten world champions were awarded beautiful deer hides. Then Todd observed "much dancing, much talking, much exchanging of addresses and much good cheer," a fitting climax to "the finest world powerlifting championships ever held."[21]

Women's Powerlifting

Also important to powerlifting's growth was the involvement of women. The idea for an "All-American Girl Power Championships" arose at the 1976 men's nationals, in Arlington, Texas. It was taken up by Joe Zarella, AAU power chairman, who staged the first such meet the next April in Nashua, New Hampshire. There were twenty-seven enthusiastic lifters, including teams from Mississippi State University and New Germany, Nova Scotia. An interesting aspect of the competition was the participation of Cindy Reinhoudt and Jan Todd, whose husbands, former superheavy champions, served as coaches. Reinhoudt won the best lifter trophy with a 360 squat, 210 bench press, and 375 deadlift, while Todd made the meet's highest total, 970 pounds. By "meet's end there wasn't an unsmiling face in the arena," noted Al Thomas. In 1978 women's powerlifting gained official status, and Zarella hosted its first nationals. There were thrice as many lifters, but the most notable change was in quality of performance. Winning totals in most classes exceeded those of the previous year. In the 123-pound class the 1977 winner would have earned eleventh place in 1978. Highlighting the competition

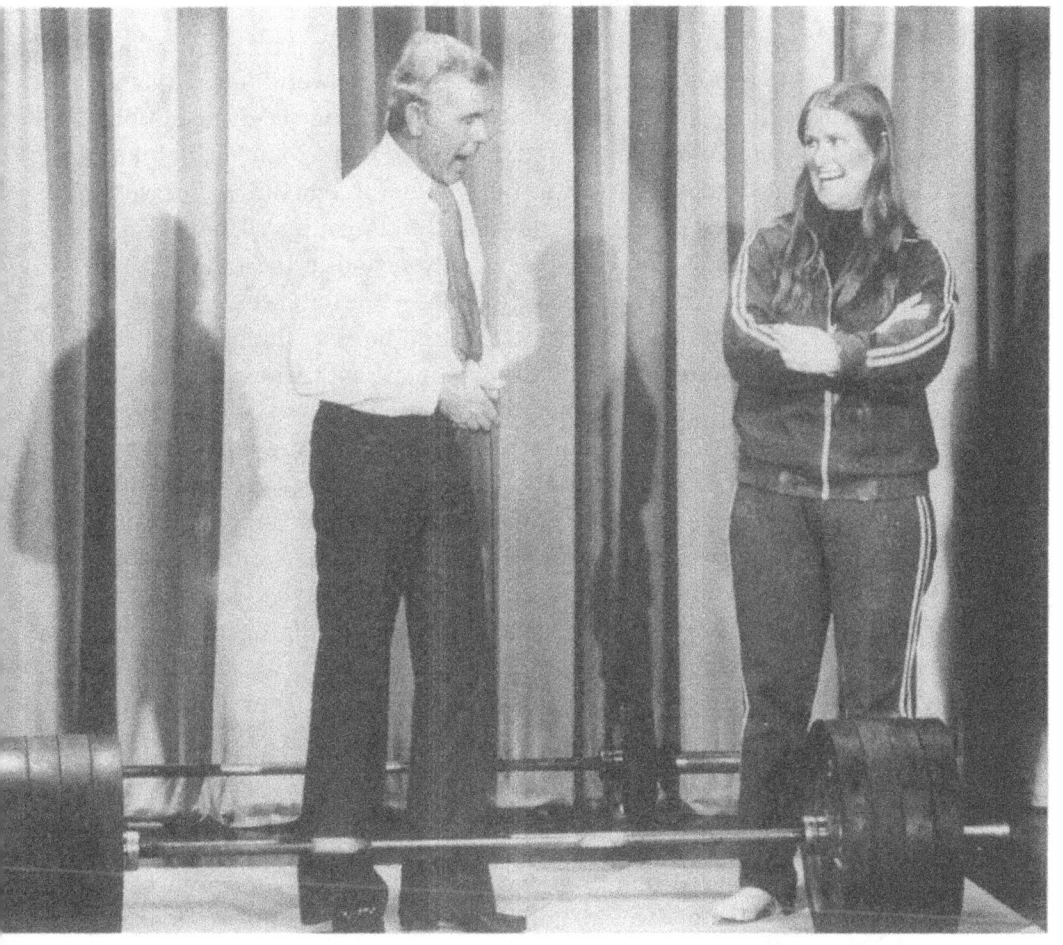

Jan Todd with *Tonight Show* host Johnny Carson in 1978. After Todd completed a deadlift of 415 pounds for eight repetitions, Carson tried, without success, to pick up the weight, at first alone and then with bandleader "Doc" Severenson. Only with the help of actor Jack Klugman were they able to negotiate the 415 to lockout position.

was Todd's record 453 deadlift. Dubbed "Super Woman," she shattered all records in her class, including an 1,128 total, and appeared on the *Tonight Show* to demonstrate the deadlift to Johnny Carson. By 1979 women, like the men, were lifting in kilos and planning a women's world championships. Their invasion of the iron game soon sparked a debate in York magazines on the place of women in sport and society. "Women today no longer accept the fact that they are the 'weaker sex,'" observed Grimek. He recommended that men be receptive to women in the formerly all-male bastions of lifting and bodybuilding.[22]

International Powerlifting Matures

Till the late 1970s national and international powerlifting survived largely through Hoffman's generosity, and when he received the bid to host the 1979 world meet in York, he vowed to make it "every bit as spectacular and successful as the one this year in Finland": "We want York to become and to remain the powerlifting center of the world." Terlazzo noted that "a few people . . . entrenched in the powerlifting organization [had] tried gradually to phase Bob out," but "when it [came] to raising funds they always turn[ed] to him." Indeed, so long as powerlifting continued to rely on Hoffman, York would control its destiny. It was fortuitous for powerlifting's future, however, that Todd, acting on behalf of the IPF, negotiated a contract for the Finland meet to be broadcast on CBS *Sports Spectacular* with proceeds being split between the IPF, the American powerlifting committee, and the Finns. Henceforth Todd would head an IPF media committee, and all future television rights would belong to the IPF. With the IPF less beholden to York, Mercer dictated more stringent requirements for the 1979 meet. He explained to Terpak that the IPF was "no longer a backyard (or Mickey Mouse) outfit" and that international meets held outside the United States had "all been of a very high standard."

> When it became known that the Championships for 79 were to be under the banner of the York organisation, many comments were made, none of them complimentary, the general opinion was that the 79 champs would be an anticlimax, after the wonderful show in Finland. . . . To be quite honest the general opinion amongst both Lifters & Officials is, that whilst we are very grateful to the York Organisation for helping to get Powerlifting off the Ground in the early stages, the Organisation of the World Champs held under your banner have been abysmal.

Mercer recommended renting Madison Square Garden as a venue and engaging a professional organizer. Not surprisingly York felt slighted. *Strength & Health* reminded its readers that York had organized the first world meets "to the satisfaction of everyone involved. Then it suddenly 'appeared' that York wasn't doing enough for the sport. . . . rather odd, we think."[23]

Unable to satisfy IPF requirements for a meet in Muscletown, Terpak arranged to cosponsor it with Larry Pacifico at the Dayton Convention

Center. York paid $10,000 in expenses, provided equipment, and advertised the meet. The results were spectacular. Pacifico not only ran it but won his ninth world title. In the bantamweights American Lamar Gant and New Zealander Precious McKenzie vied for honors, the latter making a world-record 562 squat. But Gant made a five-times-bodyweight deadlift of 617 (nearly 70 pounds above the world record!), dubbed by Tony Fitton "the greatest deadlift of all time to win." So sportsmanlike was McKenzie that he "picked the victor up in his arms and paraded him around for the cameras and audience." Even more remarkable was middleweight Mike Bridges. In an impromptu publicity display at Dayton Mall several days earlier he had violated all training conventions by performing near world-record lifts. At the meet, "[h]is squats were deep and strong, especially his World record 716 and the attempt at 755 came very close. Both the 451 and the fourth attempt 457 bench press were World records and performed with power to spare. The 644 and 661 deadlifts gave him new World record totals of 1813 and 1829 respectively, five World records in all and if that wasn't enough the total was . . . over 11 times his bodyweight—the only person to ever achieve that plateau." Ten thousand spectators watched 103 lifters from seventeen countries perform. Though steroids, supersuits, knee wraps, and other artificial aids played an important role, the United States led the world with 104 points to England's 77, Canada's 72, Finland's 68, Australia's 50, Sweden's 40, India's 30, and Japan's 28.[24] There was much for Bob to be proud of, but meet, lifters, and organization no longer belonged to York.

Powerlifting's Breakup

The most serious consequence of York's abdication of control was the emergence of a rival federation. Elements in the sport had been debating whether the United States, with such depth in this sport, should be allowed a second team. Additionally Pacifico, who was heading a new National Powerlifting Association, had failed to make the 1980 world team after missing his deadlifts at the nationals. A second team would give him a chance to win a tenth consecutive title. Responding to arguments that politics was behind Pacifico's denial, Marty Joyce argued, "No one man is bigger than our sport and our rules cannot be changed or compromised to benefit one individual no matter who that individual is." As the 1980 world meet in Arlington, Texas, approached, it was still uncertain which federation would represent the United States. Lawsuits were filed, and marshals appeared with orders to shut down the championships. At the last moment, however, a compromise was reached whereby NPA lifters could perform as "guests," unable to win titles but eligible to set world records.[25] Afterward the NPA was dissolved, but over the next decade, with the advent of drug-free powerlifting, the sport fractured into numerous factions and federations. York even lost publicity rights. In the early 1980s *Muscular Development* carried detailed powerlifting reports by Mike Lambert. But Lambert used this exposure to publicize his own fledgling publication, *Powerlifting News*. Soon it effectively replaced York's publication as the official organ for powerlifting, much as Weider magazines had done in bodybuilding. The lifeblood of manly culture at York was being siphoned into more vibrant sectors of muscledom.

A Return to Greatness?

What remained a York enclave was Olympic lifting. And the election of Murray Levin, an energetic York ally, as chairman of the national committee in 1976 held promise of new initiatives. With only $306 in the treasury, he quickly set about to cure the sport's financial ills and further lessen its reliance on Hoffman. In 1977 Sears agreed to sponsor the Junior Olympics. Television money and wise investments helped push the balance to more than $12,000 by the end of that year. But it was Levin's association with Mack Truck that brought a significant boost in funding after 1978. Levin also did much to bring weightlifting to public attention, hoping to enlist more lifters and funds. In 1977 he staged a "Record Makers" meet at the Aladdin Hotel in Las Vegas, where an enthusiastic crowd of 2,500 watched eleven lifters from six nations attempt world records. A broadcast of its highlights on CBS *Sports Spectacular* generated one of the highest ratings in that program's history. A culmination of Levin's tenure was the 1978 world championships he directed at Gettysburg, with lifters from fifty-three nations. At its conclusion York Barbell held a banquet coinciding with Hoffman's eightieth birthday. By the end of Levin's first term he could look back with satisfaction. "A Return to Greatness" was the message he conveyed in the 1979 *Rulebook:* "After a decade of crushing defeats by the countries of Eastern Europe and Cuba, the United States Federation is now regaining her status in World weightlifting." Levin aimed to link the York tradition of greatness with a "new crop of men" who were viewed as America's great hope for the 1980 Olympics.[26]

Such uplifting phrases seem remarkable in light of the dismal showing of American athletes in the late 1970s. Lee James, silver medalist at Montreal, seemed an ideal base on which to build a strong team. He was a member of the York Barbell Club and recipient of a Hoffman scholarship. Unfortunately a knee injury cut short his tenure as a serious competitor. The luster of two other American champions, Mark Cameron and Phil Grippaldi, was diminished when they tested positive for steroids at Montreal. The rationalization that "they didn't intend to 'cheat,' " that the medication was "prescribed" to allow them to compete at maximum bodyweight, had a hollow ring. Though barred from international meets for a year, it was still hoped that they would provide leadership for American lifters. At the 1977 senior nationals, however, the nation's three best lifters, Grippaldi, Cameron, and Wilhelm, were injured. Hence totals were low. The lone bright spot was flyweight Curt White, the youngest person, at fourteen, ever to win a national title. Somewhat better were performances at the 1978 seniors in York, yet the continued lack of international-caliber lifters led *Strength & Health* to speculate that the hot lights set up by the television crew might have depleted their energy. Distractions were also cited as the reason why *no* records were broken at the Record Makers meet in Las Vegas. "There was too much of everything going on, too many pretty girls parading around and too many slot machines that begged handling." Nevertheless, with sights set on the upcoming world championships on home turf in 1978, a national coaching seminar was staged in the York gym just after the nationals. Topics included injuries, camps, cluster training, kinesiology, hypnosis, the cardiovascular system, and Eastern bloc training programs. Yet nothing seemed capable of averting disaster for American lifters at Gettysburg. Kurt Setterberg placed the highest of any American at seventh in the 220-pound class. The team came in thirteenth place with 24 points, far behind the winning Russians and Cubans at 281 and 221 respectively.[27]

Strength & Health readers therefore were hard put to select a Weightlifter of the Year for 1978. Forsaking erstwhile leaders in the sport, they selected the lesser-known Paul Salisbury of upstate New York, perhaps as a result of a campaign waged by members of his local club. A former powerlifter, he exhibited exceptional strength, but what endeared Salisbury to his training partners was his modesty: "Although the walls are literally covered with newspaper articles on him and he is frequently being filmed or interviewed by our local press, he has not fallen prey to his ego." A reader from Kansas described Salisbury as "a gutsy lifter with a lot of personality. No theatrics or nastiness on stage. He's a breath of fresh air to those of us who are fed up with antics of prima donna lifters." Still, Salisbury's record, in light of America's lifting tradition and current international standards, showed more promise than achievement. At the 1978 seniors he was only a runner-up. While he did win the Pan-American portion of the mid-heavy class at the Gettysburg world championships, his 682-pound total was 50 pounds less than he had made at the nationals and got him only thirteenth of fifteen. By this time Hoffman, after two decades of disappointments, no longer expected heroics. In his report of the 1978 world meet there are few words of regret over the shortcomings of the present generation but effusive praises for the achievements of the elders who conducted the meet. At the 1979 nationals in Totowa "the overall performance of the lifters could not match the efficiency of the administrators as 21 of the 74 competing athletes bombed out." Another nineteen were only able to register two lifts for a total.[28]

As the 1980 Olympics approached, various veterans emerged from retirement to make one last stab at the most coveted of all honors. Remarkably these "old-timers" turned in performances rivaling those of the current champions, yet another indication of how little American lifting had progressed. At the 1980 nationals Fred Lowe came in third as a middleweight, Joe Puleo second as a mid-heavy, and Joe Dube third as a superheavy. Though Salisbury missed all of his clean and jerks, Brian Derwin, a bright new star on the horizon, added 115 pounds to his 1979 total, won the 220-pound class, and carried away best-lifter honors in the heavier classes. Once dismissed as a "nobody," Derwin compiled an enviable record in 1980. In addition to winning the seniors, he tied an American record in the clean and jerk, won his class at the United States—Australia meet, and came in second at the Blue Sword Invitational in East Germany. In lieu of the 1980 Olympics in Moscow, an alternative meet was arranged for boycotting nations in China. Here, and at the America's Cup meet on the homeward journey, Derwin scored impressive wins against an international field. Admittedly it included no eastern Europeans, but a Chinese official was so impressed with America's showing that he was reminded of such greats as George, Kono, Sheppard, Davis, Vinci, and Schemanski: "I believe your men will become strong once again in the world."[29] It was no surprise that Derwin was named Weightlifter of the Year, but unlike past champions, his achievements were limited to one year, and he was never tested against the world's best. After being injured, he failed to total at the 1981 nationals. That he was later named to the Weightlifting Hall of Fame, beside many former American greats, caused some to question the meaning of such honors. A comparison of world to American records from 1979 to 1980 shows respective increases of 138 and 5 pounds in aggregate totals. Some of the latter had not changed for decades.

Financial Triumphs for Weightlifting

From a financial standpoint, however, American lifting had never been healthier. By April 1981 the United States Weightlifting Federation reported assets of $80,501, and an Olympic Training Center directed by Harvey Newton was in place in Colorado Springs. He felt "strongly that U.S. lifting could move up several notches" by 1984. Others shared Newton's confidence in the center, sensing that this was a factor that propelled Communist sports programs to the forefront in the 1950s. In 1982, Miller Brewing Company donated $3 million to it. In addition to excellent training equipment, some donated by York, it had devices for monitoring endurance, growth, and stress levels on world-class athletes. Though some lifters achieved "remarkable gains," it was obvious that not everyone was benefiting from this exposure. Newton reported in 1982 that "constant time in camp seems to have taken some of the fight out of some of the lifters." A more effective use of resources, he thought, would be to bring leading lifters in "prior to major meets, rather than spending four years here doing the same routines." Manager Roger Sadecki reported that the lifters showed "insufficient cooperation, initiative, and enthusiasm" prior to the 1982 world championships in Ljublyana, Yugoslavia. He recommended extracurricular activities to alleviate boredom when not training. Levin concluded that lifters who spent extensive time at the center "became weightlifting bums and chased women at night. Not one of them has panned out."[30]

The most promising American prospect in the early 1980s was Jeff Michels. Still a teenager in 1981, he broke junior records in two classes, captured fourth at the junior world championships (best ever by an American), was junior Pan-Am champ, set an American record in the snatch, and took seventh in the world championships in Lille, France. Named Weightlifter of the Year, Michels went on to score impressive wins at the 1982 and 1983 seniors, but disaster struck when he tested positive for testosterone at the Pan-Am Games in Caracas. Consequently he was suspended for a year from international competition, and the press gave him much negative publicity. As the 1984 Olympics in Los Angeles approached, American lifting, despite able leaders and ample finances, was adrift. In light of constant unfavorable comparisons with powerlifting and bodybuilding and dismal international performances, it is not surprising that lifters struck out against their elders. Artie Dreschler, athletes representative on the national committee, informed Levin that "the athletes want a say in governing our sport." At the 1981 National Sports Festival in Syracuse, Dreschler continued, "forty athletes 'some of the best we have,' organized a formal protest. All of the athletes signed a petition supporting what they wanted and they were ready to boycott the Nationals to get it. . . . If the athletes don't see some improvement soon I think you'll have some real conflict on your hands. This may be the best of times from a money standpoint [but] it isn't from a morale one." Even more daunting to American spirit was the appearance of Naim Suleimanov, truly a "boy wonder," on the Bulgarian team. "Looks like it's time for American weightlifting to run up the 'white flag,' " was the reaction of a Michigan reader. "We are now more than accustomed to European lifters of 18 or 19 setting Junior World and near-World records and going on to even greater prominence as Senior lifters . . . but now . . . we get the ultimate insult with Bulgaria sporting a 14-year-old who sets Junior World records and attempts Senior World marks!"[31] About the same time, any hopes that York might still propel young Americans to international fame were dashed at the 1982 senior nationals when its winning streak of twenty-nine, dating back to 1952, was snapped by the Sports Palace of San Francisco and the Sayre Park team of Chicago.

York continued to field respectable teams and to sponsor local meets and clinics, but weightlifting's center of gravity shifted to the Sports Palace. Coached by Jim Schmitz and led by superheavy Mario Martinez, it won the next three nationals, but it was no more able than York to infuse life into American lifting. At the 1983 world championships in Moscow, all Americans failed to total. With the best weightlifting nations boycotting the Los Angeles Olympics in 1984, it appeared the United States might win some medals. But at the trials the team lost one of its best prospects. "Of all the lifters," noted Bruce Klemens, "Curt White seemed to have the best chance of making the team. In fact, only a bombout could keep him off . . . and, to the shock of all, that's exactly what occurred." At the games Martinez blamed the coaches for his second place behind Australia's Dean Lukin, insisting they had underestimated him in their poundage selections: "What good is six-for-six if you don't get a chance to do your best?" America finished fifth behind Romania, China, Japan, and West Germany, with only one other medal, Guy Carlton's bronze in the 110-kilogram class. Nor was television coverage provided to enhance weightlifting's image. The one gigantic benefit that came from the 1984 games was the profit accrued because of Peter Ueberroth's organizing genius. The Olympic Committee provided $656,000 to the USWF. This money was first invested in high-yield (over 12 percent) securities by Levin, then transferred to a separate foundation. In 1985 the USWF had a balance of $150,000 and the foundation $707,618. Still, American lifters were performing no better, and an American Weightlifting Association was reforming in California under longtime maverick Bob Hise II.[32]

Final Honors

Obviously all three areas of the iron game were drifting away from York, but Hoffman was at last attracting the kind of adulation and honors he had always sought. Already known as "Father of World Weightlifting" and "Living Pioneer of the Health Food Industry," he acquired a plethora of other honors: Outstanding Humanitarian, Distinguished Pennsylvanian, admission to the Softball Hall of Fame, a tribute in the *Congressional Record*, the IWF National Honor Medal, and a team trophy for fifty senior national victories. The worthiest recognition Bob received in his waning years resulted from his accomplishments in health and fitness. "Not so long ago," noted *Muscular Development*, "it was an odd spectacle to see people running or jogging along the road." Now the public was "more health and fitness conscious." In contrast to earlier eras, there was "hardly an institution that [didn't] have some form of weight training program." Bob could also bask in the attention paid him as a personality. In 1977 he rode in the Preakness Parade in Baltimore, viewed by over one hundred thousand persons. "People hailed the float, not by dancing in the streets, but by exercising." More than ever, "see and be seen" was Bob's attitude. Former mayor John Krout agrees that Hoffman was "not a shrinking violet" and that he "liked the notoriety." Infatuation with his own self-importance was obvious on a 1976 trip Bob sponsored for a York high school band to Florida. As he rode in a celebrity car, people shouted, "Hi, Bob." Not aware of the placard with his name on the side of the car, he thought they knew him by sight.[33]

The Demise of Muscletown

There were other areas where Hoffman had less cause for satisfaction. He never understood why "isometrics fell out of favor" or why drugs and other ills continued to afflict his sport and nation. Observing in the country the same "malaise" as diagnosed by President Carter after Vietnam, he remarked that "only a naive optimist could look at the happenings of our society and say that everything is going along well." The Save the United States Movement persisted into the 1980s, but Hoffman was less confident that the power of his ego and fortune could cure the nation's ills. It seemed hopeless that his group could "combat such threatening menaces as inflation, hunger and armed aggression when the great minds of our times" could not.[34] Indeed Hoffman could no longer control his own sport in his hometown. While it was true, especially in summer months, that "a lot of visitors" toured the hall of fame and others watched the lifters train on Ridge Avenue, York was invaded by the California physical-culture craze in the 1980s. Local bodybuilders Don King and Chris Conrad established a branch of Gold's Gym, the famed West Coast physique Mecca, in Muscletown, and in 1984 they staged (with York Barbell) the Gold's Classic Colonial Open at the Performing Arts Theater. Guest poser was 1983 Mr. Olympia Samir Bannout. No longer could Weider's pervasive influence in physique be ignored. Mercifully Bob was probably not aware of this extravaganza or the coverage of Weider-sponsored events in his own magazines. Perhaps nothing better illustrated the impotence of York than its failure,

Bob Hoffman's Departure

in 1984, to organize an open power meet. Despite much interest from potential participants, the meet had to be canceled, allegedly because of renovations at the York gym and concern that residue from the baby powder powerlifters used in deadlifting would ruin the concrete floor. A more likely explanation was that John Terlazzo's retirement in 1980 left no one who wanted to run it. In 1985, the year of Bob's death, there was talk about reviving the York picnic at Brookside, but Dellinger and Smitty were too busy with other company functions.[35]

The precipitous decline in Bob's capacity to manage his affairs began in 1978. When he reached eighty, an air of unreality pervaded a *Muscular Development* statement that Hoffman was "still robust and very active" and aiming "to live in three centuries." Yet Bob knew the world was passing him by. "I am close to being the last of my era," was his comment on the deaths of Otto Arco and George Hackenschmidt in 1976. By the time of his own death virtually an entire generation of associates had passed away, including Ottley Coulter ('76), Dave Asnis ('77), Frederick Tilney ('77), Paul Bragg ('77), Karo Whitfield ('77), Joe Bonomo ('78), Steve Stanko ('78), the "Mighty Atom" ('79), K. V. Iyer ('80), Johnny Krill ('80), Arthur Gay ('81), Harold Sakata ('82), Joe Miller ('83), David Matlin ('83), John Ziegler ('83), Walter Podolak ('84), Firpo Lemma ('84), Oscar State ('84), and John Davis ('85). In 1985 Grimek and Harry Utterback, two of the company's oldest employees, retired. The steady exit of old friends caused a socialization void, leaving Bob standing alone. He even lost touch with his girlfriends, whom he continued seeing until heart surgery in 1978 prevented him from driving. Then he relied on Alda. Bob had always "thought he was going to live forever, and I did too," she recalls. But in the late 1970s he deteriorated rapidly.[36]

The World's Unhealthiest Man

As his condition worsened, he needed more care. Alda vowed she would be faithful to Bob and not put him in a nursing home. But he was a big man who needed a lot of care, so she hired a battery of nurses to watch him around the clock. Their records show this former superman declining to almost total enfeeblement. "Very depressed this A.M.," was the observation on April 21, 1981. "Edema of both legs & feet. . . .

Complains he is half dead. 'Only lives half a life.'" Occasionally Bob would try to engage in purposeful activities, such as continuing his book on the Save the United States Movement, working out with dumbbells, or greeting tourists at the hall of fame, but he could not concentrate. "Confused" and "disoriented" are the words most frequently employed to describe his condition. Yet he assured his physician on August 5, 1981, that he felt "wonderful—the healthiest man in the world but also said he didn't understand any of this." On September 28 he "saw old girlfriend Helene & didn't recognize her. Later, became very agitated disoriented and admitted that he 'is bewildered.' Spoke of being very unhappy—unwanted—lack of 'sexual love.' "[37] It seemed ironic that he was plagued with complete sexual dysfunction. He was not only impotent and incontinent but had a troublesome rash that irritated his sexual organs. His daily routine consisted in getting up early and receiving treatments for his many complaints, then having the nurse drive him to the hall of fame. After lunch he would return home exhausted and rest for most of the afternoon. In the evening he would either attend a softball game or watch television. His chief pleasure in life came from the large dishes of ice cream he consumed several times daily. For a man who was a workaholic most of his life, this routine of inactivity must have been stifling.

Over the next several years Bob exhibited paranoia and fear that he was losing his faculties and fortune. Numerous nursing notes refer to his obsession with money. On April 26, 1982, Bob was very pleasant at the hall of fame until he started autographing magazines for some visitors. Then he began "accusing them [of] stealing them & he would not make any profit like that!" He was extremely restless and agitated, and resented the nurses' presence so much that he started swearing for the first time in his life. He "got very nasty around 2:00" on September 22. "Said Nurse was a stranger & to mind my own 'G D' business & he will do what he wants without any help from the damn girls. Up & down out of chair constantly." He also talked incessantly. To make life more bearable for all, the nurses administered an abundance of pharmacopoeia, including plenty of aspirin, Peri-Colase for his stool, Percodan for pain, Nitrostat for chest pain, and lots of Hoffman Rub. Often Bob complained of hurting all over. Restoril, normally given to induce sleep, was freely administered. Only with references to the past and affirmations of his ego was it possible (along with medicine) to calm him. Doctors attributed his confusion and the pain in his feet and

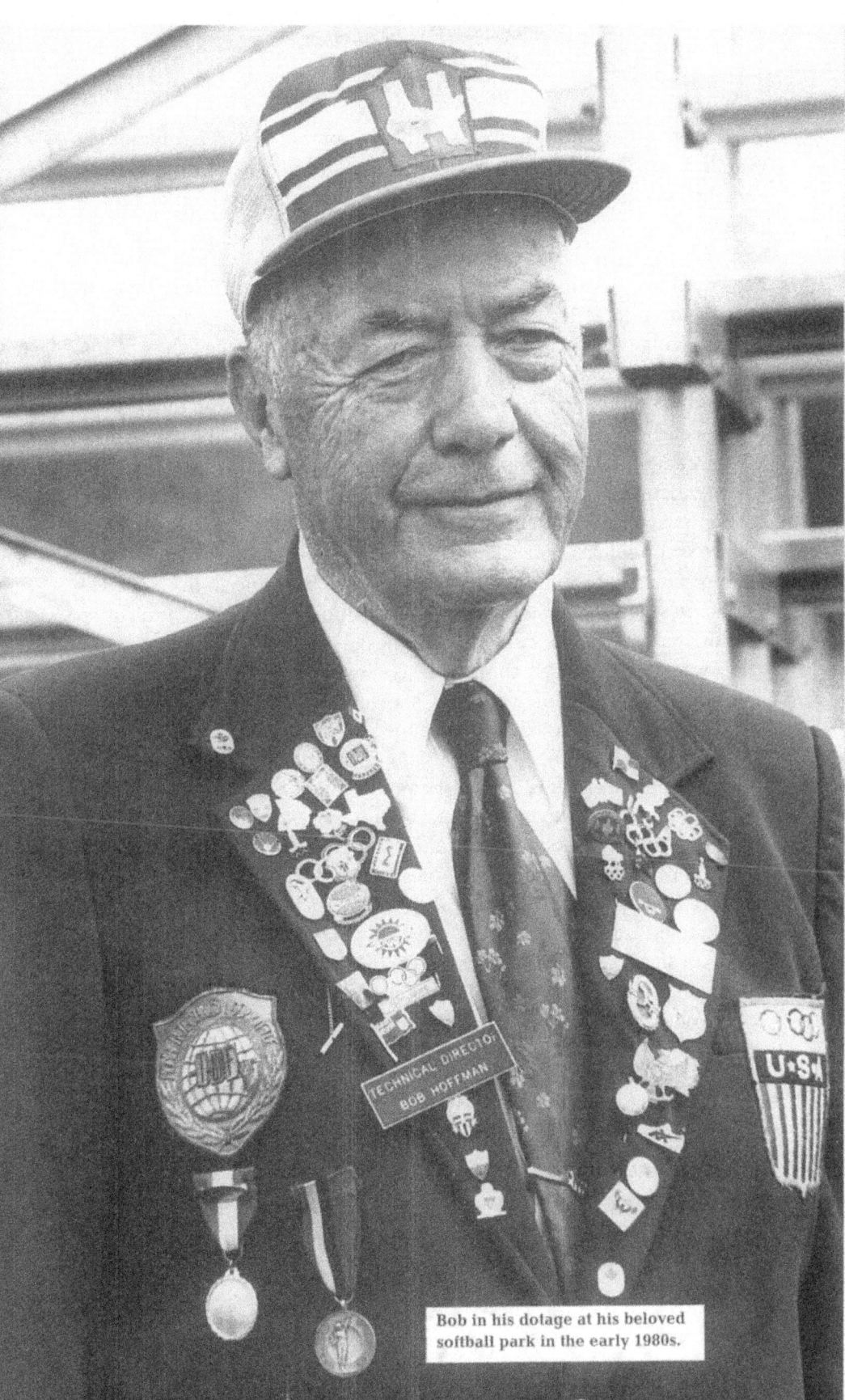

Bob in his dotage at his beloved softball park in the early 1980s.

shoulders to his high heart rate, while his paranoia was a symptom of senile dementia.[38] Hoffman, who had spent so much of his life preaching against doctors and prescription medicines, was now completely at their mercy.

"He was in such misery," recalls Alda, who believes that "you will pay double for everything you do." She thinks Bob may have "payed in suffering in his latter years" for his transgressions. He had something wrong with every part of his body. In addition to multiple aches, pains, and rashes, he was afflicted with edema in his legs and feet, seriously impairing ambulation, and at times his abdomen was distended. He was tired nearly all the time, yet he slept poorly and was always restless. In September 1983 he experienced chills, shakes, sore throat, stomach growling, and a slight temperature. His doctor explained that he probably had bacteria all through his body and that any additional fever might induce septic shock. This did not happen, but Bob was also plagued with hemorrhoids, which often caused bright red bleeding in his stool. His urine was usually a cloudy dark amber and foul smelling, indicating serious infection. He was later diagnosed as having a kidney stone. Bob was hardly ever in control of his bowels, and even with a diaper on he frequently made a mess of his clothes wherever he was sitting or standing. He wore out a succession of nurses, who had difficulty handling such a large man with so much wrong with him. More serious than his other ailments were a large cancerous sore on his forehead, which required an operation, and a stroke in November 1983, which required three weeks hospitalization. By the time of his discharge his doctors listed twelve afflictions (mostly heart-related) from which Bob suffered and for which there was no cure. Small wonder that in early December Bob stated that the "only thing left to do when old and worn out is to 'lay down and die.' " On December 23 he cried out, "Help, help, help, no one knows who I am." Nothing could have been more tragic for someone who had spent his entire life trying to become known.[39]

In January 1985 Alda placed Bob in a nursing home, where he clung tenaciously to life for another six months. After a series of strokes, his final days were spent in York Hospital. Alda recalls the last evening of his life, July 18, when she met on the elevator a United Church of Christ minister who agreed to come to Bob's room. There they joined hands with her daughter, granddaughter, and Terpak for prayer. "He fell asleep during that prayer. I think he was waiting for it." Although Hoffman's death was featured on the front page of the York papers,

Bob Hoffman's Departure

which highlighted his local philanthropy, it received surprisingly little coverage in the iron game. Bill Starr called him "the John D. Rockefeller of the sport of strength" but controversial. "He assisted, but he also controlled. He encouraged, but he also actively discouraged any competition. He supported, but a beneficiary of that support would also be the bottom line of the York Barbell Company." Terry Todd called him the most dominant iron-game figure of the twentieth century: "We would not be where we are had we not been carried forward in the arms of giants, the tallest of whom was Bob Hoffman." *Strength & Health* included various tributes to Bob, but words could not do justice to the role he had played in his community, sport, and nation over a half century. Of the many expressions of sympathy received by Alda, the one that would have most pleased Bob came from Richard Nixon, who stated that "as Vice President and later as President, there is no one for whom I had greater respect and affection." Nothing, on the other hand, would have been more likely to arouse his indignation than the flowers and note expressing "deepest sympathy" from Joe Weider.[40]

Epilogue and Conclusion

> These are perilous times to be a man in America. There are forces afoot that have changed men's sense of themselves, blurring what once seemed clear-cut modes and models of manhood. John Wayne is dead, and we have not yet picked his stand-in.
>
> —Daniel Goleman

On July 23, 1985, Hoffman was buried in Mount Rose Cemetery in one of the eighty plots he had bought to accommodate members of the York gang and their families. The inscription on Bob's tombstone included his likeness, signature, and title—"Father of World Weightlifting." "At one time I stood alone," he boasted from his grave. "I was the only believer in weight training for athletics—now there are millions." A most remarkable revelation was the size of his fortune, particularly since so much of it had already been given away, stolen, or unwisely invested. So extensive were his holdings that it took five years to settle the estate, initially valued at $11.5 million. By the time disbursements were made, including $2,616,022 to the federal government, $893,608 to the state, and $513,104 for attorney and executor fees, it was reduced to $5,758,075. Although it was feared that the federal estate tax would be so great that liquidation of the business would be required, obligations were met by selling a large portion of Hoffman's shares in the company.¹

Before his death there were 250 voting shares and 252 nonvoting shares. Hoffman virtually owned the business, holding all of the latter and 248 of the former. The only other shareholders were Dietz and Terpak, who had been given one share each of voting stock in 1965, just after Bob's first operation, thereby providing them a financial stake in the corporation and a lock on its destiny. All nonvoting stock was bequeathed to the Hoffman Foundation, while the voting stock, after one-third was used for taxes, was distributed equally to Mike, John, and Alda, who served as executors of the will and corporate directors. Thus Bob's common-law widow now had a real voice in company operations. Notwithstanding stories at York Barbell about Mike's self-serving practices, Alda believed that "if there wasn't a Mike Dietz, there wouldn't have been a company." He was the "brains of the management."² It was because of Alda's support and position as swing vote on the board that Dietz succeeded Bob as its chairman and as president of York Barbell.

Whether Mike and John, who had disliked each other for fifty years, could effectively run the business seemed doubtful. Todd thinks Bob might have kept them at odds in order to make them less of a threat to himself. In any case, "Mike and Johnny were not suited to manage a multimillion-dollar corporation." In September 1986 an upbeat article on York Barbell in the *New York Times* pictured its two chief executives with insets of their sons, John Terpak Jr. and William Dietz, now secretary and treasurer respectively: "York Barbell today employs 140 people and grosses $25 million in annual sales." Yet a 1989 article in the *Los Angeles Times* reported that the Weider empire boasted "2,000 employees worldwide and gross revenues of more than $250 million a year." What jeopardized York's position most was internal dissension. "Mike and John were like two mules pulling in separate directions," was Alda's assessment. Dellinger likens the company in the 1980s to "a third-world army": "The general got shot. We're getting shelled, but what do we do? Those under him were just caretakers."³

The greatest controversy after Hoffman's death, however, resulted not so much from management gridlock as from the terms of the founder's will. It had the effect of breaking up the York gang, the organization's nucleus for a half century. By making Dietz, Terpak, and Ketterman almost sole benefactors, it created rancor and raised

Epilogue and Conclusion

accusations that Dietz and perhaps others had changed the will as Bob was lapsing into dotage. It was not simply that many loyal individuals had contributed much to the fruition of Bob's dreams of personal and financial success, but that he had stated repeatedly his indebtedness and intention to remember them. A 1968 editorial in *Strength & Health* was often cited as proof: "When I leave this world, 51 percent of the company, according to present plans, will belong to the men who have worked so hard with me to make it what it is. John Grimek, Steve Stanko, Dick Bachtell, John Terpak, Mike Dietz, Harry Utterback and others of the old-timers, and the newer men who form such an important part of our organization, will all have a share in the York Barbell Co." Especially in light of the low salaries paid at York, these reassurances helped keep workers in line and trustful that their patriarch would look after them. What makes the final settlement so questionable is that it was drawn up and signed during a period of physical and mental decline, when Bob was facing the stress of a further operation. In addition to major disbursements to the Hoffman Foundation and the three executors, the will of March 1978 set up a $500,000 trust for allocation to five other beneficiaries named in the codicil: Helen Gemmil, 10 percent; Helene Lukens, 35 percent; Rosetta Morris, 12 percent; Harry Utterback, 33 percent; and Ruth Snellbaker, 10 percent.[4] The inclusion of Utterback, one of the few employees who got on well with Dietz, fueled suspicions that Mike had exercised a heavy hand over the codicil. Noticeably excluded were such stalwarts as Bachtell and Grimek.

It is not surprising that the will created a furor in the weightlifting world. Only Grimek had the resources and personal courage to speak out. He filed his initial complaint in December 1985. In an attempt to elicit support for Grimek, Robert Kennedy's *Musclemag International* issued "A Plea to Help the Monarch of Muscledom," hoping that more witnesses would come forward to underscore the testimony in Bob's 1968 editorial. The article contended that "Bob and John remained good friends to the very end, and Bob would never 'disown' him regardless of circumstances.... One only has to refer to Bob's many books and magazine articles... to see how he felt about Grimek.... There are some who feel it was Bob who left JCG out of his will. Grimek, however, doesn't feel this way but feels others, behind the scenes, made the change." Only Ray Degenhardt and Jim Murray testified at the May 1989 trial. They verified Hoffman's remark that "Grimek and the boys were going to be rich men when he died" and other such statements, but they were unable to state how much the claimant was to receive. Lack of specificity doomed Grimek's challenge. He appealed, but Pennsylvania's Superior Court concurred with the judgment, and the Supreme Court denied the case a hearing.[5] After five years of litigation, the Grimek case ended in October 1990, but the tragedy of his failed protest went far beyond monetary loss. Aside from Bob, Grimek most epitomized, for the many thousands who idolized him, the most manly image of York in its prime. As Murray characterized him in the trial, he was the Arnold Schwarzenegger of his day. Muscletown would never be the same.

Concurrent with the breakup of the York gang were decisive changes in the business that would imprint on York Barbell a totally new character. Its transformation from a company of jocks to a strictly business concern came about chiefly through attrition—by the death, retirement, or resignation of those who helped make York a Mecca of weightlifting and bodybuilding for nearly a half century. By the late 1980s Terpak realized, on receiving a letter from an old friend in Florida, that he was the only remaining link to the great York tradition: "After reading the names you referred to (Hoffman, T. Terlazzo, Terry, Stanko, and Davis) I was momentarily stunned—they're all dead. Of the 'old York gang' only Grimek and I remain. Sig Klein and Milo Steinborn are gone, too." The hall of fame, with its priceless memorabilia, remained, and visitors continued to be drawn to York, almost as a conditioned reflex, but the champions were gone. "We're Not Muscletown Anymore" was the heading for a local newspaper column when the Ridge Avenue gym closed its doors in October 1988.[6] As the old-timers faded away, York's magazines disappeared also. Terpak attributed the demise of *Strength & Health* in 1985 to its antisteroid stance, but the demise more likely resulted from the decline of Olympic lifting, Bob's death, and losses of $15,000 per issue. *Muscular Development* was also losing money, but when its sister magazine went under, an attempt was made to revitalize it by making it a monthly and Weiderizing its format. By June 1988 it was losing $20,000 per month. Therefore it was sold to Twin Laboratories of Ronkonkoma, New York. Soon properties on Ridge Avenue and in Greencastle, once central to the corporate mission, were sold, and the House on the Hill was divested under a lease-purchase agreement. The softball fields in Hoffman Park began to show signs of neglect. And Trudy Engel, the lobbyist on whom Bob had lavished so much attention in his latter years, found that she had no place in the new order. Excluded from the will and dismissed from her position, she did what others who left York had done in previous decades. Redman remembers watching one of President Reagan's news conferences when Trudy suddenly appeared to present him with a fitness award from Joe Weider: "It was her ultimate glory."[7]

Those who entered the company in the 1970s and 1980s were oriented more toward business. Some who were involved in sales and promotion of York products—Dellinger, Redman, and Don Hess—were sympathetic to York's glorious heritage, but no one in the corporation, aside from the elder Terpak and Dietz, was directly linked to it. Indeed the period from 1985 to 1989 was one of readjustment, and no one seemed sure how the new character of York would be defined. Most noticeable, however, was the company's deteriorating financial condition. Sales figures (with profits in parentheses) reflect this deterioration.[8]

1983—$11,558,647 (392,793)
1984—$11,869,854 (48,363)
1985—$9,999,925 (153,138)
1986—$8,166,958 (155,604)
1987—$7,158,424 (–290,243)
1988—$7,437,211 (–415,066)
1989—$6,990,594 (–557,182)

Though some of York's subsidiaries, notably U.S. Lock and Hardware, showed a profit, enormous losses from the parent company could not easily be absorbed. "For several years after Bob's death we were roaming around in the wilderness," is Dellinger's recollection of the "caretaker" years. "This place was running on its own momentum during the eighties and then headed into a downward spiral." Dietz and Terpak, of course, had to bear the responsibility for this state of affairs. Without Bob to pull the company together, the ranks became sharply divided. Plant manager Gene Heiland recalls that when he arrived in 1987 "you were either a Dietz or a Terpak." Claudia Keister confirms that "everyone was always fighting. . . . There was no management, just tension. . . . It was the worst place I had ever worked."[9] Clearly Terpak, as vice-president, was less influential. He was less concerned than Dietz with internal operations, had fewer employees answerable to him, and was outvoted on the board of directors. Johnny had always been an excellent backup man for Bob, but he was incapable of supporting his longtime adversary or exercising any independent leadership.

Mike's death in June 1988 caught both factions unawares, but they soon settled on a compromise whereby Terpak became chairman of a board consisting of himself, William Dietz, and Alda. Dietz, who held a management degree from the University of Pittsburgh and had worked at York Barbell since 1977, became president and took charge of the company's daily operations. He was the most respected of the Dietz brothers and attained his standing on the board as executor of his father's will. Terpak explains that he consented to Bill's becoming president, "aside from personal considerations, [assuming] he would do what is right for the business." Most important, Alda consented. Again she held the swing vote, and it was pointless for Terpak to oppose her. But over the next year the younger Dietz did little to cultivate Alda's favor. Not only did the company continue its downward course, but there was increasing evidence of conflicts of interest between Mike's estate and the company. Bill appeared to be positioning himself and his brothers for a takeover. The final straw dropped in November 1988, when he gave salary increases to his brothers David and Mike Jr., "despite a direct mandate to the contrary by the board of directors." This act of defiance led to a direct bid for power by the Dietzes in early December. That seemed an opportune time inasmuch as Terpak was in Indonesia attending the world championships. But Bill's raises to his brothers "rubbed a lot of people the wrong way," states Keister. Furthermore, he no longer had the support of Alda, who recalls, "Bill Dietz came out to the house with an envelope and stated that he wanted to run the company alone, 'Otherwise here's my letter of resignation.' " The next day he vacated his office.[10]

The popular interpretation of Dietz's actions is that he and his brothers believed they were indispensable. What the Dietzes had not counted on was the intervention of Vic Standish, who had provided sound management of U.S. Lock and Hardware for many years. "Mike screwed things up at York Barbell," notes Redman, "but Vic was so good with the foundry that he couldn't get his hands on that." While the parent firm was sustaining enormous losses, U.S. Lock was turning in a yearly profit and probably staving off disaster. Also, Standish, the corporate treasurer, was constantly pressing for more authority, and Terpak had been giving way to his advances. So when Dietz vacated his post as president, Vic, who possessed a degree in accounting and many years of hands-on experience in manufacturing, was the man of the hour. "All the road signs were pointing to Vic," remarks Dellinger. "He would not have been denied the top spot." John Terpak Jr. agrees that Vic was "the key person."[11] In recognition of his vital position in the new order,

Epilogue and Conclusion

Vic was made a stockholder and added, with the younger Terpak, to the board of directors.

That the Terpak faction should triumph seemed miraculous. But some major hurdles had to be cleared before the company was out of its doldrums. One was the continued possession of corporate shares by the Dietzes, who filed suit against Standish, Ketterman, and the Terpaks to overturn the reorganization. By early 1992 a settlement was reached whereby the Dietz interest was paid off with $1.2 million in cash and land. Hoffman's legacy was at last free of all claims placed on it through the vagaries of his will. But this last episode had wrought a terrible cost on the company. Keister admits that after the Dietzes left in 1988, "it was rough for a year or so, but eventually the plant got moving." Slowly the company recovered.[12] What kept the corporation afloat in these doleful times were profits from York's subsidiaries, U.S. Lock and Hardware, Swiss Automatics, and Costas-York, always insulated from the parent firm. Interestingly, after Standish left U.S. Lock in 1989, its performance weakened and that of York Barbell strengthened. For it was he, more than any other person, who revived the company's fortunes.

The death of John Terpak Sr. (1993) and the retirements of Alda Ketterman (1993) and John Terpak Jr. (1995) seemed not to upset this balance. The elevation of Standish to president and majority shareholder assured that the company would be administered by professionals according to sound business procedures. When treasurer and managerial vacancies arose, they were occupied by nonweightlifters. Nor is it surprising, given his foundry background, that Standish steered the company back to its original specialty of manufacturing cast-iron products. A new emphasis, however, was placed on marketing entire weight lines, not just weights. York now provides equipment for anaerobic fitness needs on all levels—from low-price import weights to elite weight stack units for circuit training. To maximize its total fitness approach, York is changing its marketing strategy, moving away from mail order and sporting-goods outlets and toward specialty fitness dealers. Operational levels have improved accordingly, with a doubling of plant employees and a tripling of equipment sales. "York Barbell is alive and well," boasts a recent brochure. "After twenty years of slumber, the giant has come to life."[13]

By far the most exciting development in several decades, however, is the takeover of York Barbell by a local investment group called Susquehanna Capital. President Paul Stombaugh and his associates

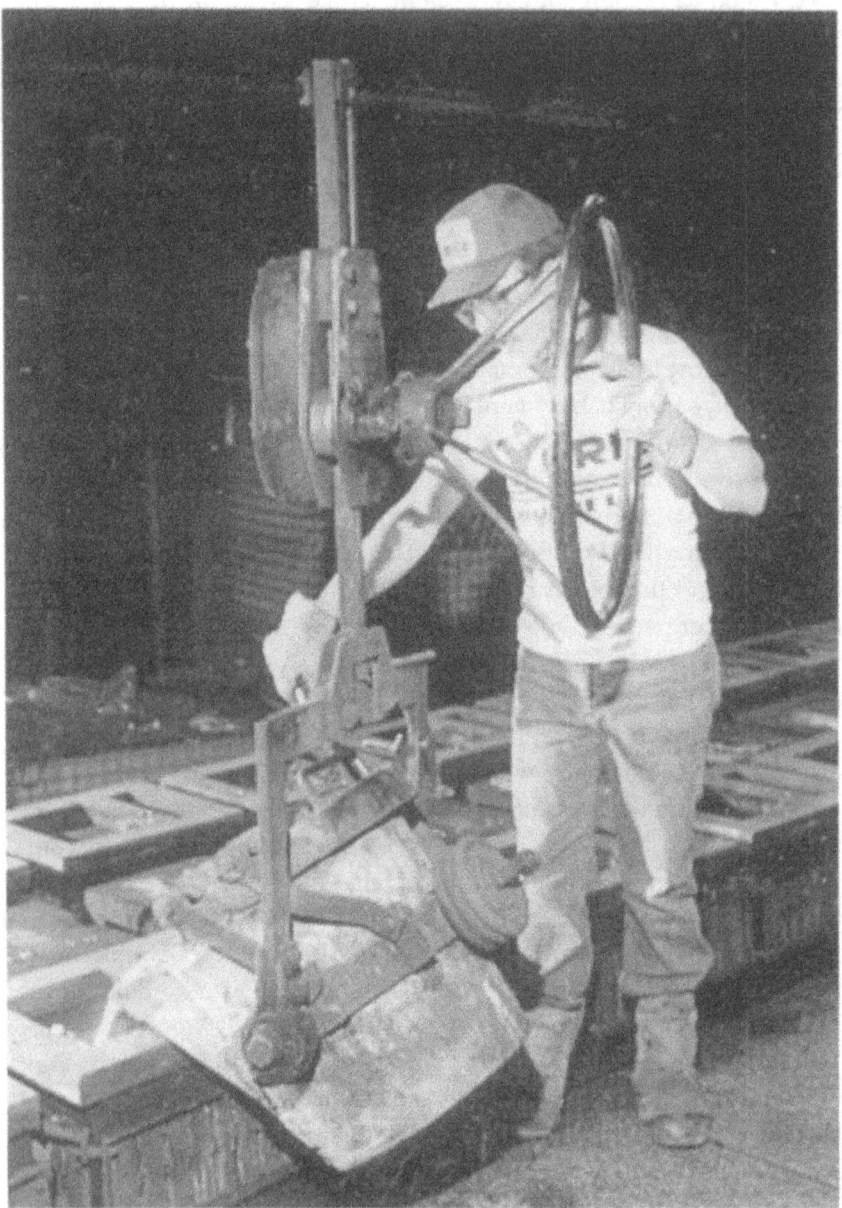

A York Barbell employee pouring molten iron at the company's foundry on the Susquehanna River.

Epilogue and Conclusion

are taking bold steps on many fronts to restore the magic and glory of the York tradition. The York Barbell Institute has been established to serve as a focal point for study of all aspects of strength training, nutrition, and techniques to enhance athletic performance. In June 1998 the company staged a revival of the annual York picnic. It was a three-day strengthfest, reminiscent of Hoffman's shows of yesteryear, where iron-game enthusiasts were treated to powerlifting and strong-man contests, celebrity appearances, hall-of-fame inductions, and audience-participation events. "We want to reestablish York as a Mecca for weightlifting, powerlifting, and bodybuilding," declares Stombaugh. That IWF certification (permitting use of York equipment in Olympic and world championships) has been restored demonstrates the new owners are serious about returning the company to its leading position.[14] Nor would it be surprising to see a reappearance of *Strength & Health*. Finally, a renewed effort is being placed on food supplements, both musclebuilding and performance enhancing, with the hope of generating the kind of income and name recognition that made York such a powerhouse under Hoffman. Susquehanna Capital, recognizing that York's future lies in its rich traditions, seems determined to give meaning to its claim to be "The Strongest Name in Fitness."

What seems remarkable in retrospect is that the company not only survived but thrived for nearly a half century during which employees were hired for athletic prowess rather than business acumen. Perhaps this is the greatest tribute that can be paid to Bob Hoffman—that he could mold a gang of weightlifters in the heart of the Great Depression into a multimillion-dollar corporation. Indeed Hoffman's foremost attribute was his promotional genius. To Donnie Warner "he was a man who could tell you how great hell was and you could hardly wait to get there." "Bob was a self-made man with a streak of eccentricity," observes John Terlazzo. "An egomaniac."[15] Hoffman has been justly criticized for his egotism and for exaggerating and falsifying claims. Yet ironically these were the qualities most vital to his success. Put simply, he believed in himself—an essential ingredient to motivation. Bob was likely overcompensating for youthful deficiencies, striving to fulfill societal expectations for masculinity at the turn of the century. According to Gregory Rochlin, the constant need for men to "prove themselves" stems from low self-esteem and uncertain identity. Anthropologist David Gilmore argues that male behavior in most societies is a response to "psychological deficits," compelling men to "impregnate

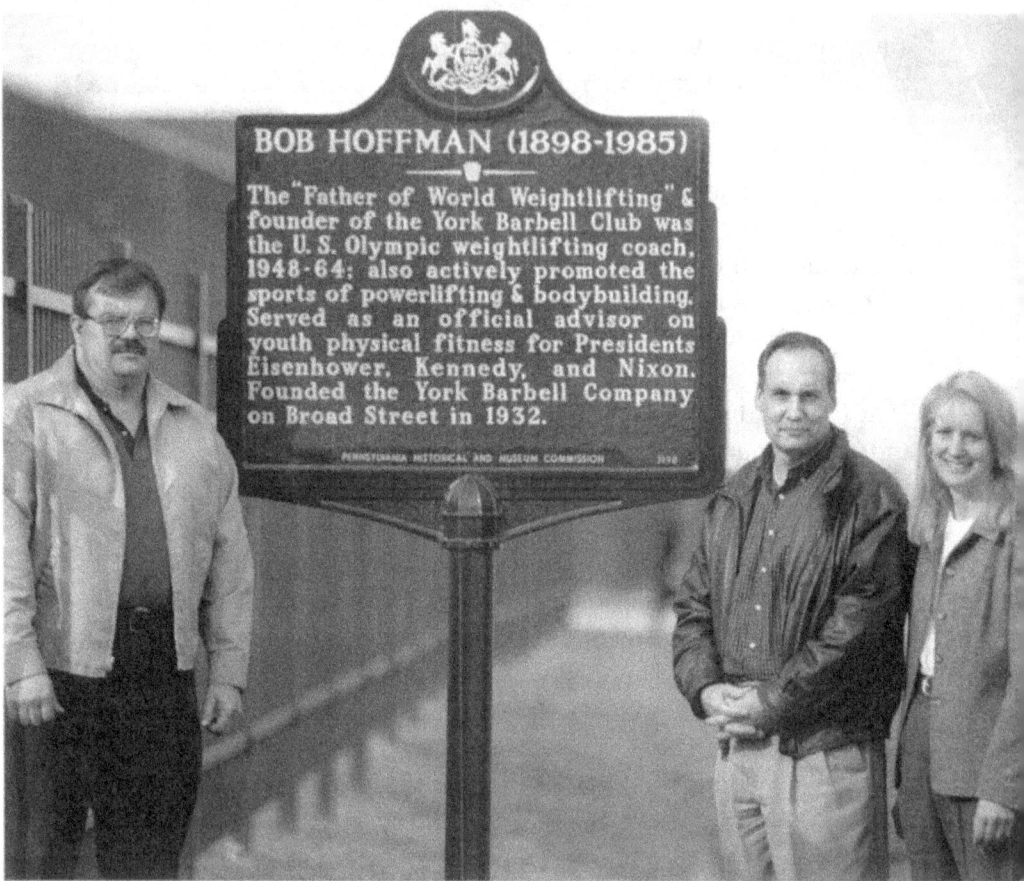

On November 9, 1998, the Pennsylvania Historical and Museum Commission erected a marker at York Barbell commemorating the centenary of Bob Hoffman's birth and his lifetime of achievement. Pictured are the three company officials—Sales Representative Jan Dellinger, President Paul Stombaugh, and Librarian/Archivist Barbara Andrelczyk, who are most involved in keeping the York tradition alive.

women, protect dependents from danger, and [make] provision [for] kith and kin." David Chapman, in his biography of Eugen Sandow, reifies this "imperative triad," concluding that "physical strength, sexual prowess, and economic success" characterized his subject's involvement in physical culture at the end of the Victorian era.[16] Hoffman too was nurtured on these cultural criteria for manhood, leading one to suspect that his aggressiveness addressed psychological needs peculiar to his gender.

Bob's self-confidence was tested first in the lakes and rivers of his native Pittsburgh and then on the battlefields of France. Later it was

Epilogue and Conclusion

manifested in his oil-burner career and, through the tutelage of George Jowett, applied to weightlifting. Hoffman's ideology of success was a unique synthesis of ego, business, and sport. He sought to inspire the building of bodies, character, and self-esteem by projecting himself and his organization as paragons of virtue in an otherwise imperfect world. Key to the success of his movement was socialization—a process encouraged by strong societal forces favoring homogeneity during the first half of the twentieth century. Toward this end he recruited some of the best-built and athletic human specimens in the world—the York gang—who epitomized manliness by winning Olympic medals and Mr. America titles. They served as models for a generation of neurasthenic and hyphenated American youth and helped Hoffman accumulate the resources to bring about a golden age for American weightlifting.

As an innovator, Bob Hoffman was far ahead of his time. More than anyone, he successfully promoted the widespread use of weights for general fitness and training for virtually all sports. He was also a pioneer in the marketing of food supplements. Hoffman was not only a patriarch of American and world weightlifting, he also did much to foster bodybuilding and powerlifting as sports. Isometrics and steroids were later innovations for which he can be held at least partly responsible. On another level, Hoffman, by his corporate socialization of weightlifters, aided in the corruption of the amateur ideal, an important aspect of the larger story of the commercialization of American sport and the nationalization of sport in other countries. He is unique in being the only person ever to realize financial success and worldwide fame just from weightlifting. That he misrepresented the accomplishments of himself and his lifters, led a scandalous sex life, misled consumers, cheated on taxes, and rarely practiced what he preached should not detract from any final estimate of his worth. However great his shortcomings, tens of thousands of persons ultimately benefited from his teachings and products. Great men rarely play by the rules.

Muscletown, at the height of its worldwide influence in the 1950s, was the place to be for youth seeking validation of their manhood. "It's hard for people around now to imagine what a potent place York was at that time," remarks Terry Todd.[17] By the mid-1960s, however, many of the ideals projected by Hoffman, based on assumptions from an earlier era, were no longer credible. The melting pot of Bob's youth was no longer melting, and the Horatio Alger pitch that had worked so effectively for so long seemed irrelevant in the fragmented cultural context of modern

America. York ceased to be a center of innovation as Bob expended his creative energies in monumental struggles with the Weiders, the Soviet Union, and his own government, none of which he could win. Although riches from the sale of Hi-Proteen put his organization on a firm financial footing, it was beset by a host of debilitating influences. Greed, jealousy, and corruption permeated the York gang, displacing the team spirit that had been so instrumental to success in the early days. In the later days the older generation guarded its power and place from incursion by any intruder. To the young, ambitious Texas types who tried to instigate a new spirit of socialization, more in tune with the times, Hoffman's Victorian construct of manliness was no longer tenable. Yet Bob, still obsessed with being the world's healthiest man and striving for immortality, refused to accept their alternative lifestyle or values and was unwilling to sanction any transfer of power to the younger generation. This denial, accompanied by the ubiquitous counterculture of the Vietnam War era, prompted a revolt in 1968 and beyond that brought an end to his manly Mecca of muscle. A resulting loss of focus led to divestment of the maturing entities of bodybuilding and powerlifting. Olympic lifting, though it gained a firmer financial base than ever, became an anachronism along with Hoffman. Pathetic attempts to regain patriarchal esteem through softball and the Nixon White House were doomed to failure as American social norms adopted a postmodern definition of manhood. It was the inability of the founding father to sustain his body of manly myths that brought an end to the York version of the American dream.

In the years following Bob's illness and death, York Barbell and American weightlifting have struggled to find new and more realistic strategies for success. So great and so lasting was Hoffman's influence over the iron game that some think that there will eventually be a second messiah, who will restore York and America to preeminence. But however considerable Hoffman's legacy might be, it is unlikely that history will repeat itself. The cultural landscape has shifted since the 1950s, more in keeping with the hegemonic formulas of the Weiders. While it is instructive to conjure the reasons for the rise and fall of manly culture at York, it must be concluded that any regeneration must proceed from a totally different set of assumptions, more in keeping with the dawn of a new century. Whether Susquehanna Capital will be able to restore York to its lofty position in the iron game has yet to be determined. But much will depend on reviving not merely the forms of greatness but the same driving force and spirit of innovation that made York such a wonder in the world of Muscledom. There may never be another Bob Hoffman, but the two most basic components of his ideology of success—socialization and individual initiative—remain as applicable today as they were fifty years ago. It was Hoffman's vision and genius in combining these timeless precepts in the York gang that brought so much glory to Muscletown, USA.

Notes

INTRODUCTION

1. Jackson Lears, *No Place of Grace: Antimodernism and the Transformation of American Culture, 1880-1920* (New York, 1981), 18. For treatments on American success ideology, see Irvin Wyllie, *The Self-Made Man in America: The Myth of Rags to Riches* (New Brunswick, N.J., 1954); Moses Rischin, ed., *The American Gospel of Success: Individualism and Beyond* (Chicago, 1965); Richard Weiss, *The American Myth of Success: From Horatio Alger to Norman Vincent Peale* (New York, 1969); and Theodore Greene, *America's Heroes: The Changing Models of Success in American Magazines* (New York, 1970).

2. Anthony Rotundo, *American Manhood: Transformations in Masculinity from the Revolution to the Modern Era* (New York, 1993), 5–6. Other works on hypermasculinity at the turn of the century include Mark Carnes and Clyde Griffen, *Meanings for Manhood: Constructions of Masculinity in Victorian America* (Chicago, 1990); Elizabeth Pleck and Joseph Pleck, *The American Man* (Englewood Cliffs, N.J., 1980); Charles Rosenberg, "Sexuality, Class, and Role in Nineteenth-Century America," *American Quarterly* 25 (May 1973): 131–53; Peter Stearns, *Be a Man! Males in Modern Society* (New York, 1979); George Sage, *Power and Ideology in American Sport: A Critical Perspective* (Champaign, Ill., 1990); and Joe Dubbert, *A Man's Place* (Englewood Cliffs, N.J., 1979).

3. Elliott Gorn, *The Manly Art: Bare-Knuckle Prize Fighting in America* (Ithaca, 1986), 142. See also Clyde Franklin, *The Changing Definition of Masculinity* (New York, 1984), 99, and Kenneth Dutton, *The Perfectible Body: The Western Ideal of Male Physical Development* (New York, 1995), 234.

4. Paul Hoch, *Rip Off the Big Game: The Exploitation of Sports by the Power Elite* (New York, 1972), 155. For a more general treatment, see Donald Sabo and Ross Runfola, *Sports and Male Identity* (Englewood Cliffs, N.J., 1980).

5. Robert Harlow, "Masculine Inadequacy and Compensatory Development of Physique," *Journal of Personality* 19 (1951): 313–14. Alan Klein, in "Pumping Irony: Crisis and Contradiction in Bodybuilding," *Sociology of Sport Journal* 3 (1986): 112–33, contends this inadequacy was even more evident in bodybuilders.

6. Robert Boyle, *Sport—Mirror of American Life* (Boston, 1963), 100. Other studies on the relationship between sport, social class, and the social mobility of fringe groups include Robert J. Havighurst and Bernice L. Neugarten, *Sport and Education* (Boston, 1957); John Loy, "The Study of Sport and Social Mobility," in *Aspects of Contemporary Sport Sociology*, ed. Gerald Kenyon (Chicago, 1968), 101–33; D. Riesman and R. Denney, "Football in America: A Study of Culture Diffusion," *American Quarterly* 3 (1951): 309–19; and John Betts, *America's Sporting Heritage* (Reading, Mass., 1974).

NOTES

7. George Kirkley, *Modern Weightlifting* (London, 1957), 21.
8. Rick Wayne, *Muscle Wars: The Behind-the-Scenes Story of Competitive Bodybuilding* (New York, 1985), 112–14.
9. William Hunt, *Body Love: The Amazing Career of Bernarr Macfadden* (Bowling Green, Ohio, 1989); Robert Ernst, *Weakness Is a Crime* (Ithaca, 1991); Alan Klein, *Little Big Men: Bodybuilding Subculture and Gender Construction* (Albany, N.Y., 1993); David Chapman, *Sandow the Magnificent: Eugen Sandow and the Beginnings of Bodybuilding* (Champaign, Ill., 1994); John Neuright and Timothy Chandler, *Making Men: Rugby and Masculine Identity* (London, 1996); and Kim Townsend, *Manhood at Harvard: William James and Others* (New York, 1996).
10. Roger Horrocks's *Male Myths and Icons: Masculinity in Popular Culture* (New York, 1995) typifies the former approach, while Robert Bly's *Iron John: A Book About Men* (Reading, Mass., 1990) and Sam Keen's *Fire in the Belly* (New York, 1991) were best-selling mythopoeic works in the early 1990s.
11. Michael Kimmel, *Manhood in America: A Cultural History* (New York, 1996), 333, and Garrison Keillor, *The Book of Guys* (New York, 1993), 11.
12. See Herbert Butterfield's classic critique *The Whig Interpretation of History* (New York, 1965).

CHAPTER 1

1. Information on Hoffman's family is drawn largely from a typescript prepared by John L. (Jack) Hoffman in December 1987; an interview with John Hoffman (Parker, Pa.); a letter from John Hoffman to the author, February 13, 1988; and a letter from J[ohn] L. Hoffman to Channing Galbreath, February 26, 1962, Hoffman Papers, hereafter cited as HP.
2. R. L. Polk and Co's *Pittsburg City Directory*, 1903–15, Carnegie Library, Pittsburgh, Pa.
3. Registrar's and Orphans' Court Records, June 1925, no. 142, Allegheny County Court House.
4. Interviews with J. Hoffman and Alda Ketterman (Dover, Pa.); *Strength & Health* (hereafter *SH*) 1 (January 1933): 3, and (February 1933): 22.
5. *Health Food Business Review*, November 1968, 13; interview with J. Hoffman; and *SH* 1 (October 1933): 8.
6. *Philadelphia Inquirer*, April 23, 1973, and *SH* 1 (February 1933): 22.
7. Typescript by Hoffman; interview with Ketterman; and *SH* 1 (January 1933): 3.
8. *SH* 3 (October 1935): 11; Bob Hoffman, *Big Arms: How to Develop Them* (York, Pa., 1939), 125; *SH* 4 (January 1936): 22; and *Polk's City Directory*, 1903–21.
9. Interview with J. Hoffman, and *SH* 12 (November 1945): 15.
10. *Pittsburg Press*, August 13 and September 24, 1916; *SH* 12 (November 1945): 15; and *SH* 1 (May 1933): 11 and 26.
11. Bob Hoffman, *I Remember the Last War* (York, Pa., 1940), 34, 58, and 59; Nat Fleischer, ed., *Ring Record Book and Boxing Encyclopedia* (New York, 1957), 114; and *SH* 2 (January 1935): 10.
12. Hoffman, *I Remember the Last War*, 54–55, 63, 80–81, 112–13, and 120–21.
13. Ibid., 118–19, 129–31, 135–36, and 139–40, and Hoffman, *Road to Super-Strength*, 23.
14. Hoffman Service Records, Department of Military Affairs, Pennsylvania State Archives, Harrisburg, and *Pennsylvania in the World War: An Illustrated History of the Twenty-Eighth Division* (Pittsburgh, 1921), 2:507 and 552–53.
15. Interview with Ketterman; Hoffman, *I Remember the Last War*, 157 and 300–301; J. Hoffman to Ketterman, August 4, 1985, HP; and *SH* 4 (June 1936): 17.
16. *SH* 4 (May 1936): 40, and *SH* 3 (March 1935): 20–21 and 46–47.

Notes

17. Interviews with J. Hoffman, Lavern Brenneman, and John Terpak Sr. (York, Pa.); *SH* 12 (November 1945): 36; and typescript by Hoffman.
18. Interview with Rosetta Morris (Fruitland, Md.), and *SH* 29 (November 1961): 4.

CHAPTER 2

1. See John Lucas and Ronald Smith, *Saga of American Sport* (Philadelphia, 1978); Donald J. Mrozek, *Sport and American Mentality: Eighteen Eighty to Nineteen Ten* (Knoxville, Tenn., 1983); and William Baker, *Sports in the Western World* (Totowa, N.J., 1982).
2. Harvey Green, *Fit for America: Health, Fitness, Sport, and American Society* (New York, 1986), 85. See also Jan Todd, *Physical Culture and the Body Beautiful: An Examination of the Role of Purposive Exercise in the Lives of American Women, 1800–1870* (Macon, 1998), and James Whorton's study *Crusaders for Fitness: The History of American Health Reformers* (Princeton, 1982).
3. Dietrich Wortmann, "History of Modern American Weightlifting and Body Building," in *1948 U.S. Olympic Team Trials, Weightlifting: Official Program of the United States Olympic Committee* (1948), 11.
4. *Mighty Men of Old: Being a Gallery of Pictures and Biographies of Outstanding Old Time Strong Men* (York, Pa., 1940).
5. Baker, *Sports in the Western World*, 215.
6. *Physical Culture* 1 (October 1898): 245–48, and *Strength* 10 (February 1926): 83.
7. *Strength* 6 (March 1922): 8–9, and (June 1922): 42.
8. *Strength* 6 (July 1922): 14–17, 56–57, and (August 1922): 6, and *Strength* 5 (July 1920): 18–19 and 32.
9. *SH* 13 (January 1946): 12, and *Strength* 5 (October 1920): 3.
10. See Donald Meyer, "The Discovery of the 'Nervous American,' " in *The Positive Thinkers: A Study of the American Quest for Health, Wealth, and Personal Power from Mary Baker Eddy to Norman Vincent Peale* (Garden City, N.Y., 1965), 21–31.
11. *Strength* 7 (February 1923): 36 and 37, and *Strength* 11 (April 1926): 58.
12. George Jowett, *Key to Might and Muscle* (Philadelphia, 1926), 7–9; Charles Smith to the author, July 26, 1989; and *Iron Master*, August 1993, 27. For a more sympathetic view of Jowett, see *Iron Game History* 3 (December 1994): 23–24, and *Iron Game History* 4 (July 1995): 21.
13. Gottfried Schodl, "Just a Look Back," *Anniversary Magazin, 1880–1980*, n.d., 2; David Webster, *The Iron Game* (Irvine, Strathclyde, 1976), 31 and 74; and Gottfried Schodl, *The Lost Past* (Budapest, 1992), 42–47 and 74–76.
14. See Joan Paul, "The Health Reformers: George Barker Windship and Boston's Strength Seekers," *Journal of Sport History* 10 (winter 1983): 41–57, and Wortmann, "History of Modern American Weightlifting," 11.
15. David Webster, *Barbells and Beefcake* (Irvine, Strathclyde, 1979), 19–20; Coulter to Webster, letter fragment [1960s], Webster Papers, Irvine, Scotland; and *Strength* 2 (January 1917): 14–15.
16. *Strength* 5 (November 1920): 23–26; Jowett to Coulter, November 9, 1920, Coulter Papers, Todd-McLean Collection, University of Texas; *Health and Life* 1 (July 1922); and *Strength* 6 (August 1922): 53–54.
17. *Strength* 9 (November 1924): 8, and (December 1924): 39.
18. *Strength* 9 (November 1924): 30, and (December 1924): 39.
19. *Pittsburg Press*, July 25, 1920; *SH* 12 (November 1945): 36–37; and Hoffman, *Road to Super-Strength*, 23.
20. *Strength* 9 (November 1924): 31 and 33; *Health and Life* 2 (May 1923): 159 and 178; and *SH* 12 (November 1945): 38–40.
21. *Strength* 12 (August 1927): 53–54; *Strength* 13 (January 1928): 49–50, and (February 1928): 74; and Bob Hoffman, *Weight Lifting* (York, Pa., 1939), 25.

NOTES

22. *SH* 13 (January 1946): 11 and 12, and (March 1946): 37; *Strength* 4 (March 1917): 13; and Autobiography and Supplement of Robert Snyder Jr., Washington County Library, Hagerstown, Md., 56–57.

23. *SH* 13 (December 1945): 14, 39–43; (January 1946): 11–12; (February 1946): 11–13, 30–32; (March 1946): 12, 33–34; and (April 1946): 22.

24. *Strength* 14 (August 1929): 55 and 67; interview with Robert Knodle (Hagerstown, Md.); and *Outlook*, June 11, 1919, 252.

25. *Strength* 16 (August 1931): 67–68 and 70, and *Strength* 17 (June 1932): 27–28.

26. Interview with J. Hoffman; *SH* 29 (November 1961): 4; and *Philadelphia Record*, August 22, 1932.

27. *SH* 13 (March 1946): 34–35; *Strong Man* 1 (November 1931); *SH* 1 (November 1933): 10; and *SH* 8 (September 1941): 27.

28. *Correct Eating and Strength* 17 (March 1932): 19, 42, and 30–31, and (April 1932): 52–53.

29. Hoffman to Good, [1932], Good Papers, West Reading, Pa.

30. *Arena–Strength* 17 (June 1932): 26–27.

31. *Arena–Strength* 17 (August 1932): 27, and Hoffman to Good, April 23, 1932, Good Papers.

32. *Correct Eating and Strength* 16 (November 1931): 21.

CHAPTER 3

1. *SH* 6 (June 1938): 21, and *SH* 7 (December 1938): 43.
2. *SH* 14 (September 1946): 28, and *York Gazette Daily*, January 4, 1932.
3. *SH* 2 (January 1934): 10–11 and 13.
4. Hoffman, *Weight Lifting*, 19; Jowett to Coulter, December 14, 1932, Coulter Papers; and *SH* 1 (February 1933): 10.
5. *SH* 1 (January 1933): 20; (February 1933): 20–21; and (December 1932): 1.
6. *SH* 1 (March 1933): 2; (April 1933): 12; and (June 1933): 8.
7. *SH* 1 (May 1933): 21, and (August 1933): 17, 27, and 28; and *SH* 2 (January 1934): 19.
8. *SH* 14 (August 1946): 20, and *SH* 2 (December 1934): 24.
9. *SH* 14 (October 1946): 19, and *SH* 1 (December 1932): 9.
10. *SH* 1 (June 1933): 8; (January 1933): 23; (June 1933): 2; and (July 1933): 12.
11. Interview with Walter Good (West Reading, Pa.), and *SH* 1 (November 1933): 8 and 9.
12. *SH* 1 (December 1932): 8; *SH* 2 (October 1934): 8; *SH* 3 (September 1935): 65; and *SH* 2 (March 1934): 2.
13. *SH* 2 (April 1934): 12 and 29; *SH* 1 (January 1933): 10; and interview with John Grimek (York, Pa.).
14. *SH* 2 (January 1934): 13; *SH* 3 (February 1935): 31, 33, and 20–21.
15. *SH* 2 (January 1934): 11, and (November 1934): 19, 38–40; *SH* 3 (December 1934): 6–7; and *SH* 2 (September 1934): 20.
16. Interviews with Dave Mayor (Philadelphia) and Weldon Bullock (Creedmore, N.C.); and *SH* 3 (July 1935): 72.
17. *SH* 2 (October 1934): 23–24; Jowett to Coulter, March 20, 1935, Coulter Papers; and *SH* 3 (December 1934): 30.
18. Jowett to Coulter, October 16, 1935, Coulter Papers, and *SH* 4 (July 1936): 30.
19. *SH* 5 (December 1936): 4; Sales Records, *Strength & Health*, 1934–36, HP; *SH* 1 (November 1933): 2; (April 1933): 10; and (July 1933), 12.
20. *SH* 2 (November 1934): 24 and 31; (May 1934): 3; (June 1934): 20; and (February 1934).
21. *SH* 3 (December 1934): 10–11; (January 1935): 14; (March 1935): 18; and (June 1935): 66–67.

Notes

22. *SH* 3 (October 1935): 41 and 44; *Weightlifting USA* 8 (1990): 18; and interview with Terpak.

23. *SH* 3 (July 1935): 78, 18, and (November 1935): 21; *SH* 4 (May 1936): 20; and *SH* 3 (November 1935): 18.

24. Interview with Jim Messer (Morristown, Pa.); *SH* 3 (June 1935): 78–80, and (July 1935): 79; and *SH* 4 (February 1936): 16–17, and (April 1936): 29.

25. *SH* 4 (April 1936): 29–30; (June 1936): 30; (June 1936): 44; and (August 1936): 29.

26. *SH* 4 (October 1936): 39 and 41, and *SH* 5 (February 1937): 4.

27. Interviews with Terpak and Grimek; *SH* 4 (October 1936): 5; *Physical Training Notes* 2 (August 1936): 2 and 20–21; and *Mark Berry v. Robert Hoffman*, May 11, 1938, Court of Common Pleas of Philadelphia County, HP.

28. *SH* 4 (May 1936): 50; (July 1936): 11, 34; and (August 1936): 31.

29. Interview with Terpak; Venables to Ward, n. d., HP; *New Yorker*, January 3, 1942, 27; and *SH* 4 (July 1936): 34.

30. *SH* 5 (September 1937): 45, and (November 1937): 35 and 46; and interview with Mayor.

31. *SH* 4 (November 1936): 14–15 and 41–42.

32. *SH* 4 (January 1936): 43; interviews with Grimek, Mayor, Messer, and Joe Bowers (Baltimore); *SH* 4 (October 1936): 8–9, and (July 1936): 13; and *SH* 5 (January 1937): 32.

33. Interview with Morris; Coulter to Jowett, February 1, 1938, and Jowett to Coulter, February 8, 1968, Coulter Papers; *SH* 5 (June 1937): 32; and R. Hoffman to B. Hoffman, November 21, 1937, HP.

34. "Connie" to Hoffman, December 1, 1937, HP; *SH* 6 (July 1938): 50; and Hoffman to Tommy Kono, September 8, 1954, HP.

35. *SH* 4 (May 1936): 39; *SH* 5 (January 1937): 8–9; (May 1937): 8–9; and (November 1937): 36 and 48–49.

36. *SH* 5 (May 1937): 8–9; (August 1937): 9; and (October 1937): 40.

37. *SH* 5 (August 1937): 9; interview with John Terlazzo (York, Pa.); and *SH* 5 (August 1937): 10.

38. *SH* 5 (July 1937): 10, and (January 1937): 45 and 42.

39. *SH* 5 (August 1937): 46, and (June 1937): 29.

40. *SH* 4 (May 1936): 36 and 46; *SH* 6 (August 1938): 24; and Bob Hoffman, *Secrets of Strength and Development* (York, Pa., 1940), 208–16.

41. *SH* 6 (March 1938): 44, and (April 1938): 29 and 41; and Hooley Schell, Itemized Expense List, March 7, 1938, HP.

42. *SH* 5 (October 1937): 8 and 10.

43. *SH* 6 (April 1938): 21, and *Iron Game History* 2 (April 1992): 8.

44. *SH* 6 (July 1938): 28, 4, and (August 1938): 6; and *SH* 7 (February 1939): 22, and (April 1939): 32–33.

45. *SH* 6 (July 1938): 28, 4–6, 35; (August 1938), 5, 6; and (September 1938): 4–5.

46. *SH* 6 (November 1938): 6; and *SH* 7 (December 1938): 4, and (January 1939): 7.

47. Interview with Brenneman; Jowett to Coulter, February 7, 1939, Coulter Papers; and Hoffman to Sam Shipley, November 1, 1938, HP.

48. Cash Book, 1939–42; Daily Receipts Books, 1935–36; Monthly Summaries Book, 1938–41; and Check Stubs, February to April, 1939, HP.

49. *SH* 7 (March 1939): 25; (August 1939): 30; and (November 1939): 43.

CHAPTER 4

1. Cash Book, 1939–42, and Monthly Summaries Book, 1938–41, HP.

2. Interview with Mayor, and Bob Hoffman, *How to Be Strong, Healthy, and Happy* (York, Pa., 1938), 16–19.

3. Hoffman, *How to Be Strong, Healthy, and Happy*, 322, 337–38, and 377.

NOTES

4. Hoffman, *Weight Lifting,* 7 and 102, and idem, *Guide to Weight Lifting Competition* (York, Pa., 1940), 91.

5. Hoffman, *Secrets of Strength and Development,* 48, 55, 69, 74, and 136.

6. Hoffman, *Big Arms,* 66, 70, and 72, and idem, *The Big Chest Book* (York, Pa., 1941), 11, 37, and 56.

7. Bob Hoffman, *Your Sex Life Before Marriage* (York, Pa., 1939), 13, 27–28, 84, 130, 137, 154–55, 158, 187–88, and 93.

8. Bob Hoffman, *Successful-Happy Marriage* (York, Pa., 1945), 144, 172, 187, and 189; idem, *The High Protein Road to Better Nutrition* (York, Pa., 1940); and *Food and Life: Yearbook of Agriculture, 1939* (Washington, 1939), 6–34.

9. Cash Book, 1939–42, HP; *SH* 8 (December 1939): 11; American News Company Distribution List, June 1941, HP; and *SH* 8 (March 1940): 5.

10. *SH* 8 (January 1940): 23, 5, and 30; interview with Bill Curry (Opelika, Ala.); and *SH* 9 (March 1941): 52.

11. *SH* 8 (December 1939): 27 and 39; (June 1940): 30; and (April 1940): 29–30 and 64.

12. *SH* 9 (January 1941): 8; (February 1941): 9; (March 1941): 14; interview with Ketterman; and *SH* 10 (July 1942): 48.

13. *SH* 8 (June 1940): 20–21, and (July 1940): 30 and 48; and *SH* 9 (July 1941): 8 and 27.

14. *SH* 9 (July 1941): 38; *SH* 8 (August 1940): 24–25, 6, and 9.

15. Interview with Jack Elder (Kilgore, Tex.), and *SH* 9 (January 1941): 47.

16. *SH* 9 (June 1941): 20 and 41.

17. *SH* 8 (May 1940): 10; Rosetta to Bob Hoffman, March 30, 1942, HP; and *SH* 9 (January 1941): 28, and (May 1941): 26.

18. *SH* 9 (June 1941): 8, 10, and 22–23; Hoffman to Eugene Wettstone, July 24, 1941, and G. Grabeel to Hoffman, October 18, 1941, HP; and *SH* 9 (February 1941): 32 and 45.

19. *SH* 10 (December 1941): 30–31, 38; (January 1942): 8; and (February 1942): 31 and 48.

20. *SH* 10 (January 1942): 15; *SH* 11 (July 1943): 10; *SH* 12 (December 1943): 20; and interview with Ketterman.

21. *SH* 8 (October 1940): 3; (September 1940): 8; (November 1940): 9, 26–27, 44, 45, and 50.

22. *SH* 9 (April 1941): 46, and (October 1941): 3; and *SH* 10 (January 1942): 22.

23. *SH* 9 (September 1941): 28 and 36; *SH* 12 (June 1944): 21 and 36–37; and *SH* 13 (March 1945): 35.

24. *SH* 10 (December 1941): 15, 39, and 40.

25. Ibid., 18; *SH* 10 (January 1942): 10; and *Bob Hoffman's Simplified System of Barbell Training* (York, Pa., 1941), 5.

26. *SH* 10 (August 1942): 37; interview with Terpak; and *SH* 11 (April 1943): 17 and 36.

27. *SH* 11 (July 1943): 28, 39, and (February 1943): 22.

28. *SH* 10 (June 1942): 10; *SH* 11 (February 1943): 15; and Terpak to Tanny, June 4, 1942, HP.

29. *SH* 10 (June 1942): 4; Hoffman to Clinton Duffy, April 20, 1944, and General Correspondence, 1941–45, HP.

30. Hoffman to the War Production Board, January 12, 1942; Hoffman to Rothensies, April 30, 1942; Hoffman to Collector of Internal Revenue, October 8, 1942; and Hoffman to York County Selective Service Board, February 29, 1944, HP.

31. "Marietta Machine Shop and York Barbell Company," October 26, 1943; Employer's Tax Returns, 1943–45, HP; *SH* 11 (September 1943): 21; and *SH* 12 (December 1943): 22–23.

32. Cash Book, 1939–42, and Daily Receipts Books, 1942–45, HP; Hoffman to Sherrill, January 30, 1945, HP; and *SH* 13 (January 1945): 17.

33. *SH* 12 (October 1944): 3; Gottlieb to Hoffman, July 20, 1945, and Terlazzo to Terpak, February 3, 1945, HP; and *SH* 13 (July 1945): 20.

34. Hoffman to T. Harrity, June 5, 1944, and Terlazzo to Terpak, January 25, 1945, HP; and *SH* 13 (June 1945): 44.

35. *SH* 12 (December 1943): 20; (August 1944): 23; and (June 1944): 23.

Notes

36. Rosetta to Bob Hoffman, June 8, 1945, HP; Jowett to Coulter, December 24, 1967, and Coulter to Jowett, December 18, 1967, Coulter Papers.

37. *SH* 12 (March 1944): 33; P. Rasch to Hoffman, April 14, 1944, HP; Smith to the author, August 13, 1990; and Ross to Terpak, August 20, 1945, HP.

38. *SH* 13 (August 1945): 33; *SH* 9 (September 1941): 8; *SH* 13 (August 1945): 47; David Matlin to Hoffman, May, 1945, HP; and *SH* 13 (September 1945): 17 and 18.

39. *SH* 12 (August 1944): 39–40, and *SH* 13 (June 1945): 3 and 48.

40. Hoffman to E. Bolton, Regional Manager Compliance Division, 1944, HP, and *SH* 13 (August 1945): 48.

CHAPTER 5

1. *SH* 13 (October 1945): 17.

2. Bill Curry to Terpak, October 6, 1945; Falcon to Terlazzo, September 22, 1945; and "Weight Lifting Activities for the Year 1945," HP; *SH* 14 (January 1946): 20–21; Casper Pinkster to Terpak, November 5, 1945, and Irwin Rosee to Hoffman, October 28, 1947, HP.

3. Money Order Books, 1942–50; Terlazzo to Terpak, January 29, 1945; Tanny to Terpak, February 18, 1945, HP; and *SH* 23 (January 1955): 4.

4. Book Sales Records, HP; *Gazette and Daily*, December 6, 1945; and Bob Hoffman, *Broad Shoulders* (York, Pa., 1946), 30 and 7.

5. *SH* 14 (December 1945): 3; *SH* 16 (March 1948): 5; and Terlazzo to Terpak, December 2, 1945, HP.

6. Giardine to Hoffman, September 23, 1945, and Spellman to Hoffman, January 2, 1946, HP; and *SH* 14 (January 1946): 45–46, and (May 1946): 46–47.

7. *SH* 14 (December 1945): 12–13, 44, and (November 1946): 16.

8. *SH* 14 (July 1946): 24, 50, and (August 1946): 16–17; and *SH* 15 (December 1946): 14, 39, and 45.

9. *SH* 15 (April 1947): 3, and (October 1947): 10; *SH* 16 (December 1947): 25; and *Fortune* 35 (February 1947): 100 and 161.

10. *Your Physique* 8 (May 1947): 24–26 and 47.

11. Wayne, *Muscle Wars*, 112–14. For biographical information on Weider, see *Your Physique* 4 (October–November 1944); *Muscle Builder* 1 (August 1953): 34, 40, and 42; *Flex* 3 (June 1985): 3, 96, and 98; David Ferrell, "Joe Weider's Iron Grip on an Empire," *Los Angeles Times*, March 2, 1989; and William Moore's bibliography, "The Joe Weider/JWFC Bibliophiles."

12. Interview with Grimek, July 11, 1990; *SH* 47 (March 1979): 40; *SH* 14 (March 1946): 9; *Muscle Builder/Power*, August 1975, 26; *SH* 14 (November 1946): 21 and 41; and *SH* 15 (February 1947): 47.

13. Stagg to Terpak, March 10, 1947, and Yarick to Terpak, June 10, 1947, HP.

14. *Your Physique* 5 (December–January 1945–46): 23; *SH* 13 (October 1945): 14–15 and 40; *Your Physique* 5 (February–March 1946); and *SH* 14 (June 1946): 12–15 and 34–37.

15. *Your Physique* 6 (August 1946): 12–15.

16. *SH* 14 (June 1946): 5, and Elder to Terpak, June 21, 1946, HP.

17. *SH* 16 (March 1948), 5, 33, and 100; Hoffman to N. Grueber, December 31, 1946, HP; *SH* 16 (December 1947): 5; *SH* 15 (February 1947): 36 and 8.

18. *SH* 15 (January 1947): 4, 15, and (August 1947): 4; Stanko to Joseph Nadzier, June 17, 1946, HP; and *SH* 15 (November 1947): 33.

19. *SH* 15 (May 1947): 8, 9, and (October 1947): 11 and 12; *Iron Man* 7 (1947): 2; *SH* 16 (September 1948): 10–11, 30–33, and (October 1948): 21.

20. *SH* (October 1948): 7, and (November 1948), 28; interview with Spellman (Pensacola, Fla.); and *SH* 16 (January 1948): 29.

21. Terpak to Sepp Manger, May 1946, HP, and *SH* 16 (October 1948): 45.

NOTES

22. *SH* 15 (February 1947): 9; *SH* 14 (July 1946): 43; and *SH* 17 (December 1948): 46–47, and (January 1949): 22.

23. *SH* 16 (February 1948): 47; (May 1948): 8, 11; (October 1948): 10–11; and *SH* 15 (February 1947): 37.

24. *SH* 17 (January 1949): 17, 37; (May 1949): 28; and (March 1949): 12.

25. Interview with E. M. Orlick (Brandywine, Md.); *Your Physique* 9 (May 1948): 26–27 and 30; interview with Phyllis Jowett (Morrisburg, Ont.); and *Flex* 3 (June 1985): 50, 96, and 98.

26. *Your Physique* 5 (February–March 1946): 36, and (December–January 1945–46): 10; and interviews with Orlick and Louis DeMarco (Courtland, Ohio).

27. *Your Physique* 10 (November 1949): 11 and 32, and (May 1950): 10.

28. *SH* 17 (January 1949): 21; *SH* 18 (January 1950): 3; (March 1950): 15, 30–31; and (March 1950): 13 and 28.

29. Meagher to Hoffman, July 2, 1947; Bradford to Hoffman, February 12, 1948; Grant to Hoffman, March 10, 1948; and Leslie to Hoffman, May 9, 1949, HP.

30. *SH* 18 (March 1950): 10–11; Joe Barker to Hoffman, December 27, 1949, HP; *SH* 19 (August 1951): 23; and *SH* 18 (May–June 1950): 40.

31. *SH* 18 (August 1950): 32; Hoffman to Barker, February 20, 1950, HP; and *SH* 17 (August 1949): 19.

32. *SH* 18 (October 1950): 19 and 40–41.

33. Hoffman to A. Yarick, January 10, 1949; Glen Waring to Hoffman, April 8, 1949; Bill Howe to Hoffman, August 8, 1949; and Hoffman to Tanny, January 19, 1949, HP.

34. *SH* 16 (March 1948): 5; *SH* 19 (December 1950): 3 and 11; and *Your Physique* 9 (May 1948): 5. York even started using the same printer as Weider, near Washington. Van Cleef to Alton Eliason, October 27, 1950, Eliason/Van Cleef Papers, Todd-McLean Collection.

35. *Gazette and Daily,* September 28, 1946, 4; Suits to Hoffman, July 16, 1948; Albert Seica to Hoffman, March 20, 1953; C. H. McCloy to Terpak, June 27, 1947; James Nesbitt to Hoffman, January 2, 1951; Phil Whiteman to Hoffman, June 6, 1953; and Kaprelion to Hoffman, November 25, 1947, HP.

36. Gerald Nagler to Hoffman, February 12, 1948, and Oscar Hostetter to Hoffman, March 29, 1948, HP; *Lufkin News,* June 4, 1947; *El Dorado Times,* March 30, 1947; *Saturday Evening Post,* July 3, 1948, 27; and Gerald Travis to Hoffman, May 1, 1953, HP.

37. *SH* 16 (March 1948): 41; *SH* 18 (October 1950): 36; and *Iron Man* 46 (September 1987): 71.

38. *SH* 19 (January 1951): 48–49, and (February 1951): 9.

39. *SH* 19 (March 1951): 3 and 5; *SH* 20 (January 1952): 5 and 49; interview with Spellman; and *SH* 20 (October 1952): 12.

40. *SH* 20 (October 1952): 5; Money Order Books, 1946–54; Book Sales Records, "September 29, 1948, Accounts Receivable"; "York Precision Company, Recapitulation of Accounts Receivable," May 1, 1949, to November 30, 1949; "Statement, Epstein and Sons," September 1, 1950; "Attachment to Credit Statement, May 1, 1951," and "Robert C. Hoffman, Statements of Financial Condition," 1950–52, HP; and interview with Spellman.

41. Van Cleef to Alton Eliason, October 27, 1948, Eliason/Van Cleef Papers; interview with Jim Murray (Morrisville, Pa.); *SH* 19 (April 1951): 5; interviews with Jules Bacon (York, Pa.), Jim Park (Ripley, W.V.), and John Terpak; and Smith to the author, October 10, 1986.

42. Interview with Dick Bachtell (York, Pa.).

43. Hoffman to Venables, January 23, 1946, and May 29, 1950, HP; interview with Murray; and *Your Physique* 15 (June 1951): 28, 30, and 45–47.

44. Sheppard to Houston, April 2, 1953, HP; *York Dispatch* and *Gazette and Daily,* April 25 and May 4, 1953; *SH* 17 (January 1949): 25; and *SH* 22 (January 1954): 42.

45. S. A. Snell to Hoffman, November 6, 1948, and Grabeel to Grimek, July 8, 1947, HP; and interviews with Murray and Park.

46. Interview with Murray; *Your Physique* 16 (November 1951): 7–9 and 30–34; and *SH* 19 (July 1951): 9 and 46.

Notes

47. *Your Physique* 16 (February 1952): 7, 46, and 47; *SH* 20 (December 1951): 35; *SH* 19 (October 1951): 10; *SH* 20 (November 1952): 25; and *Iron Game History* 1 (March 1991): 19.
48. Interview with Murray.
49. *SH* 20 (June 1952): 27 and 48, and *SH* 21 (January 1953): 15.
50. *SH* 20 (November 1952): 46, 48, and (February 1952): 28; *Muscle Power* 15 (June 1953): 38; *SH* 21 (September 1953): 43; and *SH* 22 (December 1953): 10–11 and 42.
51. *SH* 22 (November 1954): 3–4, and *SH* 23 (December 1954): 37.
52. *SH* 20 (September 1952): 30, and *SH* 19 (April 1951): 5.
53. Interview with Murray; Hoffman to Kono, September 6, 1954, HP; and *SH* 19 (September 1951): 5.
54. *SH* 20 (December 1951): 38; *SH* 21 (October 1953): 61–62; and *SH* 20 (November 1952): 17.
55. Terlazzo to Terpak, February 14, March 11, and April 18, 1953; Yacos to Terpak, April 20, 1953; and Hoffman to Don Kedney, Noah Williams, and M. G. Marsh, November 18, 1954, HP.
56. *SH* 22 (December 1953): 58 and 60, and *SH* 23 (December 1954): 60–61 and 64.
57. *SH* 23 (February 1955): 60–61; interview with Joe Pitman (Jacksonville, Fla.); *SH* 21 (May 1953): 33 and 58; and "Show Time Is Here Again," January 1953, HP.
58. *SH* 22 (October 1954): 28; *SH* 21 (April 1953): 38; *SH* 23 (February 1955): 39 and 34–35.
59. *SH* 22 (March 1954): 26.

CHAPTER 6

1. *SH* 22 (March 1954): 39, and (May 1954): 37; and interview with Jim George (Akron, Ohio).
2. *SH* 15 (January 1947); *SH* 24 (July 1956): 17; and *SH* 23 (February 1955): 61, and (January 1955): 34–35.
3. *Washington Daily News,* November 1, 1954, 30; *Sports Illustrated,* August 1, 1983, 66; and Bob Goldman, *Death in the Locker Room: Steroids and Sports* (South Bend, Ind., 1984), 1.
4. "Professional Biography of John Bosley Ziegler, M.D., " Ziegler Papers, Olney, Md.; *SH* 23 (October 1955): 44–45; Bill St. John, "Dr. John B. Ziegler" (typescript in the author's possession); and interview with John Grimek (York, Pa.).
5. B. Jeffs to Grimek, January 27, 1943, and Grimek to Ziegler, August 25, 1954, Ziegler Papers; Grimek to the author, February 15, 1990; and interview with Park.
6. *SH* 24 (May 1956): 44; *Weightlifting USA* 8 (1990): 14; and *SH* 24 (April 1956): 47, and (January 1956), 60.
7. Paul Anderson, *The World's Strongest Man* (Wheaton, Ill., 1975), 40; *SH* 23 (September 1955): 52–53; *Sport* 21 (June 1956): 86; and Norris McWhirter and Ross McWhirter, *The Guiness Book of Records* (London, 1973), 335. On the credibility of Anderson's lifts, see the debate between Bob Hise and Steve Neece in *Musclemag International* (July 1992), 137–45.
8. Anderson to the author, March 31, 1986; *SH* 23 (September 1955): 26; and *SH* 24 (March 1956): 7; (February 1956): 4; and (July 1956): 55.
9. *SH* 25 (January 1957): 10, and *SH* 26 (July 1958): 60.
10. *SH* 23 (October 1955): 61; *SH* 24 (January 1956): 49–51, and (December 1955): 66; and interview with George.
11. Interviews with George, Morris, and Ketterman; "Notice to Property Owners of New Assessment," June 11, 1956, and "Payment for Rosetta Morris," [1960], HP.
12. *SH* 24 (July 1956): 53, and (January 1956): 42; *Asahi Evening News,* June 9, 1961; interview with Dellinger (York, Pa.); and *SH* 24 (April 1956): 3.

NOTES

13. Jim Murray, *Winning Weight Training* (Chicago, 1982), xi; *SH* 24 (December 1955): 34–35; and *SH* 25 (March 1957): 9. For references to female athletes who trained with weights, see *Iron Game History* 2 (April 1992): 10–12.

14. Bob Hoffman, *Better Athletes* (York, Pa., 1959), 5, 21, and 349–52; Walter Camp, *The Daily Dozen* (New York, 1925), 27–34; and *SH* 28 (December 1959): 4.

15. Interview with Murray, and Murray to the author, August 26, 1987.

16. Murray to the author, August 26, 1987, and *SH* 24 (January 1956): 26 and 60.

17. *SH* 23 (February 1955): 49; *SH* 25 (June 1957): 56; Hoffman to Ed Jubinville, March 20, 1958, HP.

18. *SH* 26 (January 1958): 64–65, and (February 1958): 10–11; Hoffman to Matlin, July 29, 1958, HP; and interview with Terpak.

19. Hoffman to Matlin, September 30, 1957, HP; *SH* 27 (July 1959): 14–15, 60, and 4; interview with Ketterman; *SH* 27 (September 1959): 6; and Hoffman to Ackerman, November 16, 1958, HP.

20. *Iron Game History* 3 (September 1993): 18; *SH* 27 (April 1959): 44; and *SH* 28 (May 1960): 64.

21. *SH* 23 (May 1955): 42 and 44; Thomas D. Baxter to Hoffman, January 17, 1955, HP; Robert H. Griffith to Dietz, May 16, June 13, and June 25, 1956; Griffith to Hoffman, August 10, 1955, HP; interview with Park; and *SH* 23 (April 1955): 12.

22. Money Order Books and Book Sales Records, 1953–58; Financial Statements, 1958–63, HP; *SH* 25 (October 1957): 6; interview with Dick Smith (York, Pa.); and Hoffman to Ben Kahan, November 4, 1957, and Hoffman to Jowett, March 5, 1958, HP.

23. *SH* 25 (October 1957): 6–9; J. Hoffman to B. Hoffman, July 22, 1958, and Maurice Shefferman to Hoffman, March 1957, HP; and interviews with Starr (Forest Hill, Md.), Terpak, and Clarence Johnson (Baton Rouge, La.).

24. Interviews with Ketterman, Starr, Terpak, Day, Smith, and Murray; General Journal, December 31, 1957, and Winston Day to Hoffman, May 8, 1957, HP; and *SH* 14 (June 1946): 5.

25. Interviews with Terpak and Mayor; *SH* 26 (May 1958): 45; *SH* 25 (February 1957): 49, and (May 1957): 55; *SH* 27 (June 1959): 62; *SH* 28 (August 1960): 64; and interview with Bacon.

26. Jowett to Coulter, n.d., Coulter Papers, and Morris to Hoffman, October 11, 1957, HP.

27. Eleanor Pedano to Hoffman, n.d., and B. Hoffman to Rosetta Morris and C. Hoffman, n.d., HP; and interview with Smith.

28. Hoffman to Director of Internal Revenue, May 4, 1959; Hoffman to Markowitz, March 3, 1960; Markowitz to Hoffman, March 28, 1960; and Tax Court Memo 1960-160, Docket No. 64405, 925–40, HP.

29. *Mr. America* 1 (January 1958): 28–29; (February 1958): 33 and 52–54; and (March 1958): 16–17.

30. George to Hoffman, January 20, 1958, HP; *SH* 25 (June 1958): 3–4, and (November 1958): 42–43; *Weider v. Hoffman*, U.S. Middle District Court of Pennsylvania, February 4, 1965, HP; and Terpak to the author, May 8, 1991.

31. Hunter McLean to Hoffman, January 25, 1957; Lee Lamascus to Hoffman, February 14, 1958; Robert Barnett to Hoffman, June 17, 1959; Barrs to Hoffman, October 10, 1960, HP; *SH* 26 (October 1958): 53; and Liederman to Hoffman, March 12, 1959, HP.

32. Alfred Albelli, "2 Bodies Beautiful Linked in Wife Suit," *Daily News*, January 6, 1960.

33. Joseph Puntel to Dietz, April 3, 1956; Bopp to Hoffman, September 20, 1958; Akin to Hoffman, May 14, 1959; Hoffman to Akin, May 18, 1959; Pierson to Hoffman, September 11, 1959; and Hoffman to Mrs. Roy Seymour, April 7, 1960, HP.

34. Charles Snellstrom to Hoffman, July 13, and Hoffman to Snellstrom, July 23, 1957; Bates to Hoffman, November 6, and Hoffman to Bates, November 9, 1958; Myers to Hoffman, March 25, 1958; and John Murray to Terpak, September 19, 1958, HP.

35. Levin to Hoffman, June 2 and 20, 1958, HP.

Notes

36. Jones to Hoffman, July 1, 1960; Greene to Hoffman, May 2, 1956; Avant to Hoffman, March 3, 1957; Lord to Hoffman, June 10, 1957; Beaudoin to Hoffman, June 27, 1957; Loar to Hoffman, July 26, 1957; Sciaroni to Hoffman, May 5, 1959; and Crow to Hoffman, July 11, 1956, HP.

37. Edwin Resser to Hoffman, October 30, 1959; Hoffman to Matlin, February 15, 1959; Alan O'Brien to Hoffman, January 10, 1961, HP; interview with Terpak; You to Hoffman, July 14, 1960, HP; *SH* 26 (June 1958): 27; Jowett to Hoffman, "General," n.d., and March 10, 1958; Hoffman to Jowett, March 5, 1958; Sylverst to Hoffman, May 24, 1958; Edgar Snow to Hoffman, January 23, 1961; and Hoffman to Snow, February 6, 1961, HP.

38. Hoffman to Rosee, March 3 and 20, 1958, HP; *SH* 26 (February 1958): 56; *Bob Hoffman's Daily Dozen* (York, Pa., 1958); *SH* 26 (August 1958): 27 and 42; and *York Dispatch*, April 12, 1958.

39. Hoffman to Shane McCarthy, November 3, 1958, HP; *SH* 25 (July 1957): 49; *SH* 27 (July 1959): 26; Jerome Gorman to Hoffman, April 23, 1960, HP; and *SH* 28 (October 1960): 48.

40. Hoffman to Ferris and Hoffman to Bushnell, September 30, 1957; Hoffman to McCarthy, December 13, 1957; Hoffman, "The York Plan for Physical Fitness"; Hoffman to Dean Markham, May 28, 1961, HP; *Honolulu Star-Bulletin*, June 20, 1961; *SH* 29 (December 1960): 62; and Rome Olympics diary, HP.

41. David Mercer to James Simms, July 29, 1959; newspaper clipping titled "Strong Man Cited in Morals Case"; Hoffman to Berger, n.d., HP; *SH* 24 (September 1956): 49; Hoffman to Kono, February 24, 1959; "This Is Olympic Year," [1960], HP; and *SH* 28 (August 1960): 4.

42. *SH* 27 (May 1959): 4; *SH* 24 (September 1956): 49–50; *Lifting News* 7 (July 1960): 3; and Hoffman, *Better Athletes*, 307.

43. *SH* 27 (February 1959): 22; *SH* 28 (March 1960): 4; (July 1960): 4 and 6; (September 1960): 3, 4, and 43; and (March 1960): 54.

44. *Lifting News* 7 (July 1960): 1; *SH* 29 (January 1961): 19 and 56, and (February 1961): 43.

45. Hoffman to Harold Zimman, November 18, 1957, HP; *SH* 27 (January 1959): 6; and *SH* 29 (January 1961): 13.

46. *SH* 25 (December 1956): 26.

CHAPTER 7

1. *SH* 28 (January 1960): 24.

2. Bob Hoffman, *You Can Live Longer, 10–20–30 Years Longer* (York, Pa., 1960), 61–62 and 65–66.

3. Interview with Terpak, and Bob Hoffman, *Old Age Is a Slow Starvation* (York, Pa., 1960), 27 and 34.

4. Bob Hoffman, *The Protein Story* (York, Pa., 1960); idem, *Protein-Building Blocks of Life* (York, Pa., 1962); and idem, *High Protein Recipe Book* (York, Pa., n.d.). See Frederick Stare, ed., *Protein Nutrition* (New York, 1958).

5. *SH* 29 (November 1961): 30–33, and Bob Hoffman, *Functional Isometric Contraction* (York, Pa., 1962), 63, 23–26, 12, 35, 44 and 41.

6. Hoffman, *Functional Isometric Contraction*, 47; Ziegler to Grimek, January 22, 1959, Ziegler Papers; *SH* 27 (September 1959): 24–25; interview with Bill March (York, Pa.); and *SH* 29 (November 1961): 30–31.

7. Charles Kochakian, *How It Was: Anabolic Action of Steroids and Remembrances* (Birmingham, Ala., 1984), and interview with Charles Kochakian (Birmingham, Ala.)

8. Grimek to the author, February 15, 1990; Grimek to Ziegler, Wed. pm [May 11, 1960]; Grimek to Ziegler, n.d. [late June 1960], Ziegler Papers; and *SH* 44 (December 1966): 43. Garcy now admits that effects of the steroids were "immediately noticeable," but everything he said about Kono's mental coaching was true. Interview with Tony Garcy (Chicago, Ill.).

9. Grimek to Ziegler, September 7 and 15, 1960, Ziegler Papers.

NOTES

10. *SH* 32 (January 1964): 20–21; interview with Riecke (April 29, 1989, Harahan, La.); "In Flight" note, November 18, 1960, Riecke Papers, Harahan, La.; *SH* 30 (April 1962): 3; and *SH* 35 (October 1967): 9. See also *True* 48 (April 1967): 8.

11. Ziegler to Riecke, January 3 and 25 and February 1, 1961, Riecke Papers; *SH* 29 (May 1961): 27; and Riecke to Ziegler, February 5, 1961, Ziegler Papers.

12. Hoffman to Kono, April 26, 1961, HP, and interview with Riecke.

13. *SH* 29 (October 1961): 53, and *Sports Illustrated*, October 30, 1961, 19–21.

14. Interviews with March, Riecke, and George.

15. Drury to Hoffman, January 8, 1962; Goostree to Hoffman, January 29, 1962; Olson to Hoffman, July 16, 1962; Rasmusson to Hoffman, February 13, 1962; Stoller to Hoffman, February 16, 1962; Dreher to Hoffman, March 9, 1962; Stamp to Hoffman, May 9, 1962; Partridge to Hoffman, July 8, 1962; Warner to Hoffman, April 18, 1963; and Newton to Hoffman, March 24, 1963, HP.

16. *SH* 29 (November 1961): 42; *SH* 30 (June 1962): 28; *SH* 31 (July 1963): 66, and (December 1963), 34; *SH* 35 (October 1967): 34; and *SH* 34 (June 1966), 8.

17. *SH* 31 (December 1962): 42–44; *SH* 32 (December 1963): 8; and *SH* 30 (November 1962): 6.

18. *SH* 32 (December 1963): 8; *SH* 35 (July 1967): 44; *SH* 32 (March 1964): 81; *SH* 30 (January 1962): 45; and James Blake to Hoffman, July 27, 1961, and H. Hiroishi to Hoffman, November 6, 1964, HP.

19. *SH* 31(October 1963): 8, and (April 1963): 18; and *SH* 30 (October 1962): 19.

20. *Scholastic Coach* 32 (October 1962), and *Sports Illustrated*, March 12, 1962, 50–53.

21. *SH* 31 (December 1962): 44; Klein to Hoffman, November 20, 1962, HP; and Terry Todd, "Karl Klein and the Squat," *NSCA Journal*, June–July 1984, 28–29 and 67.

22. Rasch to Terpak, with draft article, December 19, 1961; Hoffman to Rasch, December 27, 1961; Rasch to Hoffman, January 2, 1962; McCabe to Hoffman, July 1, 1963; and Long to Hoffman, August 29, 1967, HP.

23. Davis to Hoffman, October 20, 1963, and Drury to Hoffman, June 24, 1963, HP; and Rieger to the author, January 21, 1994.

24. *SH* 29 (November 1961): 18; Monthly Financial Statements, 1960–67; "Thomasville Inn, Statement of Income and Expense at August 31, 1967," HP; and Board of Directors Minutes, June 8, 1965, York Barbell Company Files.

25. Elledge to Hoffman, July 10, 1962, and Hoffman to Low, June 20, 1963, HP; and interview with Terpak.

26. Walter to Hoffman, November 24, 1961; Rexroad to Hoffman, January 17, 1965; Abels to Hoffman, May 19, 1962; Corlman to Hoffman, May 20, 1962; and Miller to Hoffman, September 2, 1962, HP.

27. Hasse to Murray, February 4, 1964, Murray Papers, Morrisville, Pa., and *SH* 33 (March 1965): 7.

28. *SH* 32 (September 1964): 57; *Muscular Development* (hereafter *MD*) 2 (March 1965): 8; *SH* 33 (August 1965): 5 and 9; and *SH* 32 (October 1964): 60 and 62.

29. *SH* 33 (January 1965): 25.

30. *SH* 31 (November 1963): 9; *SH* 33 (October 1965): 15; (November 1965): 60–61; and (April 1965): 9. Modeled on the ideas of J.C. Hise and style of McCallum is Randall J. Strossen's *Super Squats: How to Gain Thirty Pounds of Muscle in Six Weeks* (Larkspur, Calif., 1989).

31. *SH* 33 (August 1965): 5, and (June 1965): 29–30 and 71; Todd to Hoffman and Terpak, n.d., HP; and *SH* 33 (January 1965): 78, and (October 1965): 76.

32. *SH* 33 (August 1965): 5 and 9; *MD* 3 (March 1966): 26–27; *SH* 33 (July 1965): 16–17 and 68; and *MD* 2 (March 1965): 27.

33. *SH* 32 (December 1963): 15; *MD* 1 (January 1964): 5; and *MD* 2 (February 1965): 7.

34. *SH* 31 (May 1963): 56–57; (May 1963): 6 and 60–61; and (October 1963): 26 and 65; and *SH* 33 (March 1965): 7.

35. *SH* 29 (October 1961): 16; Wayne, *Muscle Wars*, 40; *SH* 31 (October 1963): 62–63; and *SH* 32 (December 1963): 11, and (November 1963): 11.

Notes

36. Webster, *Barbells and Beefcake*, 107, and Wayne, *Muscle Wars*, 96.
37. *SH* 31 (August 1963): 15, and interview with Norbert Schemansky (Livonia, Mich.).
38. Interview with Joe Puleo (Livonia, Mich.).
39. Interview with Garcy; *SH* 34 (September 1966): 75; and *SH* 35 (September 1967): 70.
40. Interviews with Bill March (York, Pa.) and Gary Glenney (Livonia, Mich.).
41. *SH* 30 (March 1962): 26, and interviews with John Terlazzo (York, Pa.) and Smith; and *SH* 38 (June 1970): 44.
42. *SH* 31 (July 1963): 60, and (October 1963): 16.
43. Anderson to Hoffman, February 7, 1962, HP; *SH* 32 (August 1964): 14–15 and 8–9; *SH* 33 (October 1965): 5; and *SH* 34 (December 1965): 9.
44. *SH* 34 (March 1965): 9; D. P. Boyd to Corbett, March 8, 1965; Hoffman to Lahey Clinic Foundation, March 16, 1965; "1965 National Convention, Natural Food Associates," April 21–24, 1965, HP; and *MD* 2 (May 1965): 36.
45. Notes by Hoffman and Kimble to Ziegler, August 21, 1965, HP; *SH* 34 (April 1966): 7 and 9; Corbett to Hoffman, March 22, 1966, and Sidney Alexander to Hoffman, May 10, 1966, HP; interview with Clarence Johnson; and *SH* 34 (February 1966): 7, and (March 1966): 75.
46. *SH* 32 (September 1964): 33; *SH* 33 (July 1965): 7; *SH* 34 (August 1966): 5; *Muscle Training Illustrated* 2 (November–December 1966): 33; and *SH* 34 (April 1966): 7.
47. Interview with Tommy Kono (Baton Rouge, La.); You to Hoffman, January 11, 1966, and "Plan," June 17, 1965, HP; *MD* 1 (October 1964): 45; Ziegler to Hoffman and Terpak, December 2, 1965; copy of York contract, n.d.; and Ziegler to Hoffman, September 8, 1966, Ziegler Papers.
48. *SH* 32 (March 1964): 34–35; Bishop to Hoffman, February 20, and Fronheiser to Hoffman, February 23, 1964, HP; and *SH* 35 (April 1967): 5 and 8.
49. *SH* 35 (September 1967): 28; *MD* 1 (December 1964): 60; interview with Smith; *Sports Illustrated*, June 23, 1969, 70; and *SH* 35 (January 1967): 23.
50. Interviews with Terpak, Starr, Smith, Smith and Ketterman, Terry Todd (Austin, Tex.), and Tommy Suggs (Freeport, Tex.); and Wages Paid in Editorial Department, December 31, 1985, HP.
51. Ziegler to Sablo, November 29, and Sablo to George Thornber, December 1, 1965, HP; and interviews with Smith, Terpak, and Todd.
52. Interviews with Smith and Ketterman, Terpak, Todd (Hanks), and Todd. Ellen Todd (Hanks) confirms that both she and Terry were shocked by Ziegler's letter, that Terry did not have high blood pressure, and that his appeals to the AAU went unanswered. Interview with Todd (Hanks) (Boerne, Tex.).
53. Interview with Starr; *SH* 34 (June 1966): 22; and *SH* 35 (May 1967): 34–35.
54. *SH* 35 (March 1967): 20; (September 1967): 72; and (October 1967): 61 and 29.
55. *SH* 35 (June 1967): 74; (August 1967): 62; (September 1967): 74; and (June 1967): 24–25.
56. Interview with Starr; *SH* 35 (June 1967): 30 and 67; *SH* 34 (January 1966): 81, and (June 1966): 77; *SH* 35 (March 1967): 5, and (April 1967): 71.
57. Interview with Garcy; *SH* 32 (February 1964): 5, and interviews with Johnson and Starr.

CHAPTER 8

1. *SH* 39 (May–June 1971): 9.
2. *SH* 35 (November 1967): 80, 26, 67, 28, and 31.
3. *SH* 35 (December 1967): 24–25, and (November 1967): 9; and *SH* 36 (January 1968): 24, 64, 68, and (February 1968): 68.
4. *SH* 36 (February 1968): 77 and 72.

5. *SH* 36 (June 1968): 62, and (July 1968): 69; *SH* 37 (April 1969): 35; and interview with Starr.

6. Reed to Hoffman, May 28, 1968, HP, and *SH* 36 (March 1968): 61.

7. Interview with Day, and *SH* 36 (February 1968): 7.

8. *SH* 37 (April 1969): 77; "Park Property Transfer Ceremony and Dinner," January 9, 1969, HP; and *Congressional Record,* 110th Cong., 1st sess., House, January 9, 1969, 115, 91–1.

9. Monthly Financial Statements, 1966–72, and Terpak to Maurice Samsel, March 23, 1971, HP; and *SH* 36 (July 1968): 7–8, and (May 1968): 7.

10. Bob Hoffman, *Running for Your Life* (York, Pa., 1967), 7, 87–89, 83, and 80, and *SH* 36 (April 1968): 42.

11. *SH* 36 (April 1968): 94; Bob Hoffman, *Strength, Energy, and Endurance* (York, Pa., 1967), 129–30; and idem, *Reducing and Weight Control* (York, Pa., 1967), 67.

12. Bob Hoffman, *How to Gain Weight* (York, Pa., 1967), 15–16; idem, *Reducing and Weight Control,* 19 and 10; and *SH* 36 (December 1968): 12.

13. Bob Hoffman, *Drink More Water* (York, Pa., 1970), 7–10, 61, and 123.

14. Ibid., 13; Arnold Lorand, *Health and Longevity Through Rational Diet* (Philadelphia, 1913), 80, 78, 91, and 318; and interview with Day.

15. Interview with Starr; *SH* 36 (October 1968): 69, 36, and (November 1968): 57.

16. *SH* 36 (May 1968): 9; (July 1968): 40; and (August 1968): 69–70.

17. *SH* 36 (September 1968): 24 and 62; Yuri Brokhin, "Bednarski" (typescript in author's possession); *MD* 7 (March 1970): 50; and *SH* 36 (August 1968): 43.

18. *SH* 36 (October 1968): 35, and *MD* 5 (July 1968): 53.

19. *SH* 36 (June 1968): 54; (October 1968): 69; and (November 1968): 71–72.

20. *SH* 36 (September 1968): 12, and (October 1968): 47 and 7–8; *MD* 5 (October 1968): 58; interviews with Fred Lowe (Livonia, Mich.); Ketterman; and Starr; *MD* 5 (August 1968): 5.

21. *SH* 36 (November 1968): 76–78; *SH* 37 (January 1969): 12; *SH* 36 (March 1968): 53; and *SH* 37 (January 1969): 76, and (April 1969): 33.

22. *SH* 37 (April 1969): 18 and 55; interview with Glenney; *SH* 37 (February 1969): 5, 7, 61, and 32; and *MD* 6 (February 1969): 28.

23. Interviews with Starr and Glenney.

24. *MD* 5 (December 1968): 53; *MD* 6 (January 1969): 52; and *SH* 37 (February 1969): 55.

25. *MD* 8 (January 1971): 32 and 6. On Schwarzenegger's connections with Weider, see Wendy Leigh, *Arnold: An Unauthorized Autobiography* (Chicago, 1990), 67–95. York also failed to acquire Lou Ferrigno, later star of television's *Incredible Hulk,* despite his desire for "an exclusive tie-in with York." Irwin Rosee to Hoffman, March 3, 1976, HP.

26. Terpak to Rader, January 28, 1970, HP, and *MD* 8 (February 1971): 53–54, and (March 1971): 63.

27. *Muscle Builder* 12 (1971): 37, and Levin to Terpak, December 9, and Terpak to Levin, December 23, 1971, HP.

28. *SH* 38 (November 1970): 35 and 69.

29. Bernard Brown to Solomon Friend, with "Consent Decree of Permanent Injunction," May 31, 1968; telephone conversation between Friend and Terpak, October 15, 1968; Friend to Hoffman, November 20, 1968; and Friend to Brown, with "Consent Decree of Permanent Injunction," HP.

30. Bates to Hoffman, April 17, 1968; Bendel to Hoffman, 1970; Echternacht to Hoffman, July 1, 1969; Sathyanarayana to Hoffman, October 4, 1970; Duncan to Hoffman, March 21, 1968; Baxter to Hoffman, July 8, 1969; Seeman to Hoffman, May 15, 1970; Gans to Hoffman, January 7, 1969; and Allan to Hoffman, October 6, 1970, HP.

31. Miller to Terpak, February 4, 1970; R. Miller to Hoffman, August 9, 1970; Babinsky to Hoffman, August 26, 1970, HP; interviews with Bednarski (Springfield, Mass.) and Bacon; and Penta to Hoffman, December 9, 1970, HP.

32. E. T. to Hoffman, August 12, 1970; Ford to Hoffman, August 10, 1970; Evanich to

Notes

Hoffman, November 21, 1970; and Anonymous to Hoffman, December 7 and August 7, 1969, HP.

33. M. Schillo to Hoffman, April 2, 1968; G. MacDonald to Hoffman, February 16, 1970; Richard Reeser to Hoffman, March 3, 1970; Hal Marshall Jr. to Hoffman, October 7, 1970; Williams to Hoffman, 1970; and Feldmann to Hoffman, November 16, 1971, HP.

34. *SH* 15 (June 1947): 8; interview with Bachtell; John Kelly to Hoffman, November 13, 1970; James Lorimer to Hoffman, October 27, 1970; Ray Miller to Hoffman, April 20, 1971; Hoffman to John Stanczak, January 5, 1971; and Ashack Ahmad Sha to Hoffman, March 4, 1971, HP.

35. Morris to Hoffman, August 6, 1970, HP; *Iron Game History* 3 (September 1993): 20; and interview with Day.

36. Kono to Terpak, October 13 and 20, 1971, HP, and interview with Kono.

37. Interviews with Bednarski and Terpak, and Brokhin, "Bednarski."

38. Brokhin, "Bednarski," and interviews with Bednarski and Starr.

39. Interviews with Bednarski, Starr, and Terpak, and Brokhin, "Bednarski."

40. Interviews with DeMarco, Bednarski, John Coffee (Marietta, Ga.), Ketterman, Levin, March, Petersen, Starr, Terpak, and Warner.

41. Brokhin, "Bednarski"; and interview with Starr.

42. *SH* 37 (August 1969): 68; interview with Bednarski; and Brokhin, "Bednarski."

43. *SH* 38 (February 1970): 16–17, and (January 1970): 81 and 16.

44. *SH* 38 (September 1970): 49; (November 1970): 10; and (December 1970): 80 and 20.

45. *SH* 38 (September 1970): 44; (October 1970): 69; (December 1970): 26 and 28; interview with Bednarski; and *SH* 38 (December 1970): 75, and (November 1970), 12.

46. *MD* 6 (June 1969): 5, and *SH* 38 (January 1970): 67.

47. *SH* 38 (June 1970): 10, 28, and (September 1970): 46; Rawluk to Terpak, November 4, 1970, HP; *Weightlifting Journal* 1 (June 1972): 21; and Levin to Terpak, September 22, 1970, HP.

48. *SH* 38 (October 1970): 5, 7, and (November 1970): 7; Whitcomb to Hoffman, October 4, 1969, HP; and *SH* 39 (January 1971): 75–76.

49. Interviews with Terpak and Starr; *SH* 38 (February 1970): 75; (March 1970): 52; (October 1970): 68; (July 1970): 67; and (December 1970): 74.

50. Interviews with Starr, Terpak, Bednarski, and Yolanda Crist (Hampton, Va.).

51. *SH* 39 (February 1971): 89, 54–55, and 68–69.

52. *SH* 39 (May–June 1971): 8; (July 1971): 79; (May–June 1971): 9; (August 1971): 8; (April 1971): 32–33 and 65–66; and (May–June 1971): 11; and Levin to Terpak, n.d., HP.

53. Stevens to Viator, with attachments, October 19, 1971, HP. Viator insists, however, that he later returned the $250 to Stevens. Interview with Viator (Marietta, Ga.).

54. *SH* 39 (August 1971): 38, 73, and (November 1971): 5; and Holbrook to Hoffman, May 22, and Terpak to Kenji Onuma, September 14, 1971, HP.

55. Morris Weissbrot, "An Open Letter to George Lugrin," July 9, 1971, HP; *MD* 8 (April 1971): 43, (July 1971): 55; and (November 1971): 9 and 53.

56. *Weightlifting Journal* 1 (July 1971): 3 and 30–31; (August 1971): 3 and 30–31; (September–October 1971): 3 and 30–31; (July 1971): 30; and (August 1971): 30.

57. *SH* 37 (November 1969): 5 and 7; interview with DeMarco; and memo by Wright, November 24, 1969, and C. Hoffman to B. Hoffman, April 3, 1970, HP.

58. Interviews with DeMarco, Yolanda Crist, Starr, and Ketterman.

59. *SH* 37 (November 1969): 44; *SH* 38 (November 1970): 8; *York Daily Record,* January 30, 1971; and *SH* 38 (May 1970): 7–9.

60. "York Weightlifters with President," *York Dispatch,* clipping, HP; *SH* 38 (June 1970): 7; "Activity Report, May 1970," HP; and *SH* 38 (November 1970): 8.

61. *SH* 38 (December 1970): 10; Hoffman to Nixon, December 16, 1970, and Engel to Hoffman, February 3, 1971, HP; and interview with Day.

62. Lovell to Hoffman, February 8, 1971, and "Activity Report, April 1971," HP; and *MD* 8 (June 1971): 62.

NOTES

63. *The Times* (London), March 8, 1971; *Washington Post,* March 24, 1971; and *SH* 39 (March 1971): 7, and (July 1971): 7.

64. Hoffman to Carson, April 29, 1970; Hoffman to Bobby Seymour, November 9, 1970; and "Activity Report, June 1971," HP.

65. *MD* 8 (September 1971): 25 and 59; "Activity Report, April 1971," "Activity Report, August 1971," and Kono to Hoffman, October 20, 1971, HP; *MD* 8 (September 1971); 57; *Weightlifting Journal* 1 (August 1971): 31; and interview with Starr.

CHAPTER 9

1. *Toronto Star,* March 25, 1972.

2. *Iron Man* 31 (February–March 1972): 34–35, and (April–May 1972): 37 and 59. See also minutes by Hise, King, and Weider, n.d., Rader Papers.

3. Heidenstam to Terpak, February 15 and May 18, 1972; Terpak to Heidenstam, February 2, 1972; Matlin to Weider, January 19, 1972; and Crist to Terpak, April 12, 1972, Terpak Papers (hereafter cited as TP); Bob Hoffman, "We Ask You to Vote No," HP; Heidenstam to Terpak, December 21, 1972, TP; and interview with Starr.

4. *Weightlifting Journal* 1 (June 1972): 31, and interview with Donnie Warner (York, Pa.).

5. Interviews with Starr, Warner, and Ketterman.

6. Interviews with Ernie Petersen (York, Pa.), Warner, Terpak, and Ketterman; "Articles Removed from Hoffman Mansion"; list of suspects, n.d.; and "Bob Hoffman's War Medals Stolen," March 14, 1972, HP.

7. Interviews with Warner and DeMarco; Holbrook to Charles Roeser, March 9, 1974, TP; and *SH* 41 (October 1973): 80.

8. *SH* 41 (December 1973): 34; interviews with Warner and Terpak; "Statement of Damages," Hospitality House, June 11, 1973, TP; *SH* 41 (October 1973): 32 and 34–35; Bruce Wilhelm to Peary Rader, June 28, 1973, Rader Papers; and interview with DeMarco.

9. Interview with Ketterman; *SH* 41 (October 1973): 41 and 43; *SH* 42 (March 1974): 74; *SH* 41 (December 1973): 79; and Leon Lankford to Hoffman, May 16, 1975, HP.

10. Terpak to Crist, February 21, 1972; Kono to Terpak, July 18, 1974; and Terpak to John Boddington, August 3, 1974, TP.

11. Interview with Starr.

12. Interviews with Terpak and Starr; *SH* 43 (June–July 1975): 51; and "A Sour Note," n.d., HP.

13. Interviews with DeMarco and Terpak; Terpak to C. E. Elliott, February 28, 1974; Michael Katz to Terpak, December 2, 1974; Jacob Karno to Norman Robinson, April 2, 1975; and Stanley Fagin to Terpak, January 30, 1976, TP.

14. "York Barbell Co. Inc. vs. Jack King, Jr., Answer," July 18, 1973, and "Release of Claim After Judgment," December 10, 1979, TP; interview with Terpak; and *Iron Man* 43 (September 1984): 46–47.

15. Interview with Terpak; Matlin to Richard Krutch, December 6, 1972; Krutch to Matlin, November 28, 1972; and Matlin to Terpak, December 15, 1972, TP.

16. Jotting by Hoffman on envelope dated March 22, 1974; Charles Curran to Matlin, May 13, 1974; Matlin to Terpak, April 17, 1974; Bednarski to Terpak, August 1974; Terpak to Cramer, November 15, 1972; Pacifico to Terpak, n.d.; and "The American Weight-Lifting Association Is Formed," HP.

17. Matlin to Terpak, November 14, 1974, and Deal to Terpak, March 24, 1975, HP.

18. *SH* 40 (November 1972): 66, and (December 1972): 70 and 74; and *SH* 41 (January 1973): 8–9.

19. Interview with Crist, and Levin to Clarence Bass, February 7, 1973, TP.

20. *SH* 42 (February 1974): 41–42; "Athletes' Report of the 1973 World Weightlifting Championships," TP; *Muscle Builder/Power* 15 (July 1974): 55, 77, and 79; *SH* 42 (August–

Notes

September 1974): 8–9; Levin to Terpak, n.d., TP; and Crist to International Selection Committee, December 29, 1973, HP.

21. *SH* 43 (December–January 1974–75): 30 and 59; *SH* 44 (December–January 1975–76), 25 and 52; interview with Crist; Terpak to George, August 19, and Hise to Peter Miller, November 29, 1975, TP.

22. Interview with Clair Bollinger (York, Pa.); Hoffman to C. Carson Conrad, n.d., TP; and *SH* 40 (May 1972): 5.

23. *Softball News* 1 (April 1976): 1; interview with Bollinger; and *SH* 43 (December–January 1974–75): 64.

24. *SH* 42 (April 1974): 70; *MD* 12 (November–December 1975): 29; and interview with Crist.

25. Interview with Dellinger; and *MD* 10 (April 1973): 23, and (May 1973): 9 and 53.

26. *MD* 10 (July 1973): 68, and (December 1973): 9; and *MD* 11 (March 1974): 46.

27. *SH* 42 (March 1974): 40–41, and *MD* 11 (April 1974): 51.

28. *MD* 11 (September–October 1974): 64; *MD* 13 (November–December 1976): 9; and *MD* 12 (September–October 1975): 11, and (July–August 1975): 49.

29. *SH* 44 (February–March 1976): 5; *MD* 13 (March–April 1976): 10–11, 64, and 66.

30. Wrange to Crist, August 13, 1976, TP.

31. *Tucson Daily Citizen*, January 19, 1968; Zitko to Hoffman, September 16, 1972, HP; *SH* 42 (March 1974): 6; interviews with Ernie Petersen and Vern Weaver (York, Pa.); and *MD* 10 (April 1973): 49.

32. *SH* 43 (October–November 1975): 5 and 7; *SH* 40 (March 1972): 15; *SH* 42 (October–November 1974): 5; *SH* 41 (December 1973): 6 and 23; and *SH* 42 (June–July 1974): 69.

33. *MD* 12 (March–April 1975): 66; Bob Hoffman, *The Best Natural Food* (York, Pa., 1972), 130; idem, *Energol Germ Oil Concentrate: The Most Important Food Element* (York, Pa., 1972), 26 and 128–29; and idem, *Why Men Die Younger* (York, Pa., 1973), 13, 109, 47, and 138.

34. Bob Hoffman, *How to Keep Your Husband Alive Longer* (York, Pa., 1974), 33, 126, 131, and 6–7.

35. *New York Post*, May 6, 1973; *SH* 40 (November 1972): 5; interviews with Ketterman, Weaver, and Petersen; Bienvenu to Hoffman, September 11, 1972, HP; *MD* 12 (September–October 1975): 65; and *Washington Post*, April 29, 1976.

36. Jerold Dorfman to Hoffman, December 14, 1973, TP; Dorfman to Terpak, December 12, 1974, HP; *Natural Health World and the Naturopath* 12 (April 1973): 1; Bob Hoffman, "Round Ten in Our Battle with the FDA," HP; *If Patrick Henry Were Alive Today*, 1; and "Activity Report, July 1972," HP.

37. "Activity Report, July 1973" and "Activity Report, October 1972," HP; interview with Bollinger; Crist to Hoffman, April 29, 1975, HP; Matlin to Terpak, January 14, 1972, TP; "Activity Report, May 1973," HP; and interview with Dellinger.

38. *MD* 11 (February 1974): 16; *MD* 10 (August 1973): 28; *MD* 11 (July–August 1974): 34; and "Activity Report, July 1972," HP.

39. *Washington Star-News*, October 24, 1973; "April 1976 Activity Report," and Miller to Hoffman, March 18, 1975, HP; *St. Louis Globe-Democrat*, September 5, 1975; Bob Hoffman, "The Unholy Alliance" and "The Unholy Alliance Is Working Hard Against Us," HP.

40. "Activity Report, February 1972" and "Activity Report, January 1973," HP; *MD* 10 (July 1973): 55, and (June 1973): 67.

41. *SH* 41 (August 1973): 71; *MD* 10 (March 1973): 26; *Sunday Patriot-News*, November 11, 1973; "Activity Report, February 1972," HP; and *Cleveland Plain Dealer*, March 8, 1973.

42. *SH* 41 (August 1973), 72; *York Dispatch*, July 6, 1973; and Holt to Hoffman, August 12, 1974, HP.

43. *SH* 43 (February–March 1975): 5; Bob Hoffman, *To Save the United States Movement*, 3; *SH* 44 (December–January 1975–76); "Activity Report, July 1976," and Hoffman to Porter, April 23, 1975, HP.

44. *SH* 44 (August–September 1976): 27; "Activity Report, July 1976," HP; and Hoffman, *To Save the United States Movement*, 5.

NOTES

45. Monthly Financial Statements, 1969–76, HP; "Distributor Sales" and "Wholesale and Retail Protein Sales," R. A. Pruger, January 8, 1974, TP; *SH* 42 (March 1974): 79–80; and Board of Directors Minutes, May 6, 1974.

46. "Activity Report, May 1973," HP; Pruger to Terpak, March 22, 1972, TP; interview with Richard Pruger (Pittsburgh); and Pruger to Hoffman, January 19, 1976, HP.

47. Terpak to Matlin, April 16, 1971; Pruger to Hoffman, January 3, 1972; Levin to Terpak, March 22, 1972; Terpak to A. Hoole, June 2, 1972, TP; and interviews with Day, Ketterman, Petersen, and Dellinger.

48. Interviews with Ketterman, Petersen, Dellinger, and Bednarski, and Miller to Hoffman, July 24, 1975, HP.

49. Bobby Colak to Terpak, [1976]; John Lee to Terpak, June 26, 1976; Leroy Corbin to Hoffman, May 10 and June 18, 1974; Anonymous photocopy [1969?]; and Cynthia Steward to Hoffman, July 17, 1974, TP.

50. Mel Pratt to Hoffman, July 19, 1974, TP; Fleming to Hoffman, August 18, 1972, HP; and *SH* 42 (May 1974): 5.

51. Interview with Terpak; Terpak to Holbrook, March 21, 1974, TP; Degenhardt to Hoffman, May 20, 1974, HP; *Muscle Builder/Power* 25 (November 1975): 31 and 32; Fleming to Terpak, with enclosure, n.d., TP; and *SH* 42 (April 1974): 15.

52. *SH* 40 (March 1972): 8, and *SH* 41 (May 1973): 8, and (October 1973): 34.

53. *SH* 41 (July 1973): 45; *SH* 43 (October–November 1975): 56 and 66; *SH* 44 (October–November 1976): 57; and Kono to Members, U.S. Olympic Weightlifting Committee, October 1, 1976, HP.

54. *SH* 41 (November 1973): 25; *MD* 10 (May 1973): 57; and "Veritas," February 1975, TP; *Muscle Builder/Power* 24 (January 1974): 86; and *SH* 44 (April–May 1976): 7.

55. *Asbury Park Press*, November 2, 1975; "Veritas II," July 1975, TP; and interview with Terpak.

CHAPTER 10

1. Interview with Claudia Keister (Terpak's secretary, York, Pa.).

2. Interviews with Dellinger, Ketterman, and Petersen, and *Muscle Training Illustrated*, April 1979, 14.

3. Interviews with Terpak and Ketterman, and Friend, Perles, Dorfman, and Kleefeld to York Barbell Co., June 1, 1979.

4. Company Records, Profit and Loss, 1974–85; "Record of Minutes," April 14 and May 2, 1977, TP; and interview with Keister.

5. Interviews with Redman and Petersen, and Board of Directors Minutes, 1978–84.

6. Robert Philbin to Terpak and Redman, April 19 and June 25, 1979, and Otis Morse to Dietz, June 4, 1979, TP; and *SH* 51 (November 1983): 40.

7. *SH* 48 (September 1980): 7; K. Lohr and N. Maddock to Robert Sestero, June 20, 1980; "Hoffman's Food Products Consumer Research," September 23, 1980, 32, 54, and 12; and "Hoffman's Food Products Proposed Marketing Plan, 1981," November 24, 1980, TP.

8. Kenneth Fischer to Terpak, December 12, 1981, and Dietz to Terpak, February 28, 1984, TP.

9. Deposition Summary by Dale Hebert, in Graham Ward to Joe Puleo, October 12, 1981; Ward to Laurence Coffey, September 8, 1981; and "State of Michigan in the Circuit Court for the County of Macomb, Stipulation for Judgment," September 1, 1982, TP.

10. Pruger to Hoffman, February 8, 1977; Complaint, Answer to Complaint, Counterclaim, Trial Memorandum of Defendants, and Motion for Sanction Order, *Pruger v. York Barbell Company*, Court of Common Pleas of Allegheny County; "Richard Pruger, Statement of Estimated Income for the period March 1, 1977, through May 11, 1978; and Pruger to Terpak, May 19, 1984, TP.

Notes

11. *MD* 8 (April 1971): 7; Michael Katz vs. Strength & Health Publishing Co., October 20–21 and 26–28, 1977, Superior Court, New Haven County, Conn., transcript; and David Reif to Terpak, November 7, 1977, and Reif to John Boddington, July 25, 1979, TP.

12. "National AAU Physique Committee Minutes," April 22, 1977, Crist Papers, 19 Barnes Court, Hampton, Va., and *Iron Man* 36 (September 1977): 36–37.

13. *Iron Man* 36 (September 1977): 40; "National AAU Physique Committee Minutes," August 10, 1977, Crist Papers; *MD* 15 (December 1977): 62; and Bass to Countryman, July 19, 1977, Countryman Papers, 779 Mandana Blvd., Oakland, Calif.

14. *Muscle Training Illustrated,* January 1980, 9; interview with Dellinger; *Muscle Training Illustrated,* December 1980, 62; and *MD* 18 (December 1981): 27.

15. *Iron Man* 39 (November 1979): 28; *MD* 16 (December 1979): 29–32; and *MD* 17 (August 1980): 32, 67, and 70.

16. *Muscle Training Illustrated,* December 1979, 10; October 1980, 8 and 63; April 1980, 40–41; and May 1981, 6.

17. *Muscle Training Illustrated,* May 1981, 62, and January 1981, 10–11; *MD* 17 (December 1980): 17; Joe Henson to Jim Manion, February 6, 1981, TP; *MD* 19 (April 1982): 21, 71, 73, and (October 1982): 72–73; and *SH* 51 (July 1983): 47.

18. *Muscle and Fitness* 43 (December 1982): 203; *Flex* (April 1983): 4; and *MD* 20 (August 1983): 29.

19. *Muscle and Fitness* 43 (October 1982): 206, and Heidenstam to Grimek, December 21, 1983, TP.

20. *MD* 14 (June 1977): 9; *MD* 15 (August 1978): 28; and *Iron Man* 38 (November 1978): 46.

21. *MD* 16 (October 1978): 9 and 61–62; interview with Todd; *MD* 16 (February 1979): 70 and 72.

22. *MD* 14 (August 1977): 67; *MD* 15 (August 1978): 42–44, 67, and (October 1978): 8; and *MD* 16 (April 1979): 5.

23. *MD* 16 (April 1979): 22, and (February 1979): 9; International Powerlifting Federation Minutes, 1978 World Congress, November 1–3, 1978, and Mercer to Terpak, December 24, 1978, TP; and *SH* 47 (July 1979): 26.

24. Terpak to Pacifico, March 22, 1979, TP, and *MD* 17 (February 1980): 12 and 70.

25. *MD* 18 (February 1981): 7, and (April 1981): 9.

26. Interview with Murray Levin (York, Pa.); *SH* 46 (January 1978): 16, and (March 1978): 10; and *Weightlifting Rules* (1979), 1–2.

27. *SH* 45 (December–January 1976–77): 33, and (September 1977): 31; *SH* 46 (March 1978): 33, and (September 1978): 43; and *SH* 47 (January 1979): 21–22.

28. *SH* 47 (May 1979): 8, 22, and (September 1979): 11.

29. *SH* 49 (May 1981): 8–9.

30. Balance Sheet, United States Weightlifting Federation, April 30, 1981, and Harvey Newton, "Report to the U.S. Weightlifting Federation," June 8, 1981, TP; *SH* 50 (November 1982): 34; Newton to Terpak, October 20, 1982, and Roger Sadecki, "Report Attendance at Olympic Training Center, August 23–September 10, 1982," TP; and interview with Levin.

31. Dreschler to Levin, February 8, 1982, TP, and *SH* 51 (March 1983): 8.

32. *SH* 52 (September 1984): 14, and (November 1984), 23; interview with Levin; Levin to Finance Committee, February 28, 1985; USWF 1985 Quarterly Financial Reports; United States Amateur Weightlifting Foundation, 1985, Financial Reports; and Digest of Minutes, USWF National Convention, Board of Governors Meeting, May 6, 1985, TP.

33. *MD* 15 (August 1978): 5; *MD* 16 (October 1979): 5; *MD* 15 (October 1977): 71; and interviews with Dellinger and Krout (York, Pa.).

34. *SH* 47 (September 1979): 56, and *SH* 48 (May 1980): 5.

35. *MD* 17 (October 1980): 71; *MD* 21 (February 1984): 28; *MD* 22 (April 1985): 7; *MD* 21 (April 1984): 21; and interview with Dellinger.

36. *MD* 16 (February 1979): 71; *SH* 45 (December–January 1976–77): 5; and interview with Ketterman.

NOTES

37. Interview with Ketterman; "Progress Notes," April 21, August 5, and September 28, 1981, Notebook I, HP.
38. "Progress Notes," April 26 and June 24, 1982, Notebook II; July 8 and 9, September 22, December 3, September 15, and December 22, 1982, Notebook III, HP.
39. Interview with Ketterman; "Progress Notes," September 13, December 2 and 23, 1983, Notebook V, HP.
40. Interview with Ketterman; *Sports Fitness* 2 (January 1986): 51 and 91; *Iron Man* 45 (November 1985): 42; and Nixon to Ketterman, July 26, 1985; and note from Weider, HP.

EPILOGUE AND CONCLUSION

1. "Robert Collins Hoffman, 1898–1985," Mount Rose Cemetery, York, Pa., and Estate of Robert C. Hoffman, File 67–85-0878 in the Court of Common Pleas of York County, March 16, 1990.
2. Last Will and Testament of Robert C. Hoffman, March 21, 1978, HP, and interview with Ketterman.
3. Interview with Todd; *New York Times*, September 21, 1986; *Los Angeles Times*, March 2, 1989; and interviews with Ketterman and Dellinger.
4. *SH* 36 (July 1968): 5, and Codicil I to the Last Will and Testament of Robert C. Hoffman, April 6, 1978, HP.
5. *Musclemag International*, December 1986, 57; opinion, *John Grimek v. The Estate of Robert Hoffman, Court of Common Pleas of York County, Pa., No. 85-SU-04775-01*; and memorandum, *John Grimek v. The Estate of Robert Hoffman*, Superior Court of Pennsylvania, No. 00322 HBG 89 TP.
6. Terpak to Jim Newton, December 27, 1989, and "We're Not Muscletown Anymore," TP.
7. Terpak to John Lambrosa, January 5, 1989; *Strength & Health* Publishing Report—June 1988, Muscular Development Magazine; Asset Purchase Agreement, August 18, 1988, TP; and interviews with Terpak and Redman.
8. York Barbell Company Balance Sheets, years ending March 31, 1988, 1987, 1986, and 1985, and York Barbell Co., Inc. and Subsidiaries Consolidated Balance Sheets, December 31, 1989, and March 31, 1989, Standish Papers, York Barbell Company.
9. Interrogatory No. 6, Profitability, *William H. Dietz et al. v. John Terpak Sr. et al.*, Court of Common Pleas, York County, May 25, 1990, No. 90 SU-00894-07, TP; and interviews with Heiland (York, Pa.) and Keister.
10. Interviews with Terpak, Keister, and Ketterman, and Interrogatory No. 5, *William H. Dietz et al. v. John Terpak Sr. et al.*, Court of Common Pleas, York County, May 25, 1990, No. 90 SU-00894-07, TP.
11. Interviews with Redman, Dellinger, and John Terpak Jr. (York, Pa.).
12. "Dietz Settlement," February 14, 1992, TP; interview with Keister; and York Barbell Co. and Subsidiaries Consolidated Balance Sheets, December 31, 1989, March 31, 1989, and December 31, 1991 and 1990, TP.
13. Interviews with Redman, Standish, and Dellinger, and *Muscletown News*, 1–2.
14. Interview with Paul Stombaugh (York, Pa.).
15. Interviews with Warner and Terlazzo.
16. Gregory Rochlin, *The Masculine Dilemma: A Psychology of Masculinity* (Boston, 1980), 84–85 and 224–26; Gilmore, *Manhood in the Making* (New Haven, 1990), 222–23; and Chapman, *Sandow the Magnificent*, 189.
17. Interview with Todd.

Index

Abbenda, Joe, 201, 217, 219
Abele, Louis, 82
Abels, Arthur, 209
Abs, Carl, 28
Achles, Kenny, 126
Ackerman, Marshall, 171
Adams, Bob, xv
aging, 72, 141, 170, 184, 192–93, 228, 284, 319, 321, 341
Agnew, Spiro, 286, 289
alcoholism, 141–42, 170, 180
Alexander, Harold, 100
Alexeev, Vasily, 266, 272, 311, 335
Alger, Horatio, 2, 62, 67, 77, 386
Allan, Tony, 264
Amateur Athletic Union (AAU), 28, 34, 36–38, 43, 49, 53, 73, 82, 90, 116–17, 128, 130, 142, 145, 152, 169, 177, 184–85, 188, 192, 216, 218–19, 225, 233, 260–62, 266, 275, 277, 279–80, 286, 290, 294–96, 301, 305, 309, 316, 329, 332, 338, 345, 349–56, 358
Ameche, Alan, 166
American Continental Weight-Lifters Association (ACWLA), 29, 34, 42–44, 46–47, 49
American Federation of Bodybuilders, 354–55
American Strength and Health League, 42, 49, 115, 329
American Weightlifting Association (AWLA), 305–6, 338–39, 367
Anderson, Paul, 2, 159–60, 206, 215, 225
Andrelczyk, Barbara, xv, 384
Anello, Vince, 312, 357
Annan, Noel, 341
Anstine, James, 143
Apollo 17 launch, 325

Arax, Gregor, 321
Arco, Otto, 39, 369
Ashman, Dave, 184, 187, 222
Askew, Eric, 171
Asnis, Dave, 369
Association of Bar Bell Men (ABBM), 32, 34–35, 37
Athletes in Action, 259, 334
Atlas, Charles, 1, 3, 25, 49, 56–57, 69, 105, 116, 171, 195
Avant, Allyn, 181

Babcock, John, 28
Babinsky, J. P., 264
Bachtell, Dick, xiv, 36–37, 44–45, 50, 69, 77, 81, 89, 101, 110, 116, 141, 160, 266, 282, 377
Backus, Bob, 206
Bacon, Jules, xiv, 82, 86, 90, 94, 99, 118, 141, 149, 172, 183, 203
Baker, William, 24
"Bandsman, Rice," 16
Bannout, Samir, 368
Bard, Gracie (Gorzetski), 66–69, 81–84, 129, 143, 165
Baritz, Loren, 23
Barker, Anthony, 28, 39
Barker, Joe, 131
Barnholdt, Claude, xiv
Barnholdt, Larry, 156, 321
Barrs, John, 178
Bartholomew, Bob, 259
baseball, 24, 166, 187, 190
basketball, 24, 182
Bass, Clarence, xiv, 352–53
Bates, Frank, 263, 335
Bates, Robert, 179

INDEX

Baxter, Don, 264
Beaudoin, Robert, 181
Bednarski, Bob, xiv, 199, 237–38, 245–47, 253–59, 264, 268–73, 276, 283, 285–86, 289, 298–99, 301, 306, 333
Belknap, Tim, 353
Bendel, Bob, 263
Bennett, Sanford, 72
bent-pressing, 65, 80, 123–24, 168
Berger, Bill, 126
Berger, Isaac, 159–60, 162, 186, 190, 212, 220–21, 225, 275
Berger, Dr. Richard, 202
Bernard, Bernard, 29
Berry, Mark, 32–33, 37, 43, 53–56, 72, 83, 105, 143, 170, 213
Better Foods Foundation (Greencastle), 204, 378
Better Nutritional Aids (BNA), 149, 152
bicycling, 96
Bienvenu, Dr. Oscar, 321
Bilik, Dr. S. E., 202
Binney, Winston, 236
biorhythms, 200
Bishop, Glenn, 231
Bleeker, Doc, 30
Blymire, George, 32
bodybuilding, 1, 5, 51, 63, 77, 90–91, 96–99, 114–19, 123–33, 142, 144–45, 147–48, 152, 158, 166, 169–70, 177, 186–87, 209–10, 215–19, 232, 235, 239, 260–61, 279, 285, 293, 295, 308, 311, 316, 338, 341, 349–56, 362, 366, 368, 383, 385–86, 389
    women's, 96–98, 353
Boff, Vic, xiii—xiv, 346
Bollinger, Claire, xiv, 310
Bond, James, 220
Bonomo, Joe, 369
Bosco, 75, 130, 132, 152–53
Bowers, Joe, xiv
boxing, 4, 16, 20, 65, 144, 190, 217, 225
Boyle, Robert, 4
Bradford, James, 121, 147, 198
Bragg, Don, 166, 288, 369
Brannum, Homer, 199, 210, 236
Breitbart, Siegmund, 39
Brenneman, Lavern, xiv
Bridges, Mike, 361
British Amateur Weight-Lifters Association (BAWLA), 28–29
Brokhin, Yuri, 270
Brookside Park, 79, 86–87, 96, 171, 188, 247, 369
Brosemer, Betty, 178
Broussard, Marty, 200
Brower, Dave, 253
Brown, Francis Wm., 202
Brown, George, 44–45

Brown, Larry, 323
Bryant, Paul "Bear," 200
Buermeyer, Henry, 28
Bullock, Weldon, xiv, 65, 67
Bureau of Standards, 180
Bushnell, Asa, 184
Butterfield, Herbert, 6
Byers, Cliff, 99, 115

calisthenics, 24, 87
Calvert, Alan, 3, 25, 33, 150
Cameron, Mark, 329, 336, 363
Camp, Walter, 34, 166
Cannon, Billy, 166
canoeing, 2, 11, 15–16, 30–31, 87, 232, 251
Capsouras, Frank, 247, 254, 272
Carlton, Guy, 367
Carnegie, Andrew, 248
Carrucio, Connie, 65
Carson, Johnny, 289, 359
Carter, Jimmy, 368
Cassidy, Hopalong, 153
chain breaking, 80, 136, 183
Chandler, Timothy, 6
Chapman, David, 6, 384
Chapman, Diane, 285
Chennault, Claire, 100
Christensen, Vera, 235, 335
Christov, Valentin, 336
CIBA pharmaceuticals, 158, 195
Cirenza, William, 134
Clark, Mark, 100
Cleveland, Gary, 212, 220, 224
Coe, Boyer, 261, 265
Coffee, John, xiv
cold war, 4, 118–19, 130, 145–47
Collins, James, 12
Collins, Robert, 12
Collins, Ron, 314, 316–17, 357
Communism, 4, 118, 130, 138, 147, 187, 245, 309, 365
Connolly, Harold, 166
Conrad, Chris, 368
Cooper Athletic Club, 28
Corbett, Dr. Frank, 202, 206, 227–28, 309
Corlman, Howard, 209
Cornaro, Luigi, 72
Coster, Charles, 178
Coulter, Ottley, 28–29, 49, 97, 234
Countryman, Ralph, xv, 338, 352
Crain, Ricky, 357
Cramer, Les, 306
Crist, Bob, xiv–xv, 263, 283, 294–95, 298, 301, 308–9, 311–12, 316, 335, 338–39, 355
Crist, Yolanda, xiv, 277, 283
Crow, Phil, 181
Curry, Fred, 110
Curry, William, xiv, 76, 106

Index

Curtis, William "Father Bill," 28, 150
Cypher, Marty, 336
Cyr, Louis, 65

Daniels, Jerry, 217
Davis, John, 63, 68, 77–79, 90, 111, 120, 123, 138, 145–46, 150, 160, 365, 369, 378
Davis, Thomas, 207
Dawkins, Pete, 167
Day, Winston, xiv, 248, 252, 267, 287, 331
Dayton, Mike, 244
Deal, Gary, 272, 305–7, 349
Decola, John, 265
Degenhardt, Ray, 210, 270, 277, 306, 334, 377
Degenhardt, Sandi, 334
Dellinger, Jack, 125
Dellinger, Jan, xiv–xv, 311, 323, 331, 342, 352–53, 369, 376, 379, 380, 384
DeMarco, Lou, xiv, 270, 283, 301–3
Dennis, Frank, 33
DePietro, Joe, 110–11, 121, 138, 160
Derwin, Brian, 364–65
Desbonnet, Edmund, 28, 113
Dickerson, Chris, 218, 260, 265, 285, 323
Dietz, Mike, Jr., 380
Dietz, Mike, Sr., 61–62, 69, 141, 164, 172, 174, 208, 221, 223, 248, 267, 269, 276, 302, 310, 330–33, 345–48, 376–77, 379
Dietz, William, 376, 380–81
Dinnie, Donald, 28
Disney World, 334
Dockey, Clifford, 142
Douglas, Mike, 290
Draper, Dave, 265
Dreher, Eldon, 200
Dreschler, Artie, 366
drug culture, 232–33, 256–57, 268–70, 273–81, 283, 290, 296–301, 304, 328, 333–34, 338, 368
Drury, Francis, 200
Dryer, Paul 40
Dube, Joe, xiv, 254, 257–59, 268, 271–73, 285–86, 289–90, 336, 364
DuBois, Dick, 152
Duey, Henry, xiv
Duncan, Mrs. Frank, 264
Duval, Roy, 313

Ebersole, Frank, 65
Echternacht, Gary, 263
Eddy, Daniel, 1
Eder, Marvin, 147
Eells, Roger, 115, 213
Egan, J. C., 29
Eichelberger, Eli, 284
Eiferman, George, 125
Eisenhower, Dwight, 100, 184
Eisenhower, Julie, 326

Eisenhower, Mamie, 326
Elder, Jack, xiv, 81, 118
Elledge, Marie, 209
Elliott, Herb, 166
Emrich, Clyde, xiv, 150
Engel, Trudy, 286–89, 293–94, 317, 322–26, 328–29, 378–79
Ernst, Jack, 89
Ernst, Robert, 5
European Championships, 28, 187–88, 195
Evanich, Charles, 265

Faeth, Karl, 309
Falcon, Dick, 106
Farbotnik, John and Joan, 135
Faris, Emmett, 36, 92, 142
Farnham, Elmer, 81, 89
Federal Trade Commission (FTC), 18, 56–57, 324, 328, 343
Federation Internationale Halterophile (International Weightlifting Federation), 28, 185, 258, 261, 306
Feldmann, Hank, 266
Ferrigno, Lou, 402
Fiedler, Steve, 346
Fiorito, Anthony, 44
Fiorito, Joe, 44–45, 65, 70
Fischer, Kenneth, 347
Fitton, Tony, 361
Fleming, Tom, 334
Fletcher, Horace, 72
Food and Drug Administration (FDA), 180, 207, 231, 263, 286, 293, 322, 324–25, 328, 338, 343
food supplements, 147–52, 157, 159, 166, 171, 173, 179–82, 184, 187–88, 193, 195, 203–9, 243, 249–51, 263–65, 290, 314, 318–20, 326, 328–29, 385–86
football, 24, 100, 155, 160, 166–67, 182, 200, 206, 285
Ford, Gerald, 328
Ford, Henry, 100
Fortney, David, xiv
Four Hundred Pound Club, 64
Fox, Jim, 353
Fox, Richard Kyle, 28
Franklin, Win, 321
Frenn, George, 261–62, 282, 301–2
Friend, Solomon, 263
Fritsche, John, 110
Fronheiser, Larry, 232

Gajda, Bob, 129, 203, 217, 219, 236
Gans, Bob, 264
Gant, Lamar, 357, 361
Garcia, Tim, 299, 301
Garcy, Tony, xiv, 196, 199, 202, 210, 212, 219, 221–22, 238, 399

INDEX

Gay, Arthur, 36, 369
Gemmil, Helen, 377
gender studies, 5–6
General Assembly of International Sports Federations (GAIF), 294–95, 316
George, Jim, xiv, 156, 159, 164, 186–87, 200, 203
George, Pete, 110–11, 120, 122, 123, 142, 145–46, 156, 159, 162, 177, 191, 202–3, 224–25, 309, 365
German-American Athletic Club, 28, 34, 36–37, 40, 43, 54
Giardine, Frank, 108
Gibson, Harold, 354
Gilbert III (artwork), 216, 353
Gilmore, David, 375
Gironda, Vince, 115
Giroux, Arthur, 32
Glenney, Gary, xiv, 202, 222, 247, 256, 258
Glick, Harry, 40
Glossbrenner, Herb, 307
Gold's Gym, 2, 350, 352, 368
Goleman, Daniel, 375
golf, 24, 155
Good, Harry, 42–44, 46, 62
Good, Walter, xiv, 36–37, 44–45, 55, 65
Good, William, 36, 44–46, 55, 62, 65
Goodling, George, 248, 286
Goodrich, Bert, 125, 128, 350
Goostree, Jim, 200
Gourgott, John, 203, 229, 254, 302–4
Grabeel, Orville, 83–84, 144
Grant, Bill, 350
Graves, Jack, 67
Great Depression, 3, 39
Green, Charles, 180
Green, Harvey, 23
Greenawalt, Richard, 123
Grimek, John, xiii–xiv, 2, 46, 55, 58, 63, 67, 69–70, 76–77, 79–83, 87, 90, 96–97, 99, 108–9, 112, 116–18, 125–26, 128, 138, 141–44, 149, 158–59, 171, 184, 194–97, 203, 206, 212, 215–16, 219, 221, 257, 265–66, 273, 282, 349, 352–53, 359, 369
Grippaldi, Phil, 235–36, 245, 247, 254, 259, 272–73, 336, 363, 377–78
Gubner, Gary, xiv, 225, 237–38, 245
gymnastics, 24, 65, 100

Hackenschmidt, George, 26, 83, 369
Hadley, Hopten, 42
Haines, Mahlon, 192
Hale America Program, 87, 94
Hall, Dave, 229
Hall, Harry, 32
Halsey, William, 100
handbalancing, 2, 65
handball, 50–51, 58, 64
Hanneman, Larry, 276, 302–3

Harley, Bob, 65
Harlow, Robert, 3
Harris, Carleton, 64–65
Hasse, Bob, 191, 198, 210, 217
Health, Education, and Welfare, Department of, 215
Health and Life, 29
Health & Strength, 29, 42
Heidenstam, Oscar, 219, 260, 295–96, 316, 356
Heiland, Gene, xiv, 379
Henderson, John, 347–48
Henry, Franklin, 99
Henry, Patrick, 322
Henry, Sid, 211
Hepburn, Doug, 147, 160
Hercules, 171, 220
Hercules Athletic Club, 28
Hess, Don, xiv, 379
Higgins, Bob, 110
hiking, 24, 87, 123
Hill, Jack, Jr., 244
Hilligenn, Roy, 144
Hise, Bob, 236, 294–96, 298, 304, 308–9, 336, 367, 397
Hise, Bob, III, 244, 254, 256, 259, 270, 280, 298
Hise, J. C., 213, 400
Hitchens, Jake, 184, 196
Hitler, Adolf, 54, 68, 86
Hoch, Paul, 3
Hoffman, Abraham, 12
Hoffman, Addison Frederick, 12–14, 16
Hoffman, Bertha Leone, 12–13
Hoffman, Bob, 1–6, 34, 138
 ancestry, 11–12, 44, 390
 and aquatics, 2, 11, 15–16, 30–31, 33, 123
 and Atlas, Charles, 56–57
 and Bard, Gracie, 66–69, 81–84, 129, 143, 165
 and *The Best Natural Food*, 319
 and *Better Athletes Through Weight Training*, 166–67
 and *Better Nutrition*, 75
 and *Big Arms*, 73, 108
 and *The Big Chest Book*, 73, 108
 birth of, 11
 childhood of, 12–16
 and consumers, 180–81, 264–65, 331, 333–35, 385
 and the *Daily Dozen*, 182, 184, 193, 286
 death of, 372–73, 375–76, 386
 divorce of, 97
 and *Drink More Water*, 251
 and drugs, 159, 188, 243, 252, 256–57, 277–78, 321, 328, 333–34, 338
 early jobs, 14–15, 20
 early years in York, 20–22
 and *Energol Germ Oil Concentrate*, 319
 financial affairs, 69, 72, 94–95, 107, 113, 118,

Index

133, 140–41, 172–77, 208, 249, 267, 329–33, 343–45, 375–76
first weightlifting contest, 31–32
and functional isometric contraction, 194–202, 207–8, 238, 368, 385
and *Guide to Weight Lifting Competition*, 73, 194
and health food industry, 209, 227, 285–86, 290, 322–26, 345, 367
and health problems, 227–28, 249–52, 283, 321, 341–43, 348, 369–72
and *High Protein Recipe Book*, 193
and Hi-Proteen, 147–52, 157, 159, 162, 169, 173, 179–82, 184, 187–88, 190, 193, 195, 205–6, 208, 224, 249, 251, 264, 314, 321, 338, 343, 347, 386
and Hi-Proteen Fudge Bars, 179, 181, 237
and Hi-Proteen Honey Fudge, 205
and *How to Be Strong, Healthy, and Happy*, 72–73, 75, 166, 214
and *How to Gain Weight*, 250
and *How to Keep Your Husband Alive Longer*, 320
and *I Remember the Last War*, 75
and investments, 181–82, 204–5, 231, 284, 305–7
and Jowett, George, 27, 29, 42
and Ketterman, Alda, 84–86, 94, 96, 129, 143, 149, 165, 171, 174, 176, 208, 266, 283, 315, 319–21, 326, 331–32, 343, 369, 372–73
and Lehman, Dorcas, 84–86, 94, 96–97, 129, 132–33, 136, 141, 143, 165, 176
management practices, 61–62, 87–89, 168, 172–77, 179, 302–4, 330–33, 345
marketing techniques, 26, 39–40, 49–52, 83, 86–87, 107–8, 118, 129, 131–35, 166–67, 173, 178–81, 194, 198–99, 203–5, 213, 238, 243, 249–52, 281, 329–31, 341, 345–48
marriage of, 21, 58–61, 165
and the medical profession, 203, 206, 229–30, 232–34, 281, 304, 321–22, 324
and *Mighty Men of Old*, 24
national heavyweight champion, 32–33
and old age, 238, 284, 306, 321, 341–43, 369–72
and *Old Age Is a Slow Starvation*, 193
and old-fashioned views, 247, 252–53, 260, 262, 274, 280, 297, 334, 338–39
and Olympics, 53–56, 61
philanthropy of, 77, 146, 184, 202, 220–21, 229, 243, 248–49, 266, 291, 308, 310, 314, 360, 373
and political involvements, 243, 248, 285–91, 293–94, 322–29
and powerlifting, 293, 311–17
and *Protein-Building Blocks of Life*, 193
and *The Protein Story*, 193
and *Reducing and Weight Control*, 250, 264

and *Road to Super-Strength*, 11
and *Running for Your Life*, 249
and the Save the United States movement, 294, 328–29, 368, 370
and science, 171, 179–80, 192, 194–208, 215, 231, 233, 238, 244, 304, 318
and *Secrets of Strength and Development*, 73
and *Sex Technique*, 75, 108
socialization techniques, 46–49, 63–69, 79–83, 87–88, 96–97, 106, 108, 110–14, 120–25, 137–38, 156, 186–90, 219–27, 236, 281, 290, 385, 387
and softball, 284–85, 293, 310, 319, 326, 329, 335, 342, 367, 371
and *Strength, Energy, and Endurance*, 250
and *Successful-Happy Marriage*, 75, 108
and Terpak, John, 52, 62
training courses, 41, 89, 125, 155, 166, 250
and water business, 204–5, 231, 249, 251–52, 265
and Weider challenge, 97, 99, 114–19, 143–45, 177–78
and *Weight Lifting*, 73
and *Why Men Die Younger*, 319
and will of, 376–78, 381
and world trip, 162–63
in World War I, 16–19, 290
and World War II, 71, 87–90, 92–97, 100–101
and York Gang, 76, 89–90
and York Oil Burner Athletic Club, 35–38
and *You Can Live Longer, 10–20—30 Years Longer*, 192
and youth rebellion, 277–81, 285, 290–91, 296–301
Hoffman, Charles (Chuck), 12–13, 21, 176, 283, 319
Hoffman, Eleanor (Booch), 12–13, 18, 80, 176
Hoffman, Ellen Shanor, 12
Hoffman, Florence, 12
Hoffman Foundation, 171, 203–4, 211, 229–30, 232, 234, 247–48, 376–77
Hoffman, John, 12
Hoffman, John L. (Jack), xiv, 11–13, 15–16, 19, 21
Hoffman Laboratories, 343
Hoffman (Morris), Rosetta Snell, xiv, 13, 21–22, 33, 35, 40, 46–49, 58–61, 66–67, 69, 83, 97, 129, 143, 165, 175–76, 266–67, 377
Hoffman's Rub, 132
Hoffman's Sun Tan Lotion, 131–32, 179, 181
Hogan, Hulk, 2
Holbrook, Dede, 280
Holbrook, Rick, 244, 254, 256, 272–73, 298, 300–301
Holbrook, Tom, 280, 299, 307, 334–35
Homola, Samuel, 206
homosexuality, 93, 209, 297
Horvath, Barton, 178

INDEX

Hosmer, Craig, 322
"House on the Hill," 35–36, 58–61, 97, 140, 143, 171, 267, 320, 378
Howard, Richard, 310
Howard, Rufus, 355
Huberman, Max, 323
Hugo, Victor, 202
Hunt, William, 5
Huska, Mihaly, xiv, 244
hypnotism, 200

ice fishing, 334
Imahara, Walter, 245
immigrants, 3–4, 23–24, 26, 28, 39, 43–44, 46, 63–64, 69–70, 99, 120–23, 152, 156, 160–61, 187–88, 389
Internal Revenue Service, 94, 141, 175–77, 182
International Federation of Body Builders (IFBB), 128, 130, 261–62, 265, 294–96, 316, 349–56
International Powerlifting Federation (IPF), 312, 316, 357, 360
Ishikawa, Emerick, 99, 101, 136
isometrics, 194–202, 207–8, 223, 238, 368, 385
isotron, 200, 231
Iuspa, Angelo, xiv
Ivanchencko, Genadij, 299
Iyer, K. V., 369

Jahn, Father Friedrich Ludwig, 4, 71
James, Lee, 336–37, 363
Jensen, Jackie, 166
Jesus Christ, 145, 209
Johns, Dave, 350–51
Johnson, Clarence, xiv, 142, 185, 202, 239, 258
Johnson, Erwin (Rheo Blair), 147–48
Johnson, Ralph, 295
Jones, Allen, 180
Jones, Bob, 50, 65, 110
Jones, Jerry, 311
Jowett, George Fiusdale, 24, 26–30, 32, 34, 42, 44, 46, 49–50, 57, 114–16, 128, 175, 182, 329, 385, 391
Jowett, Phyllis, xiv, 128
Joyce, Marty, 361
Jubinville, Ed, 352, 354
juggling, 2

Karchut, Mike, 236, 254, 272–73, 306–7
Karpinski, Dennis, 335
Karpovich, Peter, 321
Karras, Alex, 335
Katz, Mike, 349–50
Kay, Frank, 90, 92, 110–11
Keen, Sam, 191
Keillor, Garrison, 6
Keister, Claudia, xiv, 345, 379–80
Kelly, Jack, Jr., 294–308

Kelly, Jack, Sr., 87
Kennedy, John F., 185, 193, 290
Kennedy, Robert, 290, 377
Ketterman, Alda, xiv, 7, 13, 79, 84–86, 94, 96, 110, 143, 149, 165, 171, 174, 176, 234, 267, 283, 297–98, 301, 315, 320–21, 326, 331–32, 343, 369, 372–73, 376, 380–81
kickboxing, 334
Kiiha, Osmo, xiv
Kimmel, Michael, 6
King, Billie Jean, 335
King, Don, 368
King, Ernest, 100
King, Jack, 245, 276, 295, 302, 304
Kipling, Rudyard, 60
Kirkley, George, 5
Kissinger, Henry, 318, 326
Klein, Alan, 5, 293
Klein, Karl, 206
Klein, Siegmund, 3, 33, 51, 65, 75, 79, 116–17, 206, 378
Klemens, Bruce, 367
Klisanin, Steve, 170
Klugman, Jack, 359
Knauer, Virginia, 286
Knipp, Russ, 222, 236, 247, 254, 259, 272, 307
Knodle, Robert, xiv, 34
Kolchakian, Charles, xiv
Kolotov, Vasilij, 299
Kono, Tommy, xiv, 121, 123, 139, 142, 145–46, 150, 159, 162–64, 186–87, 190–91, 196, 198–99, 220, 224–25, 229, 267, 275–76, 290, 302, 336, 365, 399
Korean War, 138, 147
Kraber, Ed, 21, 69
Kratkowski, Stan, 53, 55, 68
Krill, Johnny, 369
Krol, John Cardinal, 326
Krout, John, xiv, 368
Krutch, Richard, 305
Kuc, John, 357
Ku Klux Klan, 79
Kurinov, Alexander, 224
Kurtz, Tommy, 260, 274
Kuzuhara, Yas, 159

Labor, Department of, 179
LaLanne, Jack, 115, 125
Lambert, Mike, 362
Landis, Dick, 247
Latissimus Q. Superpex, 153
Lauda, Robert, 285
Lauriano, Joe, 99
Leader, Charles, 173
Le Havre incident, 55–56
Lehman, Dorcas, 84–86, 94, 96–97, 132–33, 136, 141, 143, 165, 176
Lemma, Firpo, 369

Index

Leonard, Benny, 40
Leonard, Gary, 354
Levan, Art, 44–46, 51, 65, 70
Levin, Ezra, 180
Levin, Murray, xiv, 262, 274, 309, 331, 338, 362–63, 365, 367
Liederman, Earle, 3, 25, 40, 115–16, 178
Lincoln, Abraham, 64, 322
Loar, Rev. M. D., 181
Long, Senator Edward, 207
Loprinzi, Sam, 116
Lorand, Arnold, 193, 252
Lord, Edward, 181
Los Angeles Athletic Club, 25, 31, 36
Louie, Gloria, 281
Louis, Joe, 217
Lovell, James, 287
Low, Milton, 209
Lowe, Fred, xiv, 244, 253, 257, 259, 272–73, 307, 364
Lugrin, George, 254, 260, 279–80, 303, 313
Luke the Gook, 153
Lukens, Helene, 370, 377
Lukin, Dean, 367
Lurie, Dan, 90–91, 97, 99, 116–18, 125, 260, 352–53
Lyon, Lisa, 353

MacArthur, Douglas, 100
McCabe, Gerald, 207
McCallum, John, 212–13, 235, 400
McCarthy, Dr. Shane, 184–85
McCloy, C. H., 195
McCollum, Elmer, 193
McCune, Bob, 126
McDougald, Gil, 166
Macfadden, Bernarr, 3, 5, 24–25, 49, 116, 155, 243
Mack, "Teddy," 32
McKee, Bob, 312
McKenzie, Precious, 361
McLauqhlin, Harry, 210
MacMahon, Charles, 25, 40
Macy's department store, 134, 180
Magnuson, Warren, 322
Manger, Albert, 33
Manger, Josef, 68
Manion, Jim, 355
Maniscalco, Tony, 45
March, Bill, xiv, 195–200, 209–10, 219, 222–23, 231, 253, 276
Marcyan, Walter, 107, 125
Markowitz, Arthur, 176
Martinez, Mario, 366–67
masculinity, 2–6, 13, 16–17, 23, 25, 29–30, 32, 38, 40, 47, 50–52, 61, 67–69, 71, 75–77, 82–83, 97, 100–101, 106, 108, 119, 123–24, 144, 155, 165, 184, 192, 238, 244, 274, 320, 322, 335, 375, 383–85, 386, 389–90
Mathias, Bob, 166
Matlin, Dave, 170, 185, 216, 295, 305–6, 323, 331
Matthes, Oscar, 32
Matysek, Antone, 39
Mayor, Dave, xiv, 48, 53, 55, 57, 63, 65, 67, 69–70, 72, 295, 336
melting-pot effect, 25, 54, 63–64, 69–70, 86–87, 120–23, 145, 160, 386
Mencken, H. L., 39
Mercer, Vic, 357, 360
Merriwell, Frank, 67, 167
Messer, James, xiv, 53
Metropolitan Weight Lifting Committee, 34
Michalik, Steve, 323
Michels, Jeff, 366
Michener Associates, 345–46
Middle Atlantic Championships, 78
Mielec, Roman, 253, 260
"Mighty Atom" (Joseph Greenstein), 369
Miller, Carl, 336
Miller, Clinton, 323–24
Miller, Donald, 210
Miller, Joe, 41, 44–45, 55, 62, 65
Miller, Pete, 295
Miller, Ronald, 264
Miller, Warren, 264
Mills, Billy, 250
Mills, Joe, 237
Milo Barbell Company, 25, 35, 40, 49–50, 56, 89, 150
Minichiello, Tom, 354
Mirkin, Gabe, xiv
Miss America, 86, 260
Mr. America (AAU), 2, 76, 87, 96, 125, 128, 137, 149, 152, 155, 166, 216, 219, 223, 235, 260, 266, 280, 295, 349, 353, 355–56, 385
1939: 69, 350
1940: 79–80
1941: 79
1942: 79, 90
1943: 94, 260
1945: 97
1946: 119, 227
1951: 144
1952: 141, 148
1954: 152
1960: 216
1961: 216
1962: 201, 217
1963: 203, 217
1965: 217
1966: 129, 203
1968: 253
1970: 218, 260, 323
1971: 279, 290

INDEX

1972: 323
1976: 316
1977: 350–51
1978: 352–53
1979: 353
1980: 354
1981: 353
Mr. America (teenage), 235, 244
Mr. America (Lurie), 260
Mr. America (Weider), 215, 349
Mr. Olympia, 2, 215, 260
Mr. Olympus, 260
Mr. Universe, 149, 166, 172, 331
   AAU, 260–61
   IWF, 219, 231
   NABBA, 118, 125–26, 144, 219, 260–61, 295, 355–56
   Weider, 215, 316, 354
Mr. World, 149, 313–14, 316
Mitchell, Bob, 45, 53, 55, 62, 138
Mitchell Field, 87
Mitchell, Martha, 286
Mizell, Christy, 323
Modica, Gus, 44
Moerke, Carl, 32
Montgomery, Bernard, 100
Moore, Kenny, 254
Moore, William, xv
Morris, Elmer, 175–76
Moss, Charles, 138
Moyer, Gerald, 245, 254
Mozee, Gene, 210
Muhammed Ali, 217
Muller, E. A., 194
Murray, Jim, xiv, 141–43, 145, 148, 157, 166–68, 191, 210, 377
Muscle Beach, 125–26, 169, 186
muscle-bound myth, 24, 51, 56, 318
Muscular Development, 6, 215–16, 223, 227, 232, 265, 280, 289, 311, 333, 335, 349, 353, 362, 369, 378

Nader, Ralph, 262
Nasser, Gamel Abdel, 290
national championship (senior), 38, 53–54, 62, 66, 90, 92, 96, 99, 101, 110, 118, 132, 143, 152, 183–84, 196, 199, 207, 219–20, 223–24, 233, 235–36, 238, 253–57, 268, 272–73, 277, 282–83, 298–301, 307, 335–36, 345–46, 363–64, 366
national championship (junior), 52, 76, 215
nationalism, 23, 71, 138
   American, 4, 29, 67–70, 86–87, 100–101, 106, 119
   German, 4, 54, 64
National Press Club, 325
National Sports Act, 350, 356
Neece, Steve, 397

neurastenic youth, 3–4, 14, 24, 26, 30, 45–47, 52–53, 63–64, 69–70, 93, 99, 114, 156, 160, 161, 389
Neuright, John, 6
Newton, Harvey, 202, 365
New York Athletic Club, 28
Nickol, Donald, 203–4, 248
Nicoletti, Vic, 229
Nixon, Pat, 322, 325–26
Nixon, Richard, 162, 193, 248, 265, 285–87, 289, 319, 324–29, 338, 373, 386
Njord, Val, 129
Nootens, Chuck, 236
Norberg, Karl, 82
Novak, Gregory, 156
Nubret, Serge, 352, 356

O'Brien, Michael, 282
Oerter, Al, 166
oil-burner business, 3, 21, 35, 40, 44, 49, 57–58, 69, 385
Oliva, Sergio, 216–17, 219, 265
Olsen, James, 105
Olson, Norm, 200
Olympic games, 3–4, 15, 142, 145, 187–88, 224, 245, 335, 383
   Amsterdam (1928), 33
   Antwerp (1920), 28
   Athens (1896), 28
   Berlin (1936), 53–55, 61–62, 64
   Helsinki (1952), 145–46, 183
   London (1948), 120–21, 123, 183, 225
   Los Angeles (1932), 42
   Los Angeles (1984), 366
   Melbourne (1956), 162, 166, 187
   Munich (1972), 298, 307, 325
   Rome (1960), 180, 185–86, 188–89, 190, 194–97, 220, 236–37
   Tokyo (1964), 220, 225, 236–37, 267
   Mexico City (1968), 236, 246, 253–54, 257–59, 267–68, 271, 273
   Montreal (1976), 336–37
Orlick, Emmanuel, xiv, 128–29
Osborne, Ramey, 281
O'Shea, Pat, 202
Otott, George, 210, 259

Pacifico, Larry, 306, 357, 360–61
Page, Floyd, 125
Pan American Games, 244–46, 268, 308, 313, 364, 366
Park, Jim, xiv, 141, 148–49, 159, 172
Park, Reg, 125, 219, 261
Partridge, R. W., 202
Paschall, Harry, 33, 75, 90, 118, 130, 132, 137–38, 143–44, 149, 152, 161, 167–70, 178, 190, 210, 274, 334
Patera, Ken, 271–72, 307, 311

Index

Patterson, Clay, 313, 338
Pearl, Bill, 219, 261, 265
Pearson, Tony, 353
Pedersen, Eric, 125
Pennsylvania, 1, 2, 367
Penta, Vincent, 264
Pentz, Bob, 45
Peoples, Bob, 160
Peripheral Heart Action (PHA), 203
Pershing, General John, 18
Petersen, Ernie, xiv, 321, 330–31, 342, 349
Phantom, 152
Physical Culture, 24, 49
Physical Preparedness Campaign, 87
Physical Training Notes, 53, 55
Pickett, Ernie, 245, 253, 259, 268, 276
Pierson, William, 179
Pitman, Joe, xiv, 123, 138, 140, 162–63
Pitts, Don, 32
Pittsburgh, City of, 12, 14–16, 20, 205, 248
Platz, Tom, 353
Podolak, Walter, 117, 369
Police Gazette, 28
polka dancing, 165, 313, 315
Polo, Eddie, 147
Poole, Harold, 216–19, 265
powerlifting, 1, 187, 214–16, 261–63, 265, 282, 293, 308, 311–17, 338, 341, 356–62, 363, 366, 369, 383, 385–86
    for women, 358–59
Presley, Elvis, 238
"Protein from the Sea," 205
Proxmire, William, 324
Pruden, Bonnie, 182
Pruger, Richard, xiv, 330–31, 336, 348–50
Puleo, Joe, xiv, 212, 219–21, 253–54, 259, 272, 299, 364
Pulskamp, John, 203, 206, 212

Quinn, Roger, 298
quoits, 64

Rader, Peary, 120, 134, 187–88, 213, 261–62, 296, 352
Randall, Bruce, 331
Rasch, Philip, 206
Rasmusson, Jim, 200
Rawluk, Peter, 254, 274
Reagan, Ronald, 379
Reding, Serge, 258, 321
Redman, Phil, xiv, 342–43, 345, 379
Reed, Don, 247, 260
Reeves, Steve, 125–26, 128, 135, 220
Reinhoudt, Cindy, 358
Reinhoudt, Don, 357
Revolution of 1848, 23
Rexroad, Joseph, 209
Reynolds, Bill, 347

Richards, Rev. Bob, 166
Rider, General, 100
Riecke, Louis, xiv, 196–200, 224–26, 231
Rieger, Jon, xiv, 208
Ridge Corporation, 343
Riggs, Bobby, 335
Roark, Joe, xiii
Roberson, Gene, 215
Roberts, Randy, 105
Robinson, Robby, 350–51
Rochlin, Gregory, 383
Rockefeller, John D., 373
Rogers, Paul, 324
Roosevelt, Theodore, 4
Rosa, Ken "Leo," 144
Rosee, Irwin, 182
Roselli, Pete, 254
Ross, Clarence, 97, 99, 125–28, 261
Ross (Weider), Diana, 115, 178
Rosset, Jules, 28
Rouledge, Ray, 219
Roy, Alvin, 113, 200
Ryun, Jim, 250

Sablo, Rudy, 217, 295, 335
Sadecki, Roger, 365
St. Jean, Pierre, 222
St. John, Bill, xiv
Sakata, Harold, 220, 369
Salisbury, Paul, 363
Sandow, Eugen, 24, 28, 57, 214, 384
Sathyanarayana, H. V., 264
Saunders, Frank, 254
Save the United States movement, 294, 328–29, 368, 372
Saxon, Arthur, 161
Schemansky, Norbert, xiv, 121, 138, 145–46, 160, 191, 198, 219–21, 237, 239, 244–45, 275, 365
Schiemann, Arnold, 36
Schmitz, Jim, 366
Schutz, Fred, 236, 299
Schwarzenegger, Arnold, 1, 5, 219, 261, 357, 378, 402
Schweiker, Richard, 323
Schell, Hooley, 65, 298
Schell, Lou, 44–45, 65
Schofro, Frank, 110
Schultz, Roger, 269–70, 297
Schwartz, Reed, 45
Sciaroni, Mrs. Robert, 181
Scott, Larry, 219, 265
See, Leon, 111
Seeman, Ed, 264
self-made manhood, 2, 6, 40, 100–101, 167, 192, 275, 383
Senay, Dennis, 299, 301
Setterberg, Kurt, 363

INDEX

Severenson, "Doc," 359
sex and sexuality, 2–3, 21, 59–61, 74–75, 93, 97, 108, 129, 135, 159, 165, 178, 180, 186, 193, 209–10, 267, 270, 276–77, 280, 290, 297, 320, 323, 328, 342, 369–70, 385
Shafer, Raymond, 248
Shah of Iran, 155, 162–63, 193
Shakespeare, William, 59, 318
Shandor, George, 110, 138, 174–75
Sharp, Bill, 250
Sheppard, Dave, 112, 123, 142, 150, 159, 163–64, 186, 221
Shields, Charlie, xiv, 260, 305–6, 338–39
Shipley, Thomas, 69
Shusterich, Lud, 352
Sipes, Chuck, 265
skiing, 24
Smith, Carl, 285
Smith, Charles A., 26, 97, 123, 141, 178
Smith, Dick, xiv, 176, 195, 199, 222–24, 233–34, 254, 276, 299
Smith, John, 32
Smith, Wilbur, 117, 142–43
Snellbaker, Ruth, 377
Snyder, Robert, 33, 392
Social Darwinism, 2
socialization practices, 46–49, 63–70, 79–83, 87–88, 96–97, 106, 108, 110–14, 120–23, 137–38, 156, 164–65, 186–90, 219–27, 235–39, 244–47, 252–60, 276, 369, 385, 387
Soviet Union, 4–5, 106, 111, 118–19, 138, 145–47, 150, 152, 156–57, 162, 164, 166, 187–88, 190, 196, 220, 224–25, 227, 271, 275, 293, 329, 363
Spack, Joseph S., 312
Spellman, Frank, xiv, 110–11, 120, 122–23, 138, 140, 142, 336
Spellman, Joyce, 142
Spencer, Charles, xv
Sprague, Ken, 350, 352–54
Springfield College, 87, 194
Stagg (Yarick), Alyce, 115, 125
Stalin, Joe, 144
Stamp, Gordon, 200
Standish, Vic, xiv, 380–81
Stanczyk, Stan, 110–12, 123, 132–33, 138–39, 145, 162, 163–64
Stanko, Steve, 46, 63, 67–70, 76–77, 81, 87, 90, 94, 99, 110, 116, 118, 125, 138, 149, 266, 282, 369, 377–78
Starr, Bill, xiv, 223, 234–39, 244–47, 252–53, 256–57, 260, 270–73, 275–83, 290, 294, 296, 299, 301–3, 305–6, 331, 334, 373
Starr, Marlene, 277
State, Oscar, 145, 295, 369
Stefan, Jacob, 306, 308
Steinborn, Henry, 32, 74, 378
Stephen, Alan, 119, 125, 227

Stern, Leo, 115, 125
steroids, 188, 195–98, 200, 224, 232–34, 236, 252, 263, 268–69, 270, 275–80, 304, 321, 385, 399
Stevens, Bill, 279
Stilwell, Joe, 100
Stockton, Abbye "Pudgy," 96, 125, 129
Stockton, Les, 125
softball, 284–85, 310, 319, 326, 329, 335, 342, 367, 371, 378
Stogov, Vladimir, 159
Stoller, Ken, 200
Stombaugh, Paul, xiv, 381, 383, 384
Strength, 24–26, 28–30, 32–38, 49, 53
Strength & Health, xiv, 1, 6, 47–52, 62, 66, 72, 75–77, 82–84, 87, 90, 92, 94–98, 107–10, 114–16, 125, 130–32, 134, 140–42, 151, 155, 160, 162, 166–67, 169, 171, 182, 194–95, 198–99, 203, 210–16, 225, 229, 233–35, 237, 244, 246, 248, 253, 258, 260, 262, 265, 274, 277–79, 281, 284–85, 297, 302–3, 308, 326–28, 334–35, 338, 360, 363, 373, 377–78
founding of, 38, 42
Strength and Health picnic, 211, 369, 383
Strongfort, Lionel, 25, 39
strong-man era, 24
Strossen, Randall, xiv, 213
success ideology, 2, 50–51, 71, 77, 99, 120, 293, 385, 387, 389
Suggs, Kay, 211, 256
Suggs, Tommy, 210–12, 232–38, 244–47, 254, 256, 259, 270, 276, 302–3
Suleimanov, Naim, 366
Sundberg, Arnie, 33, 36
Superman, 152
Susann, Jaqueline, 257
Susquehanna Capital, xiv, 381, 383, 386
swimming, 334
Swiss Automatic, 343, 381
Szkalak, Kalman, 316

Taggert, Everill, 282
Talts, Jan, 271
Talluto, Pete, 220
Tanny, Armand, 51
Tanny, Vic, 51, 92, 107, 125–26, 128, 133
Taormine, Angelo, 44
Tart, Gail, 276, 285
tennis, 24, 155, 171, 335
Terlazzo, John, xiv, 215, 221, 223, 254, 360, 369, 383
Terlazzo, Tony, 36, 44, 54–55, 62, 65, 68–70, 76, 81–82, 89–90, 94–95, 101, 107–8, 110, 137, 144, 149, 203, 205, 229, 246, 378
Terpak, John, Jr., xiv, 205, 342, 376, 380–81
Terpak, John, Sr., xiv, 7, 46, 52, 55, 62, 65, 67–70, 76, 81–82, 87, 89–90, 94–95, 97, 99, 101, 110–11, 113, 115, 123, 132, 138, 141, 149,

Index

163, 170, 174, 182, 193–94, 203, 205, 209, 220–21, 233–34, 239, 246, 249, 257, 259, 261–62, 267–68, 269–70, 274–76, 280, 286, 294–95, 297–99, 301–7, 309, 323, 329, 331, 334, 341–43, 345–50, 352, 360, 372, 376–81
Terry, John, 55, 64, 68, 77, 81, 89, 110, 138, 160, 378
testosterone, 157–59
Texas connection, 210–12, 214–15, 233–35, 259–60, 303, 311, 313, 315, 386
Thomas, Al, 358
Thomas, John, 166
Thomasillo, Harry, 44–45
Thomasville Inn, 208, 298
Three Hundred Pound Club, 44, 50
Tilney, Frederick, 49, 51, 56, 115, 129, 202, 369
Tinsman, Paul, 347
Titus, Professor Henry, 39
tobogganing, 24
Todd (Hanks), Ellen, xiv, 211, 214, 233, 401
Todd, Jan, xiv–xv, 66, 358–59
Todd, Terry, xiv–xv, 171, 203, 206, 211–15, 233–34, 248, 311–14, 316, 357–58, 360, 373, 385, 401
Todd-McLean Collection, 234
Tom, Richard, 110, 183
Tomita, Richard, 183
Touni, Khadr El, 111
Townsend, Kim, 6
track and field, 2, 24, 28, 166, 190, 200, 206, 250, 261
Travis, Warren Lincoln, 3, 171
Treloar, Al, 25
Tucker, John, 115
tumbling, 2
Tunney, Gene, 17
Tunney, John, 338
Turnvereins, 24, 28

Ueberroth, Peter, 367
U.S. Lock & Hardware, 379–81
United States Weightlifting Federation, 363, 365, 367
Utterback, Harry, xiv, 89, 369, 377

Van Cleef, Ray, 108, 141, 185, 187, 191, 228–29, 234
Vasilieff, Val, xiv
Venables, Gordon, 51–52, 65, 67, 69–70, 75, 81, 86, 89–90, 94, 118, 141–42, 175, 191, 290, 321
Venus de Milo, 84, 86
Vesper Boat Club, 205
Viator, Casey, xiv, 265, 279
Vietnam War, 265, 275–76, 297, 303, 326, 342, 365, 368, 386
Vinci, Charles, 159–60, 162–64, 186–87, 189, 220, 272, 275

Vlasov, Yuri, 188, 225
Vorobiev, Arkady, 150, 157, 188
Voyages, Kimon, 99, 116

Waller, Ken, 265
Walsh, George, 130
Walter, Dick, 209
Warner, Donnie, xiv, 297, 299, 383
Warner, Robert, 202
Washington, Walter, 323
Watergate, 306, 322, 324, 326–28
Wayne, John, 375
Wayne, Rick, 114, 217
Weaver, George, 129
Weaver, Vern, xiv, 184, 217, 222
Webster, David, xiv–xv, 295
Weider, Ben, 5, 128, 262, 294–96, 338, 341, 349–55, 386
Weider, Joe, 5, 97, 99, 105–6, 108, 114–19, 125, 127–36, 142–45, 150, 152, 172–73, 177–78, 180, 182, 187, 190, 208–10, 215–16, 219–20, 228, 260–62, 265, 293–97, 301, 316, 334, 338, 341, 347–50, 352–55, 368, 373, 376, 378–79, 386, 395, 402
Weider Publications, 2, 97, 108, 114–15, 117–18, 126, 128–29, 134, 142–43, 173, 177–78, 216, 261–62, 353–55, 362, 396
weightlifting, 1–2, 4–5, 22, 24, 28–29, 31–38, 40–43, 52, 58, 61–62, 64–69, 72–73, 75, 77–79, 90, 92, 96, 99–101, 107, 110–14, 116, 118–23, 135–38, 144–47, 149–50, 152, 155–66, 168, 170–71, 173, 181, 186–90, 192, 194, 202, 207–8, 214–17, 219–27, 235–39, 244–47, 253–60, 262–63, 266–78, 281–85, 289–90, 293–96, 298–301, 307–9, 313–14, 335–39, 345–46, 357–58, 362–67, 375, 378, 381, 383, 385–86
for females, 48, 84–86, 96, 318, 335, 397
weight training, 1, 30, 57, 66, 87, 90, 94–95, 100, 106–8, 115, 133, 151, 156, 205–6, 212, 231, 250, 319, 348, 397
weight training for athletes, 155, 166–69, 190, 205, 212, 318, 335, 375
Weissbrot, Morris, 244, 280, 311, 335
Wells, Melvin, 124–25
West, Mae, 351–52
West Point, 87, 167
Whitcomb, Barry, 247, 253, 275
White, Curt, 363, 367
White, Jo Jo, 357
Whitehead, Dr. Craig, 203, 215, 229–30, 280–81
Whitfield, Karo, 81, 369
Whitfield, Mal, 166
Wilhelm, Bruce, 299, 336, 357, 363
Williams, Jim, 266
Willkie, Wendell, 81
Willoughby, David, 25, 29, 31, 129
Windship, George Barker, 28

INDEX

World Amateur Bodybuilder's Association, 355–56
World Body Building Guild, 260
world championships , 219–20, 224, 383
   Budapest (1962), 220, 224
   Columbus (1970), 258, 266, 272–73, 335
   Milan (1951), 145
   Paris (1937), 67
   Paris (1946), 111, 113, 118, 120, 156
   Paris (1950), 138
   Philadelphia (1947), 119–20
   The Hague (1949), 121
   Lima (1971), 266, 273
   Ljublyana (1982), 365
   Manila (1974), 309, 321
   Moscow (1975), 309, 336
   Moscow (1983), 367
   Munich (1955), 152, 157, 159–61, 163–64
   Stockholm (1953), 147, 150, 156
   Stockholm (1958), 187
   Stockholm (1963), 220
   Vienna (1898), 28
   Vienna (1938), 68, 77
   Vienna (1954), 150, 152, 157–58
   Vienna (1961), 224
   Warsaw (1959), 187
   Warsaw (1969), 271–72
World University, 293, 317–18
World War I, 16–19, 24, 28, 176, 202, 290
World War II, 71, 87–90, 92–97, 100–101, 105–7, 114, 121, 155–58, 248, 276, 288
Wortmann, Dietrich, 34, 37, 43, 53, 55, 105, 142
Wrange, Tom, 316
wrestling, 2, 4, 190, 225
Wright, Dennis, 314
Wright, Dr. Richard, 229
Wright, Dr. Russell, 202, 205, 229
wristwrestling, 335

Yacos, George, 149
Yarick, Ed, 115, 125
YMCA (York), 30, 31, 46, 60–61, 76, 110, 184, 248
York Athletic Supply, 72
York Barbell, 1–3, 5, 7, 57, 72, 87–89, 112–13, 138–42, 148–49, 160, 164, 172–77, 179– 81, 184, 208, 231, 243, 249, 258–59, 267, 269, 282, 294, 302–6, 308, 311, 323, 329– 33, 341–49, 350, 355, 357, 360, 362, 366–70, 373, 376–87
   on Broad Street, 7, 35, 61–61, 65, 120, 136–40, 142, 159, 168, 171
   financial data, 69, 118, 138, 140–41, 172–77, 208, 249, 267, 329–33, 343–45, 375–76, 379
   foundry operations, 88–89, 94, 101, 140, 172, 379–82
   on Ridge Avenue, 7, 171, 203, 222, 244–47, 261, 368, 378
   at Emigsville, 7, 204, 239, 310, 330, 344, 346
York Barbell Club, xiii–xiv, 96, 99, 101, 110, 119, 136–38, 183, 267, 272, 274, 301, 313, 336, 345–46, 363, 366
York Barbell Institute, 383
York, City of, 1, 20–21, 61, 94, 97, 114, 118–20, 143, 147, 182–84, 202, 222, 244, 267–68, 285, 372
York Enterprises, 331
York gang, xiii–xiv, 3, 6, 36–37, 39–40, 43–46, 49, 51, 57, 63–71, 73, 76, 81, 83, 87, 89–90, 100–101, 107, 110, 141, 159–60, 164, 168, 174, 183–84, 191, 194, 203, 219–20, 223, 225, 235, 256, 264, 276, 280, 282, 297, 310, 313, 375, 378, 386–87
York gang, "new," 191, 199, 210, 234–39, 243–47, 252–60, 291, 297, 328
York (Junior) College, 203, 220, 235, 244, 247, 266
York Light House, 175, 205
York Oil Burner Athletic Club (YOBAC), 35–38, 44, 191
York Precision Company, 133, 140, 175, 205, 343
York Victory Barbell, 89, 94
You, Dr. Richard, 181–83, 188, 202, 229, 302
Young, Noah, 25
youth rebellion, 277–81, 285, 290–91, 296–301

Zagurski, Joe, 260
Zagurski, Wally, 37, 44–46, 51, 62, 170
Zane, Frank, 265
Zarella, Joe, 358
Zbyszko, Stanislaus, 39, 83
Zhabotinski, Leonid, 225, 238, 258, 268
Ziegler, Dr. John, 157–59, 194–203, 205, 215, 222–23, 229, 232–34, 238, 247, 268, 369, 401
Ziegman, Steve, 274
Zimmerman, Dick, 51–52
Zitko, John, 318

www.ingramcontent.com/pod-product-compliance
Lightning Source LLC
Chambersburg PA
CBHW072117290426
44111CB00012B/1691